Small Animal Emergency And Critical Care

A Manual for the Veterinary Technician

W.B. Saunders Company
A Harcourt Health Sciences Company

The Curtis Center
Independence Square West
Philadelphia, Pennsylvania 19106

Editor-in-Chief: Andrew Allen
Editorial Manager: Linda Duncan
Developmental Editor: Peg Waltner
Project Manager: Catherine Jackson
Production Editor: Jeff Patterson
Design Coordinator: Judi Lang
Designer: Graphic World Publishing Services
Cover Designer: Rokusek Design
Cover images courtesy of the College of Veterinary Medicine, University of Missouri—Columbia.

Library of Congress Cataloging-in-Publication Data

Battaglia, Andrea.
Small animal emergency and critical care : a manual for the veterinary technician / Andrea Battaglia.

p. cm.

Includes bibliographical references.

ISBN 0-7216-7773-8

1. Veterinary emergencies—Handbooks, manuals, etc. 2. Veterinary critical care—Handbooks, manuals, etc. I. Title.

SF778.B38 2000

636.089'6025—dc21 00-058817

ISBN 0-7216-7773-8

SMALL ANIMAL EMERGENCY AND CRITICAL CARE: A MANUAL FOR THE VETERINARY TECHNICIAN

Printed in the United States of America

Last digit is the print number: 9 8 7 6 5 4 3 2 1

Small Animal Emergency and Critical Care

A Manual for the Veterinary Technician

Andrea M. Battaglia, LVT
Ithaca, New York

W.B. SAUNDERS COMPANY
A Harcourt Health Sciences Company
Philadelphia London Montreal St. Louis Sydney Tokyo Toronto

To my greatest teachers, my daughters,
Audrey Rae and Hannah Lorraine

Contributors

Jody Brooks, RVT†
Carson-Tahoe Veterinary Hospital
Carson City, Nevada

Craig Cornell, RVT, VTS (Emergency and Critical Care)
Animal Health Technician
Anesthesia Department
Veterinary Teaching Hospital
University of California, Davis
Davis, California

Dennis T. (Tim) Crowe, Jr., DVM, Dipl ACVS, Dipl ACV (Emergency and Critical Care)
Western Nevada Veterinary Specialist
Chief of Surgery
Director of Interns/Residents
Carson-Tahoe Veterinary Hospital
Carson City, Nevada

Harold Davis, BA, RVT, VTS (Emergency and Critical Care)
Supervisor, Emergency Nursing Service
Coordinator, Hospital Practices Course
Veterinary Medical Teaching Hospital
University of California, Davis
Davis, California

Jennifer Devey, DVM
Diplomate, American College of Veterinary Emergency and Critical Care
Carson-Tahoe Veterinary Hospital
Carson City, Nevada

Pam Dickens, CVT
Sunshine Animal Hospital
Animal Eye Clinic
Opthalmology Technician
Tampa, Florida

Rick Glass, MS, DVM, Diplomate ACVIM (Neurology), AVMA
Staff Neurologist and Neurosurgeon
Neurology and Neurosurgery
Red Bank Veterinary Hospital
Red Bank, New Jersey

Nyki Gorichs
Carson-Tahoe Veterinary Hospital
Carson City, Nevada

Adam Hulme
Pet Network of North Lake Tahoe
Incline Village, Nevada

Kenneth Kalthoff
TriCity Veterinary Clinic
Vista, California

Linda Katchatoorian
Animal Referral Center
Fountain Valley, California

Marc Kent, DVM, DACVIM
Clinical Assistant Faculty
Tufts University
School of Veterinary Medicine
North Grafton, Massachusetts

Peter W.M. Kronen, DVM
Postdoctorate Associate in Anesthesiology
College of Veterinary Medicine
Cornell University
Ithaca, New York

Midora Mower, VT
Emergency Critical Care Unit
Angel Memorial Hospital
Boston, Massachusetts

†Deceased

Donna Oakley, CVT, VTS (Emergency and Critical Care)
Director of Nursing
Director, Penn Animal Blood Bank
University of Pennsylvania
School of Veterinary Medicine
Philadelphia, Pennsylvania

Linda Porter, AHT
Carson-Tahoe Veterinary Hospital
Carson City, Nevada

Richard W. Reid, DVM, Dipl. ACVIM (Internal Medicine)
Chief Medical Officer
Veterinary Internal Medicine Specialists
Plainville, New York

Nancy Shaffran, RVT, VTS (Emergency and Critical Care)
Director, Staff Development and Education at the Veterinary Referral Centre
Charter Member and Board of Regents—Avecct
Academy of Veterinary Emergency and Critical Care Technicians
Little Falls, New Jersey

Donald M. Shawver, CRTT, MS
Technical Representative
Regional Manager
Cook Veterinary Products
New Buffalo, Michigan

Jona Spano, RVT
Veterinary Medical Teaching Hospital
University of California, Davis
Davis, California

Preface

The veterinary technician involved in emergency and critical care medicine must understand the vital role he or she plays. Many times it is the veterinary technician who begins the life-saving procedures before the veterinarian on duty has a chance to join the team.

Small Animal Emergency and Critical Care: A Manual for the Veterinary Technician was written to provide a valuable resource for veterinary technicians and students interested in this specialized area. Many life-saving procedures are detailed through diagrams and step-by-step descriptions. Common drugs used to stabilize and maintain the critically ill or injured small animal are discussed, including information about the mode of action and dosage. Chapters dedicated to shock, cardiopulmonary resuscitation, and trauma introduce the emergency section and provide the reader with information on how to assess and stabilize the critically ill or injured small animal.

The book is divided into three sections. The first section focuses on critical care techniques. Many supportive therapies are discussed. A procedure is highlighted in each chapter and described in a Technical Tip.

The second section focuses on specific types of emergencies. Each chapter details specific types of situations one encounters in the emergency room. The type of emergency is defined. A checklist is provided with information on how to equip the emergency room with the proper drugs and items needed for the specific emergency. Clinical signs, most common treatment protocols, and Technical Tips are given.

The technician involved in emergency and critical care medicine often is required to work inconsistent hours and night shifts. Scheduling is a big challenge in any 24-hour facility. The final section provides scheduling solutions and suggestions for adapting to shift changes. This will create a healthier work environment and reduce staff turnover.

My hope is for the reader to use this book as another tool in providing the best possible care for the critically ill or injured small animal. Veterinary medicine continues to evolve in all areas, so no single resource should be considered the final word on any subject. We as veterinary technicians should continue to educate ourselves on a daily basis through publications, continuing education seminars, and practical experience. Our best resources for learning will continue to be the animals we interact with and other members of our team. We must continue to learn more and be willing to share what we have learned. The animals we work with deserve our best effort.

Andrea M. Battaglia, LVT

Acknowledgments

When I announced to a published author that WB Saunders had accepted my proposal for this book, the reply was, "Oh, I will be there if you need support." Three years later I fully understand his statement and realize that it takes a strong, committed team of people to create a book.

There are so many people I would like to recognize for their positive influence on my career and indirect influence on the creation of this book. I would need to write another manual to include everyone.

I do want to thank the contributors who dedicated valuable time and effort to complete this project. You have provided me with many more essential tools to be a better veterinary technician, and I am glad others will have the opportunity to benefit from your knowledge.

A million thanks to Peg Waltner, the developmental editor. Without your constant encouragement, support, and persistence this work would not have been finished.

I would also like to express my appreciation for Dr. Steve Olender, Dr. Jack Dwyer, and Deb Johnson, LVT. Your patience during my entrance into the world of veterinary medicine and encouragement to follow my dream stayed with me over the years.

I am also very grateful for the role Dr. Melvin Chambliss played in my life during the Delhi days. You always believed in me and opened my eyes to so many possibilities in veterinary technology.

I cannot forget to thank Dr. Sue Dougherty. You introduced me to the art of critical care and made my work as a critical care technician much more fulfilling.

I would also like to thank many at Cornell University who challenged and encouraged me during my years of service and the Veterinary Emergency and Critical Care Society for the inspiration to accomplish my goals.

Special thanks to my parents, Dr. Donald and Joan Battaglia. You taught me the value of a strong work ethic and always encouraged me to reach high.

Special thanks to the many feathered, furred, and scaled creatures that passed through my hands, leaving me more experienced to better care for those who would follow.

Contents

Section I

Critically Ill Small Animals

This section introduces many technical skills needed to care for the critically ill small animal. Commonly used supportive therapies and procedures for maintaining the critically ill patient through anesthesia are included.

Chapter 1

The Skill of Observation

Veterinary emergency and critical care medicine continues to evolve, providing higher levels of care. Many 24-hour emergency and critical care facilities have been established throughout the United States, and many more are in various stages of planning and development. The veterinary technician involved in emergency or critical care must keep his or her skills current in this ever-changing profession. Many types of equipment and procedures are available to provide optimal patient care. In this age of advanced technology the hands-on skills of observation and monitoring continue to play a crucial role in treatment.

When the critically ill or injured small animal patient arrives, the initial assessment is made by checking the vital signs and obtaining a history from the owner. It is important to know the normal parameters for the dog and cat to assess what is abnormal (Color plates 1 to 3 and Table 1-1). Variations in the normal values may occur depending on the breed, size, or age of the animal. On physical examination, an obvious problem may draw attention from something less obvious. For this reason, it is important to do complete physical examinations on every patient when the patient has been initially stabilized (Figure 1-1).

Once it has been determined that the animal needs to be admitted and the owner has agreed to treat the condition, the owner should fill out the necessary forms. While the owner completes the forms, the emergency critical care team can do the necessary procedures to stabilize the animal. Readiness is the key to efficient and successful stabilization. All stations and carts should be restocked during each shift, with all equipment and oxygen sources fully functional and ready to go.

Do not hesitate to bring the owner into the hospital to alleviate any anxiety that he or she may experience upon the separation from his or her pet. This helps develop mutual trust, fosters a positive working relationship, and allows the staff to meet the owner. Encouraging visitation conveys a perception that the owner is a valued member of the treatment team. The small animal patient is now commonly recognized as a family member.

Before leaving the facility, the owner should understand the procedures that may be performed, the risks involved, and the severity of the animal's condition. A copy of the plan should be available for the owner to take home. The owner also must decide whether the animal is to be given cardiopulmonary resuscitation if an arrest occurs. The team is notified, and the order is recorded on the chart.

Treating and monitoring critically ill small animal patients often involve various drug and fluid therapies. Throughout the day, staff members monitor the patient and assess treatment response. Verbal communication and recordkeeping play a very important role. The veterinary technicians need to communicate throughout their shifts. This can be accomplished through written communication highlighting important changes that have occurred. The information is shared during shift changes.

Veterinary technicians can help create the optimum emergency and critical care center by acting as team players, educating themselves, and

TABLE 1-1 Normal Parameters

	Canine	Feline
Temperature (° F)	99.5-102.5	100-102.5
Heart rate (beats/min)	70-180	145-200
Respiratory rate (breaths/min)	20-40	20-40
Capillary refill time (seconds)	<1.5	<1.5
Mucous membrane color	Pink	Pink
Blood pressure (mm Hg)		
Systolic	100-150	100-150
Diastolic	60-110	60-110
Mean arterial	80-120	80-120
Packed cell volume (%)	35-54	27-46
Total plasma protein (g/100 ml)	5.7-7.3	6.3-8.3
Blood glucose (mg/dl)	70-118	73-134
Blood urea nitrogen (mg/dl)	8-25	15-35
Urine output (ml/kg/hr)	1-2	1-2

From Jhock: Recognition, treatment, and monitoring. *Veterinary Technician,* vol. 18, no. 3, 1997, p. 169.

sharing with the entire staff new information that they have obtained through continuing education seminars, journals, and other sources. Maintaining good communication skills (verbal and written) is essential to providing the best care for the critically ill small animal.

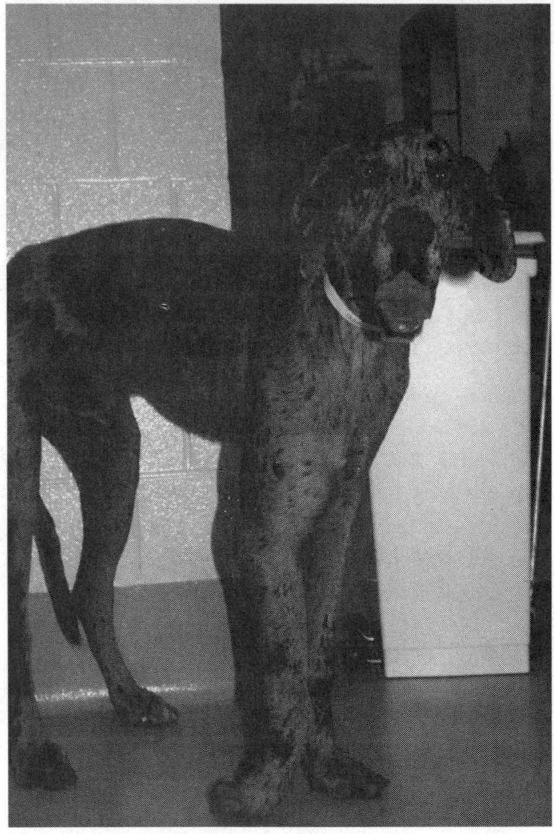

Figure 1-1

Nine-month-old Great Dane that presented with a dislocated shoulder as the primary concern. A pneumothorax was discovered upon examination.

Chapter 2

Basic Laboratory Equipment for the Emergency and Critical Care Hospital

The animal in the critical care unit needs accurate and continuous monitoring. Monitoring can be done by looking, listening, or feeling, or with the use of machines. This chapter covers the types of monitoring essential for a positive outcome and the types of equipment necessary for accurate results.

The type of equipment used must complement the team of people working in the facility. The machines should be chosen for their efficiency and ease of use. The company providing the equipment should have a 24-hour technical service representative available. Many veterinarians have in-house laboratories and can provide much information based on hands-on experience. Used equipment dealers provide many of the same benefits as new equipment providers. Hospitals must review warranties and service options carefully when purchasing all equipment.

One person should be appointed to maintain these machines, but all staff members should have the manuals available to them in case of breakdowns. Because each piece of machinery is different, staff training should include how to work and maintain all monitoring equipment.

Accurate recordkeeping also is essential for optimal monitoring. Trends should be noted and time should be taken before each shift change to describe the various monitoring techniques that were used on the previous shift and the results. The animal may become more comfortable with one type of procedure or position than another. This is critical information to be shared if trends are to be a consistent means of evaluating the animal's status.

This chapter is dedicated to the memory of Jody Brooks.

BLOOD TESTS USING CENTRIFUGES AND ANALYZERS

Sample collection is as important to accurate results as the function of the analyzers. Hemolysis, which can interfere with a number of blood tests, can be avoided by proper technique. A clean, venipuncture and light suction on the syringe are essential. Animals in the critical care setting usually need multiple blood sample evaluations. Central lines (placed in the jugular vein, medial saphenous vein, or lateral saphenous vein) can provide the technician with a sampling port. These central lines can be maintained for many days and avoid the discomfort of multiple venipunctures (Technical Tip Box 2-1).

PROCESSING BLOOD SAMPLES

After the sample is collected, it should be processed immediately. Proper handling of the sample depends on the tests being run, and it should always be checked with a laboratory reference to avoid laboratory error. For instance, blood intended for nonclotted samples should be placed in the

Box 2-1 Technical Tip: *Blood Sample Collection from Central Venous Catheters or Arterial Catheters*

Items needed: Three syringes with needles attached

Syringe #1: 0.5 ml heparinized saline
Syringe #2: empty sample syringe
Syringe #3: flush syringe with 1-3 ml heparinized saline (depending on catheter length)

1. Attach syringe #1 to female port of catheter and aspirate 1-1.5 ml blood. Cap, rotate, and set aside.
2. Attach syringe #2 to female port and aspirate the amount of blood necessary for the test.
3. Attach syringe #1 and return mixed blood sample to patient.
4. Attach syringe #3 and flush.

Note: The size of the animal must be considered when taking blood samples and flushing catheters. If an animal is already anemic, the amount of the blood loss from sample taking can be significant and can be detrimental.

appropriate tubes (calcium ethylenediamine tetraacetic acid, sodium heparin, or sodium citrate) immediately after the blood is drawn. If a packed cell volume is indicated, the blood should be transferred to capillary tubes immediately. Once the sample is placed in the tube it should be rotated gently approximately 10 times to mix the anticoagulant with the blood. Care should be taken to ensure that the right amount of blood is placed into vacutainer tubes because too little blood can lead to false results secondary to dilution. Certain tests such as blood gases, ammonia, and whole blood glucose levels must be run immediately because false values will result if the sample is allowed to sit.

For certain tests, such as packed cell volumes and tests run on serum or plasma, the blood sample must be spun in a centrifuge. The centrifuge should always be balanced by a sample of similar volume on the opposite side. This prevents uneven wear on the motor, which eventually will cause vibration. The correct speed should be selected depending on the sample being spun. Samples should not be removed from the centrifuge until it has come to a complete stop. The brake should not be used when the head is still rotating at high speeds because this causes excessive wear.

Serum or plasma should always be evaluated and the results recorded because they can give important clues about the patient's disease process. Abnormal serum can interfere with other blood tests, so it is important to note the color. The characteristics of serum are as follows:

- *Clear.*
- *Lipemic* (white, turbid). This occurs if the animal has eaten recently, or it can be associated with various diseases such as pancreatitis, diabetes, hypothyroidism, liver disease, and primary lipid disorders. The technician may need to repeat the test after withholding food for 12 hours (if appropriate).
- *Icteric* (yellow). This occurs most commonly with liver disease or hemolytic anemia.
- *Hemolyzed* (red). This occurs usually as a result of poor sampling technique and handling; however, it also can be an indicator of intravascular hemolysis associated with hemolytic anemia.

REFERENCE VALUES AND VALUES OUT OF THE NORMAL RANGE

The reference values for the individual machine should be used because machines vary significantly. Laboratory reference books should be consulted to determine the list of rule-outs for abnormal blood values for chemistries and electrolytes.

PACKED CELL VOLUME

The packed cell volume (PCV) is an important tool in patient evaluation and diagnosis. A low PCV indicates anemia, which may result in tissue hypoxia. A high PCV may indicate dehydration or polycythemia secondary to an underlying disease. The total solids should always be recorded in

TABLE 2-1 PCV Interpretation

	Canine	Feline
Normal	37%-55%	27%-45%
Mild anemia	30%-37%	20%-26%
Moderate anemia	20%-29%	14%-19%
Severe anemia	13%-19%	10%-13%
Very severe anemia	<13%	<10%

conjunction with the PCV to aid in interpreting the PCV.

The tools needed for a PCV are a centrifuge, a supply of capillary tubes, and a microhematocrit tube reader. Any centrifuge that has a microhematocrit speed is acceptable. Capillary tubes come with or without anticoagulant. If nonheparinized blood samples are being collected, then anticoagulated capillary tubes should be used. Capillary tubes must be sealed with clay after the sample is inserted and before they are placed in the centrifuge. The clay end should face outward.

After the sample is spun, three layers will be evident. The PCV is closest to the clay. The buffy coat is a white or turbid layer just above the PCV. This is composed of white cells and platelets. The third layer is the plasma protein layer.

Once the plasma is evaluated, the PCV is read using a microhematocrit tube reader, which is a slide rule used to estimate the PCV volume by percentage of total blood volume. The line where the clay meets the red cell mass is placed on the zero line of the reader. Slide the tube until the top line of the reader is flush with the top of the plasma, making sure that the bottom line is still in position. After the top and bottom are lined up correctly, look at where the red cells meet the buffy coat. This is the PCV. The buffy coat percentage also should be read and recorded (Table 2-1 and Figure 2-1).

Anemia classification schemes are arbitrary and do not necessarily correlate with the patient's status. Patients who live at high altitudes generally need a higher PCV, and this classification may not be appropriate. Dehydration affects the classification. In addition, a patient who experiences a rapid decrease in PCV from 55% to 30% may be in a critical state, whereas a patient with a chronic anemia may be stable with a PCV of 8%.

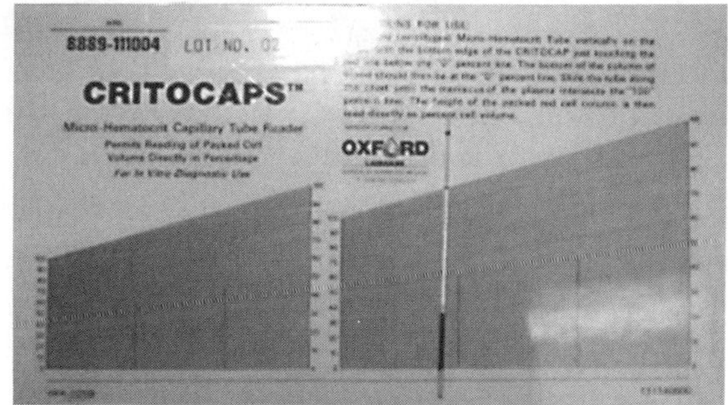

Figure 2-1
The tube must be positioned properly on the microhematocrit tube reader to ensure accurate PCV readings.

A refractometer is a device used to determine the total plasma protein. The capillary tube is split above the buffy coat, and the plasma protein is pipetted onto the surface of the refractometer. The refractometer is read by looking into the instrument and looking at the column on the grid labeled "g/dl." The line where the shaded area meets the light area is the total plasma protein. The refractometer should be calibrated regularly using distilled water.

ELECTROLYTE AND CHEMISTRY ANALYZERS

An electrolyte analyzer and a chemistry analyzer are essential for a veterinary critical care laboratory. These valuable pieces of equipment allow users to obtain rapid electrolyte and chemistry values. The laboratory technician must recognize abnormal values and bring them to the clinician's attention. This is especially important with parameters that are potentially life threatening, such as electrolyte, glucose, and phosphorus abnormalities.

There are many electrolyte analyzers on the market, so a unit should be chosen to fit the hospital's needs. Most analyzers run sodium, chloride, and potassium. Many analyzers run ionized calcium, and ionized magnesium can now be evaluated with some machines. Some chemistry analyzers run electrolytes and some do not. Some machines run electrolytes and blood gases from the same sample. The user must research all of his or her options when choosing equipment.

The main function of any critical care laboratory's electrolyte analyzer is to provide rapid and accurate electrolyte results at a reasonable cost. The buyer must take all of this into account before making a purchase. It is important to research not only the unit itself but also its associated costs such as reagents, standards, electrodes, annual maintenance, cleaning solutions, and conditioning solutions. After the final decision is made on what type of electrolyte analyzer to use, a technical manual should be acquired and read thoroughly. A maintenance protocol and cleaning schedule should be established. Keep a technical support number close to the unit in plain view for unfamiliar users. All the unit's maintenance records must be kept, as well as detailed notes of technical support remedies to technical problems that arise, so that the next time the problem occurs it can be dealt with more rapidly. A critical care laboratory must be accurate and able to produce results in a timely manner. Laboratory equipment should be down for no longer than 15 minutes.

The sampling needed for most electrolyte analyzers is heparinized blood or serum. Electrolyte analysis can be run on urine or pleural or peritoneal fluid if needed. The sampling requirements for each individual electrolyte analyzer must be referred to consistently and good sample handling techniques must be practiced. Good sample handling techniques are essential to avoid artifacts or damage to the analyzer, such as destruction of an electrode.

Ideally electrolyte panels should be run at least every 24 hours on critically ill or injured patients. Presurgical screens should include electrolytes.

A variety of chemistry analyzers are available for in-house use. Factors that influence the choice of analyzer include anticipated number of panels, whether individual chemistries or full panels are needed, reagent shelf life, and overall costs.

COMPLETE HEMATOLOGY CELL COUNTERS

Being able to quantify white blood cell numbers, platelet numbers, red blood cell numbers, and red blood cell indices are important for the critically ill patient. A variety of automated hematology cell counters are available. Some just provide white blood cell counts, and some provide red blood cell counts and platelet counts. Some provide numerical results only, and some provide graphic results. As with any machine, the equipment should be well researched before purchase because each machine offers something different. Veterinary machines are recommended over human machines because the variation in cell sizes can alter machine readouts significantly if they are not calibrated for that species. No machine currently can replace a manual differential, and blood smears always should be evaluated.

BLOOD GAS ANALYZERS

In today's critical care veterinary setting, blood gases are an important tool in patient evaluation and treatment because most critically ill or injured patients can have significant disturbances in their pulmonary and acid-base statuses. Blood gases enable the veterinarian to determine a range of factors including pH, partial pressures of oxygen and carbon dioxide, and bicarbonate levels.

When considering blood gas equipment, reliability and ease of use are the first priorities. No matter what the cost, if you cannot provide accurate and timely blood gas results you are not providing adequate patient care. Both handheld and larger machines are available. Most are easy to use, but among electrolyte analyzers, more maintenance is needed for the larger machines than for handheld units. However, handheld units tend to be less cost-effective than the larger units if a large number of samples is being run. Different machines may analyze only blood gases or may analyze blood gases and electrolytes or blood gases, electrolytes, and chemistries on a single blood sample.

Instruct all users in the sampling and sample input procedures for the machine. If a larger machine is in place, assign one person to be in charge of blood gas equipment maintenance. This can be done only by reading the technical manual and developing a close relationship with the provider's technical support branch. All maintenance instructions should be followed precisely, and if calibrations are needed, these must be done daily.

There are two kinds of blood gas sampling: arterial and venous. The major difference between the two is the lack of correlation between arterial oxygen pressures and venous oxygen pressures. Assuming normal perfusion to the area being sampled, venous samples generally correlate fairly well with arterial samples for all other parameters. The venous sampling should be done via heparinized syringe, or the blood sample should be placed into a lithium heparin vacutainer tube or lithium heparin capillary tubes. Care should be taken to ensure that the sample is not diluted. If the transfer is done quickly enough, samples can be analyzed immediately without heparinization, but this generally is not recommended because blood clots can form quickly and this can lead to erroneous results or a clogged machine. It should be kept in mind that the venous sample reflects the status of the tissues in the area from which the blood was sampled. Therefore if a patient has a traumatized distal limb and a venous sample is taken from the affected limb (cephalic or saphenous), the venous gas is likely to be very different from that of a sample taken from the jugular vein. This is important if an attempt is being made to extrapolate the venous sample to an arterial blood gas because it is unlikely to correlate, but it is very relevant if perfusion to the distal limb is being assessed.

Arterial sampling should be done via arterial puncture or arterial catheter. A 1-ml syringe is filled with heparin (1000 U/ml) and the heparin is expelled. If a direct arterial puncture is being attempted, a 25-gauge needle should be used. The sample is drawn into the syringe and analyzed. Most machines use 0.125 to 0.3 ml blood. Exposure to room air should be avoided. Either the sample should be analyzed immediately or the needle should be placed into a rubber stopper or capped with a tight-fitting cap. Ideally samples should be analyzed within 15 to 30 minutes if stored at room temperature or within 2 hours if stored in an ice bath (Tables 2-2 and 2-3).

COLLOID OSMOTIC PRESSURE

Colloids are large molecules that generally do not pass across a semipermeable membrane. The colloid osmotic pressure (COP) is the pressure exerted by these molecules across the semipermeable membrane. The blood COP is a measurement of the pressure across the vascular endothelium that is exerted by intravascular colloids, which are mostly plasma proteins. These proteins help maintain intravascular water and crystalloids. A loss of

TABLE 2-2 Normal Blood Gas Values

	pH	Pco_2 (mm Hg)	Hco_3 (mm Hg)	Po_2 (mm Hg)
Dog venous	7.32-7.40	33-50	18-26	
Dog arterial	7.36-7.44	36-44	18-26	85-100
Cat venous	7.28-7.41	33-45	18-23	
Cat arterial	7.36-7.44	28-32	17-22	85-100

Note: In-house normal values should be established if the machine does not come with a published reference range.
From Willard MD, Tvedten H, Turnwald GH: *Small animal clinical diagnosis by laboratory methods,* ed. 3, Philadelphia, 1999, WB Saunders, p. 103.

TABLE 2-3 Assessment of Abnormal Blood Gas Values

pH	<7.36	=	Acidemia
pH	>7.44	=	Alkalemia
P_{CO_2}	>44 mm Hg (canine), 32 mm Hg (feline)	=	Respiratory acidosis
P_{CO_2}	<36 mm Hg (canine), 28 mm Hg (feline)	=	Respiratory alkalosis
H_{CO_3}	<18 (canine), 17 (feline)	=	Metabolic acidosis
H_{CO_3}	>26 (canine), 22 (feline)	=	Metabolic alkalosis

COP tends to lead to tissue edema because fluid is no longer kept as effectively in the intravascular space. COP can be very important in critically ill or injured patients because fluid balance is important to survival. Although the COP may correlate in normal patients with serum or plasma protein levels, this is rarely the case in the ill patient. The decision to use crystalloid or colloid fluid therapy is most accurately determined if the COP is known. It is also the only way to determine the adequacy of therapy with synthetic colloids such as hetastarch and dextrans.

A colloid osmometer (Wescor 4400 Colloid Osmometer, Wescor Inc., Logan, Utah) measures the COP of blood, plasma, or serum. The machine uses a semipermeable membrane that separates the plasma entry port from a protein-free solution. It is recommended to use heparinized whole blood samples for clinical ease. The machine must be well maintained to ensure accurate results. It must be calibrated every day with solutions of a known COP, and it must be flushed with saline daily and zeroed with saline before and after each use.

Normal values of whole blood range from 15.3 to 26.3 (mean 19.95 ± 2.21) mm Hg in dogs and 17.6 to 33.1 (mean 24.7 ± 3.7) mm Hg in cats.

LACTATE

Lactate concentrations have been shown to have important prognostic value in critically ill patients. During anaerobic conditions the body produces lactate. Elevated lactate levels can be an indication of tissue hypoxia and usually are associated with acidemia. This can occur with patients in shock as well as in patients with an increase in anaerobic metabolism, as occurs with heavy exercise or seizures. Other conditions, such as dextrose infusions and sepsis without decreased perfusion, can increase lactate levels.

Lactate can be measured using venous or arterial blood samples. The samples must be analyzed within 30 minutes. Both handheld (designed for use by athletes; Accusport, Boehringer Mannheim Corporation, Indianapolis, Indiana) and benchtop machines are available to measure lactate levels.

COAGULATION TESTS

Coagulation abnormalities are common in critically ill patients. Coagulopathies can be associated with trauma and sepsis, inherited conditions, and anticoagulant rodenticide toxicity. Without an accurate means of determining the coagulation status of a patient, important decisions on the use of blood products cannot be made in a timely manner, which can increase morbidity and mortality rates.

Tests of the patient's coagulation status that can be performed on site in the veterinary hospital include one stage prothrombin time (PT), activated partial thromboplastin time (aPTT), activated clotting time (ACT), buccal mucosal bleeding time (BMBT), and platelet counts. Samples must be taken correctly for accurate coagulation tests.

A new handheld device is available to analyze the PT and PTT on fresh whole blood or citrated whole blood (SCA2000, Symbiotics, San Diego, California). The blood is placed immediately into a cartridge or collected into a sodium citrate tube. If samples are collected into vacutainer tubes, the

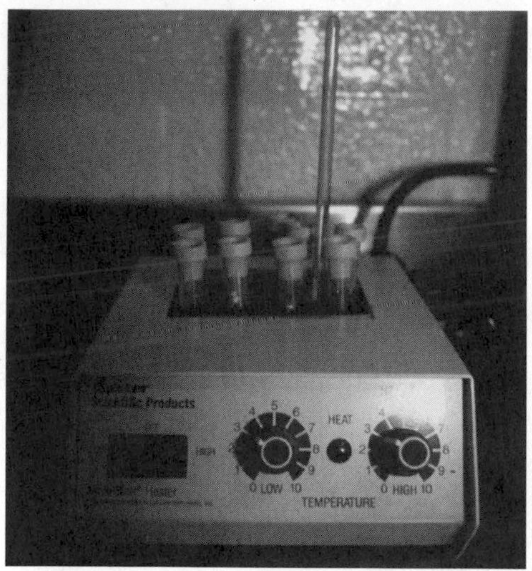

Figure 2-2

Heating blocks are used for the ACT measurement. The tube can be placed under the arm if a block is not available.

tubes must be filled with the correct amount of blood to avoid dilution.

The ACT is run using 3 ml whole blood. The venipuncture must be clean and blood must flow readily into the syringe. A venipuncture is performed and the first 1 ml is drawn and discarded. A new syringe is attached to the needle and 2 ml is drawn and placed directly into the ACT tube, which is a vacutainer tube filled with diatomaceous earth (ACT tubes, Becton Dickinson). (Because drawing 3 ml often is not feasible because of concerns for iatrogenic blood loss, the first step often is omitted.) The tube is rotated five times to ensure that the sample is mixed well. The tube is then placed in a heating block at 37° C, and the time to formation of a clot is noted. The first reading is taken at 60 seconds. This is done by rotating the tube and doing a visual check for clot formation. If a clot is not present, the tube is replaced in the heating block and checked every 5 seconds until a clot is noted. Normal values are 90 to 120 seconds for dogs and 60 to 90 seconds for cats (Figure 2-2). Significant thrombocytopenia may artificially prolong the activated clotting time.

The BMBT can be used in determining platelet function. It is the test of choice if there is any concern that a dog has Von Willebrand disease. It should be performed using a spring-loaded device (Simplate, Organon Teknika Corporation, Durham, North Carolina) because this standardizes the size of the incision. The Simplate is a disposable device with a retractable blade that cuts two uniform incisions. The site used is the labial mucosa, which is exposed by folding the dorsal lip upward. A piece of gauze tied lightly around the muzzle can hold the lip back and increase venous hydrostatic pressure. The Simplate is placed over the site and the trigger is released. Timing of the test begins at this time. Coffee filter paper or gauze is held close to the incision site to absorb the blood. Do not touch the actual incision site because this will interfere with the test results. Timing is stopped once the flow has stopped. The normal range is 1.7 to 4.2 minutes for dogs and 1.0 to 3.2 minutes for cats. Thrombocytopenia may prolong the BMBT.

BASIC TOOLS FOR MONITORING IN THE INTENSIVE CARE UNIT

Nothing can replace the human being in patient monitoring. Tools and machines may provide information that a physical examination or laboratory parameter cannot, but it is the human being who assesses the information, determines its validity, and develops a diagnostic or treatment plan based on the findings. Machines can err, and all unexpected abnormalities should be confirmed before treatment is adjusted. Confirming results may be as simple as getting another reading, but it may also involve performing a second test. For instance, if the pulse oximeter is reading 75% but the patient has pink mucous membranes and is breathing normally, the probe position should be checked before this patient can be assessed as being severely hypoxic.

A thorough physical examination is irreplaceable as a monitoring tool. Temperature monitoring is important. An elevated temperature may indicate hyperthermia, infection, or inflammation. A subnormal temperature may indicate environmental hypothermia, poor perfusion, or a decreased metabolic rate secondary to medications (e.g., opioids) or disease (e.g., hypoglycemia or hypothyroidism). Because metabolic rates are associated closely with temperature, it is vital to know the patient's temperature at all times. This can be especially important in shock states or in anesthetized patients, in whom vital organs systems such as ventilation, cardiac function, and coagulation can be adversely affected by hypothermia. Continuous temperature monitoring should be performed in anesthetized patients. Temperature can be taken using aural, esophageal, or rectal thermometers. Ear infections, long ear canals, and environmental temperature can reduce the accuracy of aural thermometer readings. Rectal temperature may not reflect core temperature in poorly perfusing patients. Core temperature probes can be purchased commercially from medical companies for use with certain multifunction monitoring machines, or simple indoor/outdoor thermometers can be purchased from electronic equipment stores.

The stethoscope is a vital extension of the technician's ears and eyes. Abnormal breathing patterns, abnormal audible sounds, and coughing are indications for auscultation of the larynx, trachea, lungs, and heart. Obtain baseline values at the time of admission or at the beginning of each shift to assess changes in the patient's condition. If gastrointestinal function is abnormal, gut sounds should be auscultated regularly. A lack of sounds indicates the possibility of ileus. An esophageal stethoscope is a useful tool in the anesthetized patient or with long-term ventilator use. It allows clear auscultation of the lungs and heart and may allow early detection of abnormalities such as pulmonary crackles and heart murmurs.

ELECTROCARDIOGRAM MONITORING

The electrocardiogram (ECG) is a record of the electrical potential of the heart muscle. A normal tracing shows a P wave, QRS complex, and T wave, which correspond to atrial depolarization (P wave), ventricular depolarization (QRS complex), and ventricular repolarization (T wave). Normal complexes do not necessarily correlate with normal muscle function.

Each wave has a normal duration (milliseconds) and height (millivolts) as well as a normal interval between waves. These measurements are useful in determining the health of the electrical conduction system. Abnormalities are associated with conduction disturbances and can be associated with changes in the heart muscle or pericardial space. Measurements can be taken only from printouts.

INDICATIONS

ECGs are used as a diagnostic or monitoring tool. Anything other than a normal sinus rhythm indicates cardiac disease or dysfunction. The ECG is used during cardiopulmonary resuscitation (CPR) to determine the arrest rhythm, which dictates the type of CPR to be performed. Asystole, ventricular fibrillation, and electromechanical dissociation are all treated differently. Without the use of an ECG, it is impossible during closed-chest CPR to determine whether the use of a defibrillator is indicated. In addition, it can be very difficult to determine whether defibrillation has been successful unless an ECG is available. ECGs are useful in anesthetized patients and those with trauma, sepsis, syncope, or pulmonary or cardiac disorders. Ventricular premature contractions (VPCs) are not uncommon with myocardial contusions, myocardial hypoxia, splenic disease, or other primary cardiac muscle diseases. It is important to be aware of VPCs because they are associated with cardiac muscle dysfunction and can lead to life-threatening arrhythmias. Continuous ECG monitoring is recommended in all critically ill patients with signs of VPCs. Primary cardiac disease can be associated with a variety of abnormal rhythms that dictate the kind of treatment needed. Diagnostic or continuous ECGs may be indicated for these patients. Drug toxicities and other poisonings may be associated with cardiac arrhythmias and are another indication for an ECG.

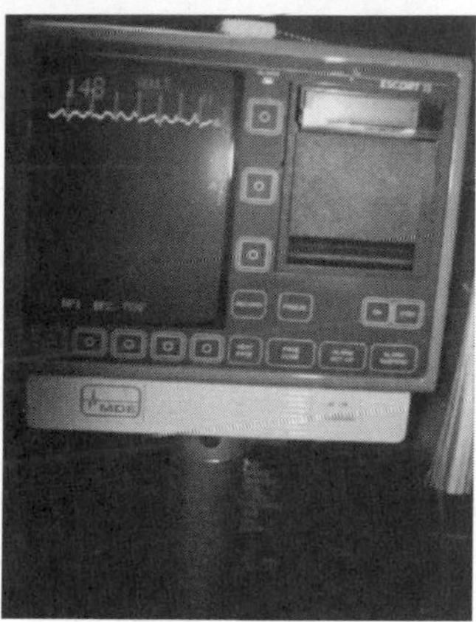

Figure 2-3

Many ECG types are available. Printing capabilities are needed to maintain complete records of abnormalities and to measure complexes.

Most ECG monitors have an audible sound associated with each heart beat. This can be useful in an intensive care unit (ICU), where the sound may alert the nurse or doctor of a change in the patient's condition (Figure 2-3).

TECHNIQUE

The standard lead II or six-lead ECG is recorded using four electrodes that are attached to the patient. There are usually five leads or electrodes that are color coded and labeled based on human anatomy: right foreleg (RA), white lead; left foreleg (LA), black lead; right hind leg (RL), green lead; left hind leg (LL), red lead; and the V lead (C), which is an exploring lead and is brown.

The leads can be attached most rapidly by using the copper clips at the skin fold near the junction of the limb and the trunk. If the pet has long or thick hair, the ECG connection sites should be shaved. An alcohol-soaked cotton swab can be used to clean the area for 10 seconds or ECG paste can be applied to the skin. Alcohol should not be used if the leads are being attached during CPR and a defibrillator may be used. In these cases, ECG paste must be applied.

Alternatively, ECG patches can be applied to the skin. To improve adhesion, the skin should be well shaved and cleaned with alcohol and dried before patch placement. Tissue glue can be used sparingly if needed. In recumbent patients the patches can be placed on the metacarpal and metatarsal pads and held in place using tape placed circumferentially.

Another means of attaching leads involves the use of 4-0 wire suture. A 20- or 22-gauge hypodermic needle is passed through the skin in the desired location and the wire is threaded through the needle. The needle is removed, leaving the wire in place. The ends of the wire are twisted together to prevent inadvertent removal. It is advisable to place tape around the ends of the wire for safety and as a visual reminder that wires have been placed. The ECG clips then are attached to the wires. This is more comfortable for long-term use and avoids skin damage from the clamping effect of the alligator clips. In an emergency, the alligator clips can be attached directly to a hypodermic needle that has been inserted through the skin. For safety reasons this is not advised except in emergencies.

Occasionally there will be problems getting a clear tracing. Usually these are caused by contact problems or patient-related problems. If there is electrical interference or no tracing, the leads should be checked to ensure they are attached to skin (or to wires or patches) and not fur. If patches are being used, it should be ascertained that the patch is still firmly adhered to the patient. Additional alcohol or ECG paste should be applied as needed. Next, the leads should be checked to ensure that they are still firmly attached to the cable. Other electrical equipment may cause 60-Hz interference, which can lead to poor tracing quality. Patient shivering can lead to similar problems. If there is significant undulation of the baseline, the most likely problem is that the patient's breathing pattern is interfering with the tracing. In the case of a shifting baseline or shivering, the leads should be attached at a more peripheral location. This will help avoid the problems caused by patient movement.

Equipment

A variety of ECG machines is available. A continuous screen readout is most useful in the ICU if continuous ECG monitoring is being used. Printout capabilities are needed to document abnormalities and measure the complexes. Machines that provide a printout only are useful for diagnostic purposes but are less useful for recording irregularities appearing over an extended time because of the large amount of paper needed. Most ECG machines must be attached to the ECG leads; however, for some monitors this is not necessary. Telemetry allows hands-off monitoring and is useful when multiple patients need ECG monitoring simultaneously. The ECG leads are attached to the patient and to a small box that is taped or bandaged to the patient and transmits data via radio signals to a main monitor. Many multichannel monitors are available. These devices can monitor any combination of ECG, oximetry, capnometry, blood pressure, and temperature.

Handheld monitors are available that do not use leads. These small devices are held against the patient's chest and a tracing is obtained. Most models have some memory capabilities to store tracings and some have printout capabilities. Although the quality of these tracings often is not equal to that obtained with regular ECG leads, the quality of the machines is improving constantly, and the major advantage is that a quick rhythm strip can be obtained in the examination room or at the patient's cage.

Esophageal ECG devices are available for use in anesthetized patients. These devices tend not to be affected by other electronic monitoring equipment, as are external devices. They should not be used in combination with electrosurgery.

PHOTODETECTOR PULSE MONITOR

The photodetector pulse monitor has a small probe that is placed on the tongue, ear, toe webbing, or inguinal or vulva skin fold. The automated device emits a beam of light directed to an area of high capillary blood flow. On the opposite side of the capillary bed a photodetector analyzes light transmitted through the capillary bed. The pulse is computed and displayed on a screen.

PULSE OXIMETRY

Pulse oximetry measures the level of hemoglobin saturation (Spo_2). A probe that emits light in the infrared and red wavelengths is attached to the patient. Saturated hemoglobin absorbs more infrared light than desaturated hemoglobin, which absorbs more red light. A photodetector receives the light signal and the oximeter senses the intensity of each wavelength received. The oximeter analyzes the information and displays the saturated hemoglobin as a percentage of total hemoglobin.

Pulse oximeters display the strength of the pulsatile signal either in a waveform or as a bar code. This signal must remain strong because the accuracy of the oximeter decreases when pulsatile flow is not detected or is poorly detected. Most oximeters give a continuous display of the pulse rate. This should correspond to the palpable pulse to ensure accuracy of the monitor.

Indications

Pulse oximetry should be monitored whenever hypoxia or hypoxemia is a concern. The Spo_2 correlates with the partial pressure of arterial oxygen (Pao_2) based on the oxygen hemoglobin dissociation curve. Normal Spo_2 at room air should be 96% to 99%. This correlates to a Pao_2 of approximately 90 to 100 mm Hg. An Spo_2 of 90% to 92% is equivalent to a Pao_2 of approximately 60 mm Hg. This is the level at which cyanosis becomes detectable in most patients (assuming adequate peripheral perfusion and a hemoglobin level greater than 5 g/dl) and is an indicator of tissue hypoxia. Oxygen should be supplemented if the Spo_2 is less than 94%. If a patient who is being provided with supplemental oxygen has an Spo_2 of 90% to 92% and is showing signs of respiratory distress, positive-pressure ventilation may be indicated. Because of problems with pulse oximetry in the awake patient, abnormal readings should be confirmed with an arterial blood gas reading.

Once the hemoglobin is 100% saturated (at a Pao_2 of approximately 100 mm Hg), pulse oximetry cannot detect changes in arterial oxygenation until a significant change has occurred, which is a serious limitation when the patient is being supplemented with high levels of oxygen. For instance, on 100% oxygen (e.g., general anesthesia) the Pao_2 should be approximately 450 to 500 mm Hg. The oximetry reading will not drop below 100% until the Pao_2 has decreased below approximately 100 mm Hg, by which time the patient may be in serious trouble. Therefore the best time to monitor patients with a pulse oximeter is when they are not on high levels of supplemental oxygen (e.g., patients with respiratory compromise being supplemented with nasal oxygen, anesthetized patients during the recovery period, or patients on ventilators when the clinician is trying to decrease the level of inspired oxygen.)

Technique

The accuracy of the pulse oximeter is affected by tissue perfusion, the thickness of the tissue through which the light must be emitted, tissue pigmentation, tissue movement (shaking or shivering), and strong overhead fluorescent lighting. The probe should be attached in a location where pulsatile blood flow can be detected readily. The ideal location is the tongue. Other locations include the lip, tail, toe web, inguinal skin fold, and skin fold in the region of the Achilles tendon. Fur should be shaved where appropriate to reduce interference with signal transmission. If the patient is shivering or shaking, an inaccurate reading may result because the sensor may not be able to detect the pulse accurately.

Equipment

Pulse oximeters come as handheld portable monitors or tabletop monitors. Either is acceptable; however, the waveform analysis that is available with the larger models helps ensure accuracy of the digital display. Many multichannel monitors are available. These devices can monitor any combination of ECG, oximetry, capnometry, blood pressure, and temperature.

Most pulse oximetry probes are transmittance probes. A diode emits a signal that is transmitted across a tissue bed and received by a photodetector. These are the standard clip-type probes. When reflectance probes, such as rectal probes, are used, the light signal is reflected back to the probe.

Troubleshooting

Low saturation may indicate a physiologic problem or a false reading related to the probe's ability to detect blood flow. Mucous membrane color should be assessed whenever a low reading is obtained. If the patient is severely anemic (hematocrit less than 10%) or if blood flow to the area is poor (e.g., low blood pressure or hypothermia), then the probe may not provide an accurate reading. If the probe is on the tongue, it should be repositioned every 5 to 10 minutes because the clips can occlude flow to the area. If the probe is located at any site other than the tongue, it should be repositioned, and if the reading is still considered inaccurate it should be moved to a different location. Whenever low readings are obtained but the reading does not match the patient's clinical status, an arterial blood gas should be evaluated.

Aberrantly high readings may result from high carboxyhemoglobin or methemoglobin levels. In addition, intense fluorescent lights can lead to falsely elevated readings.

CAPNOMETRY

Capnometry is a recording of the end exhalation or end-tidal carbon dioxide concentration ($ETco_2$). It provides a noninvasive means of measuring arterial carbon dioxide pressure ($Paco_2$).

The $ETco_2$ measurements are approximately 4 to 5 mm Hg less than the $Paco_2$ in the patient with normal pulmonary function. This means that an $ETco_2$ measurement of 36 mm Hg corresponds to a $Paco_2$ of approximately 40 mm Hg. Measurements higher than 40 mm Hg indicate hypoventilation or excessive rebreathing of the carbon dioxide. Measurements lower than 32 mm Hg indicate hyperventilation. An $ETco_2$ of 25 mm or less (assuming normal pulmonary function) indicates a $Paco_2$ low enough to cause cerebral vasoconstriction and decreased cerebral blood flow.

The $ETco_2$ does not correlate with the $Paco_2$ in patients with significant ventilation-perfusion mismatches or in patients with airway obstructions.

INDICATIONS

Capnometry is recommended any time ventilation monitoring is indicated. The three primary indications for capnometry are in general anesthesia, in the patient in the ICU who is on a ventilator, and during cardiopulmonary resuscitation.

All general anesthetic agents and many analgesics such as narcotics cause respiratory depression. This leads to a buildup of CO_2 or a respiratory acidosis. As the pH decreases, metabolic functions can be affected. Acidosis leads to vasodilation, decreased muscle contractility (including respiratory and cardiac muscles), and interference with normal metabolic functions such as coagulation. This can cause serious morbidity. The only means of determining the level of hypoventilation is to monitor the CO_2 levels. Ideally, capnometry should always be monitored in the patient under anesthesia. This can be especially important during the recovery period before the patient is extubated because this is often the time at which supportive measures (such as assisting ventilation) are discontinued, yet the patient may not be awake enough for all positive-pressure ventilatory support to be discontinued.

Close monitoring of the patient on a ventilator is needed to ensure that the machine is performing the functions that the lungs would normally perform. In other words, the ventilator must ensure that CO_2 that is being produced by the body is being exchanged at the alveolus.

During CPR it is essential to know whether the carbon dioxide that is being produced by the body is making it to the alveolus for exchange. If pulmonary blood flow is inadequate, then the CO_2 levels will be far below normal (<15 mm Hg). As cardiac compressions become more effective, pulmonary blood flow will increase and the $ETco_2$ levels should rise.

TECHNIQUE

A detector is inserted between the endotracheal tube and the anesthetic circuit. The detector is connected to the capnometer via tubing. Moisture in the sensor or the tubing will interfere with readings. For this reason, the sensor should always be in an upright position so that moisture coming from the patient's airway via the endotracheal tube does not accumulate in the sensor or tubing. The waveform or capnogram produced by exhaled carbon dioxide has a unique shape. The capnogram should be analyzed for the following characteristics:

- Height: height depends on the $ETco_2$ concentration.
- Baseline: baseline should be zero for both spontaneous and mechanical ventilation.
- Frequency and rhythm: frequency and rhythm are determined by respiratory rate and effort.
- Shape: the capnogram has an ascending limb, plateau, and descending limb.

EQUIPMENT

Capnometers come as handheld monitors or larger tabletop monitors. Waveform analysis, which is an important part of capnometry, is not available with the handheld monitors. Many multichannel monitors are available. These monitors are able to monitor any combination of ECG, oximetry, capnometry, blood pressure, and temperature.

BLOOD PRESSURE

Arterial blood pressure consists of three values: systolic, diastolic, and mean arterial pressures. Systolic pressure is the pressure generated when the heart contracts. Diastolic pressure is the pressure between contractions. Mean arterial pressure is calculated as one third the systolic pressure plus two thirds the diastolic pressure. Organ function may be compromised when mean arterial pressures fall below certain numbers. For instance, renal function decreases when the mean arterial pressure falls below 60 mm Hg. Hypertension also can lead to organ dysfunction. It is very important in most disease processes to monitor the patient's blood pressure because this will affect fluid therapy, choice of medications, and prognosis.

INDICATIONS

Blood pressure monitoring is indicated during shock states, under anesthesia, during CPR, and in all cases in which aberrations of blood pressure may exist secondary to the underlying disease (e.g., hyperadrenocorticism, hyperthyroidism, heart disease, renal failure). During anesthesia determine whether the anesthetic agents are inducing significant hypotension and determine whether fluid support or hemodynamic support is indicated. Blood pressure should be monitored not only during anesthesia but also during induction and recovery. A Doppler flow probe is especially useful because it allows the anesthetist to monitor easily for anesthetic agent–induced vagal episodes and induction-induced hypotension. During recovery it allows monitoring of similar events.

TECHNIQUE

Direct Arterial Pressure Monitoring. Direct measurements generally are made using an arterial catheter that is hooked up to a transducer. The transducer is connected to a monitor that gives a readout of systolic, diastolic, and mean arterial pressure. In addition, most monitors display a waveform analysis that provides vital information about the patient and indicates whether the readings are accurate. Direct arterial pressure monitoring is the gold standard for blood pressure measurement; however, often it is not used because of technical difficulties in placing and maintaining arterial catheters as well as lack of equipment. The availability of used monitoring equipment and transducers has substantially reduced costs and makes it affordable for any hospital dealing with critically ill or injured patients.

The catheter can be placed in any artery; however, the most commonly used are the dorsal metatarsal and the femoral arteries. The femoral artery should be used with caution in patients with coagulopathies because hemorrhage can be significant if the vessel is disrupted or the catheter is dislodged inadvertently. Special arterial catheters are available, but the same catheters that are used for venous access can be used for arterial access. Percutaneous methods or cutdown methods can be used to place the catheters. Short (1.5- to 2-inch) over-the-needle catheters tend to be difficult to maintain for longer periods of time because they tend to kink. Longer catheters (arterial, through-the-needle, or those placed by Seldinger technique) tend to last longer. Once the catheters are placed, they must be secured well to prevent inadvertent dislodging and kinking.

Arterial catheters are prone to thrombosis and must be flushed regularly with heparinized saline. Flushing can be accomplished manually by flushing with heparinized saline every hour. Alternatively, the catheters can be connected to a constant rate infusion of heparinized saline. This can be set at a drip rate controlled by a fluid infusor pump, or the bag of heparinized fluids can be placed under pressure. When the pressurized systems are connected to a commercial transducer system, they will flow at a set low rate to help maintain catheter patency.

If a transducer system is not available, blood pressure can be measured directly using the same method as for measuring central venous pressure. A catheter or needle is placed into the artery. One or two extension sets filled with fluid are attached to the needle or catheter. The end of the fluid line is exposed to the air. The height of the fluid line can then be measured using the base of the heart as the zero mark. Centimeters of water pressure can be converted to millimeters of mercury by dividing the number by 1.36. This measurement will correlate with the mean arterial pressure. Mean arterial pressure can be calculated from these two measurements. Although this is a crude means of measuring pressure, it can provide valuable information. If a needle was used, it must be removed at the end of the procedure.

Indirect Blood Pressure Monitoring. Blood pressure is measured indirectly using either an oscillometric device or a Doppler ultrasound flow detector. Both instruments have their advantages and disadvantages, and although both can be used to determine pressures, indirect measurements can be significantly different from direct measurements. For this reason, measurements always should be interpreted with caution, and a trend of measurements may be more important than actual readings. Both methods entail placing a blood pressure cuff. The cuffs can be placed over any accessible artery and generally are placed around the limb distal to the elbow or hock or around the base of the tail. The brachium is a useful location for a cuff in cats and small dogs if the instrument cannot detect a pulse more distally. A variety of cuffs is available commercially. The cuff should be approximately 40% of the circumference of the limb (or tail) around which it is being placed. Many cuffs have markings on them to indicate whether the fit is appropriate as the cuff is being placed. A cuff that is too large can lead to artificially low readings and a cuff that is too small can lead to artificially elevated readings. It may be necessary to tape cuffs to prevent the Velcro from coming undone when the cuff is inflated, but care must be taken to ensure that the tape is not too tight because this can affect readings. Some cuffs have markings on them indicating where the artery must come in contact with the cuff.

Oscillometric Devices. Oscillometric devices work by picking up pulsation under a cuff placed over an artery. The cuff is connected to a pressure cable that is connected to the monitor. The monitor inflates the cuff until flow is occluded and then slowly deflates the cuff. As the pulse returns the monitor displays the systolic, diastolic, and mean arterial blood pressures as well as a heart rate. Poor pulse signals from poor flow, small arteries, shaking, and shivering will interfere with the accuracy of the oscillometric device.

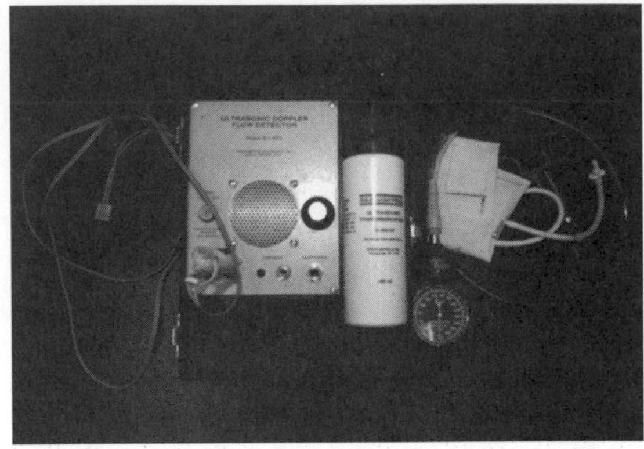

Figure 2-4

Doppler flow detectors allow the clinician to hear blood flow.

Doppler Ultrasound Flow Detectors. Doppler ultrasound flow detectors involve an ultrasonic probe placed over an artery (Figure 2-4). The most common locations are the palmar arterial arches of the forelimb and hindlimb. The most common factor that interferes with Doppler signals is poor contact between the probe and the vessel. The area is shaved and a generous amount of ultrasonic gel is placed over the artery. If the skin is very dry, it is helpful to rub a small amount of gel in first and then apply more. The probe is placed over the vessels and secured in place with tape. If the patient has a very deep groove in the location of the arch, the probe can be secured better by placing a gauze square or cotton ball over the top of the probe before taping it in place. If the tape is placed too loosely, the signal may be weak. In small patients the lack of a signal may indicate that the tape has been placed too tightly.

A blood pressure cuff is placed above the ultrasonic probe and inflated using a sphygmomanometer. Then the cuff is allowed to deflate slowly. The measurement at which the sound of the blood flow first is audible is the systolic pressure. The level at which the second sound is heard is the diastolic pressure. Although it has been shown that diastolic pressure correlates with directly measured diastolic blood pressure, the second sound cannot be heard in all patients.

Ideally the cuff should be placed immediately above the probe. In other words, it should not be above the metacarpal or metatarsal joint. This is especially important in larger patients. When the cuff is inflated above the metacarpal or metatarsal joint, it redirects blood flow into vessels in between the bones, and the pressure in the cuff forces blood under high pressure down into the foot. Therefore the first sound that is heard may be an erroneously high reading that does not actually correlate with systolic blood pressure but correlates with the flow under high pressure. In this case, three sounds should be listened for. The first is the erroneous reading. The second is the systolic pressure and the third sound is the diastolic pressure. This erroneous reading can be avoided by placing the cuff either directly above the probe but below the joint or directly over the top of the probe.

One of the significant advantages of the Doppler ultrasound flow detector over an oscillometric device is that the flow can be heard. Blood pressure does not always correlate with flow. A severely constricted vessel may indicate good blood pressure but poor overall flow into the tissue bed. By attuning his or her ear to the Doppler sounds, the technician can make a subjective assessment of flow into the area in question.

Doppler flow detectors can be used to determine the presence of flow in distal limbs whenever there is concern about circulatory disturbances. In the patient with a severely traumatized limb proximally, amputation may be needed if there is no flow distally. A Doppler ultrasonic probe allows detection of flow or lack of flow. In cats with saddle thrombi and a lack of a femoral pulse, a Doppler flow probe should be placed over the femoral artery to assess flow because this is a much more sensitive indicator of flow than digital palpation.

Certain arrhythmias also can be determined using Doppler flow probes. Irregularities in the pulse signal or rate can be an indicator of atrial fibrillation, ventricular premature contractions, sinus arrest, or heart block.

During CPR Doppler flow probe can be placed on the surface of the cornea (after placing ultrasonic gel) to monitor for the presence of blood flow to the head. Although this has not been proven to correlate with brain blood flow, the lack of an audible flow signal indicates totally inadequate forward blood flow during closed chest compressions or open-chest cardiac massage.

Lack of perfusion or very poor pulses, severe vasoconstriction, and poor probe contact can lead to an absent or very weak signal. During anesthesia the concurrent use of other electrical equipment, especially electrosurgical equipment, can interfere with the flow signal.

The gel on the ultrasonic probes should be wiped off with water after each use. Disconnecting the probe from the flow detector should be avoided because this can weaken the connections and lead to a poor signal quality.

CONCLUSION

It is very easy to rely on video monitoring of patients. The beeps and buzzers can give technicians a false sense of security. Use monitoring as another tool to assist in caring for the critically ill patient, not as the sole resource for evaluating its progress or decline. Equipment can fail through mechanical dysfunction or user errors. Machines cannot replace visual and tactile monitoring.

BIBLIOGRAPHY

Culp AM, Clay ME, Baylor IA, et al: Colloid osmotic pressure (COP) and total solids (TS) measurement in normal dogs and cats. Fourth International Veterinary Emergency and Critical Care Symposium, San Antonio, Tx, 1994, Omnipress (abstract).

Hughes D: Lactate measurement: diagnostic, therapeutic, and prognostic implications. In Bonagura JD, ed: *Kirk's current veterinary therapy XIII,* Philadelphia, 2000, WB Saunders.

King LG: Colloid osmometry. In Bonagura JD, ed: *Kirk's current veterinary therapy XIII,* Philadelphia, 2000, WB Saunders.

Willard MD, Tvedten H, Turnwald GH: *Small animal clinical diagnosis by laboratory methods,* ed 3, Philadelphia, 1999, WB Saunders.

in the cat or small dog. Radiographs can be taken to determine whether the catheter is placed properly.

VASCULAR ACCESS POINTS

The best vascular access point to use on the small animal patient depends on many factors. The treatment plan and accessibility are primary concerns. The most common access points are the right and left cephalic, right and left lateral saphenous, right and left medial saphenous, and right and left jugular veins.

The jugular vessels are the best site if a patient needs prolonged fluid therapy or if multiple blood samples must be drawn. Avoid placing catheters in the jugular vessels of animals with suspected coagulopathies. It is very difficult to control hemorrhage at the insertion site. Peripherally inserted central catheters (PICCs) are available for those situations when a central line is necessary but the jugular vessel is not an option for access.

PLACEMENT

Correct placement of intravenous catheter units entails an understanding of catheter mechanics. All materials, including the catheter unit, heparinized saline, triple-antibiotic ointment to cover the insertion site, and the materials needed to stabilize the unit, are readily available.

Placing over-the-needle catheters involves a four-step process after the site is shaved and surgically scrubbed. If the catheter is being placed in a limb, it is important to create a sterile field in which to work. This is accomplished by wrapping a sterile bandage around the distal portion of the catheter site. The unit is placed into the vessel. Once a flashback is observed, the entire unit is advanced into the vein slightly to ensure that the stylet is placed in the vessel properly. The catheter is then fed off the stylet into the vein. The stylet must be stabilized and not allowed to advance with the catheter. The stylet is then removed and the catheter is capped and flushed with heparinized saline unless intravenous fluid therapy is started immediately through this catheter.

Placing a catheter into the jugular vessel is a team effort. The person restraining and positioning the animal must work with the person placing the catheter. The animal usually is placed in lateral recumbence for this procedure, with the neck extended. A rolled towel placed under the neck can assist in visualizing the vessel. It may be necessary to try different angles of the head and extensions of the neck before the vessel can be visualized or palpated. A cat's vessels can be palpated and visualized easily when the neck is extended and the head rotated outward.

Placing obese animals or breeds with thick necks in a sitting position, with the head slightly elevated and turned away from the venopuncture site, facilitates access to the jugular vessel. This position is useful for any patient with respiratory complications.

Technical Tip Box 3-1 illustrates a six-step process that involves the use of a Peel-away sheath needle.

Technical Tip Box 3-2 illustrates a six-step process called the guidewire technique (also called the Seldinger technique). An introducer (hypodermic needle), stylet, dilator, and catheter are used.

Technical Tip Box 3-3 on p. 28 illustrates a six-step process that involves the use of a catheter placement unit (through-the-needle catheter) that is contained in a sterile covering.

Technical Tip Box 3-4 on p. 32 describes a technique that uses a feeding tube and an over-the-needle catheter.

STABILIZATION

Once the catheter is in place, it must be stabilized properly. The wrap should provide additional catheter stabilization, increase patient comfort, and protect the insertion site. Multilayered wraps should be avoided in patients receiving cancer chemotherapy intravenously. The insertion site

Text continued on p. 31

Box 3-1 Technical Tip: *Peel-Away Sheath Technique*

Note that gloves and surgical drapes were omitted from illustrations so that positioning of hands and catheter could be shown. Gloves must be worn and a sterile field provided.

Items needed:

Items for prepping, drape, and sterile surgical gloves
Peel-away sheath introducer with catheter
Heparinized saline
Injection cap with extension line
Triple-antibiotic ointment
Materials needed for stabilization

Shave and surgically prep site. Drape around site. Sterile surgical gloves must be worn. Perform a small skin nick incision.

1. Insert over-the-needle sheath through the small nick in the skin into the vessel.

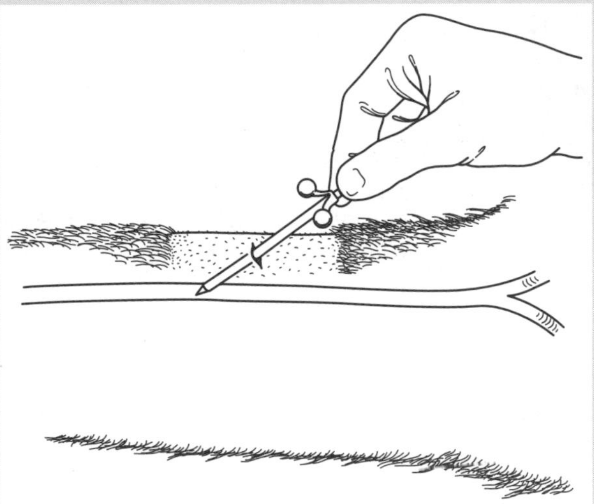

2. Advance needle sheath slightly to ensure that the sheath as well as the needle is seated in the vessel.
3. Stabilize the needle and advance the sheath, slightly rotating it back and forth, into the vessel.

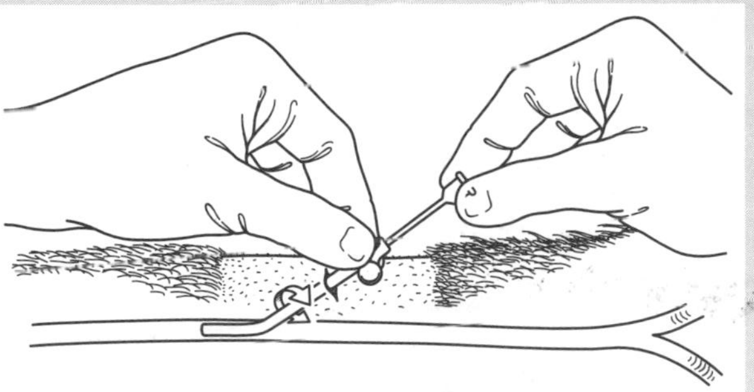

Continued

Box 3-1 Technical Tip: *Peel-Away Sheath Technique—cont'd*

4. Remove needle and place finger over the opening to prevent excessive hemorrhage.

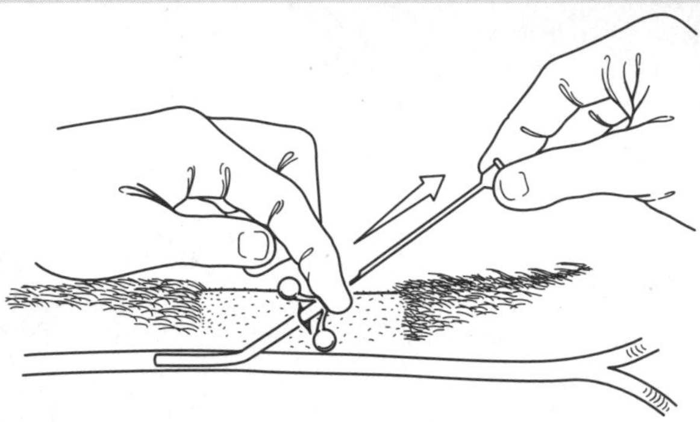

5. Insert catheter through sheath.

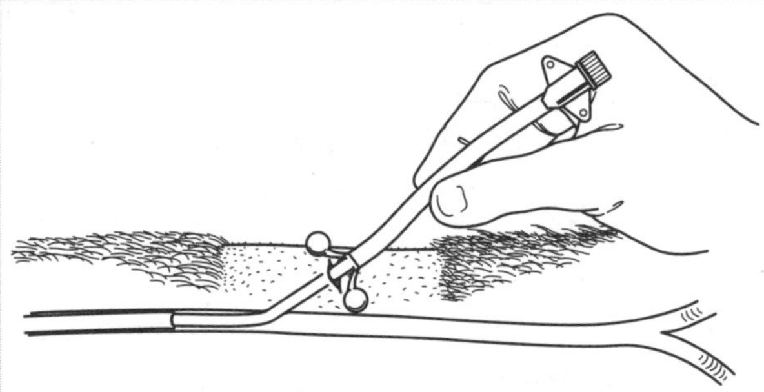

6. Cap and flush catheter with heparinized saline. Pull up and out on tabs of sheath. There will be slight hemorrhaging around the site.

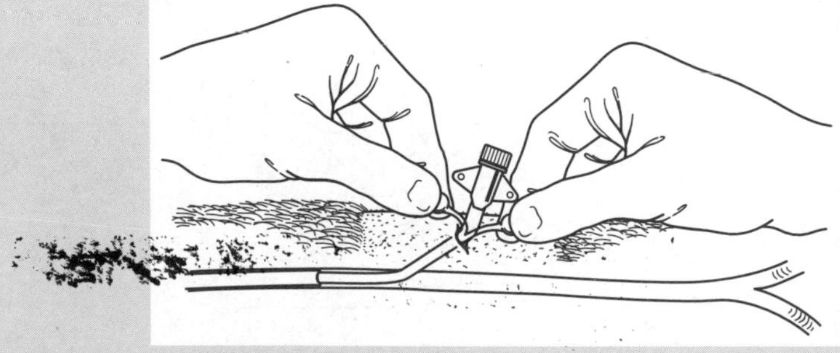

Box 3-2 Technical Tip: *Guidewire (Seldinger) Technique*

Note that gloves and surgical drapes were omitted from illustrations so that positioning of hands and catheter could be shown. Gloves must be worn and a sterile field provided.

Items needed:

Items for prepping, drape, and sterile surgical gloves.
(The following four items are available in kits made by Arrow, Mila, and Cook Veterinary Products.)
Hypodermic needle
Guidewire
Dilator
Polyurethane intravenous catheter
Heparinized saline
Injection cap with extension line
Triple-antibiotic ointment
Materials for stabilization

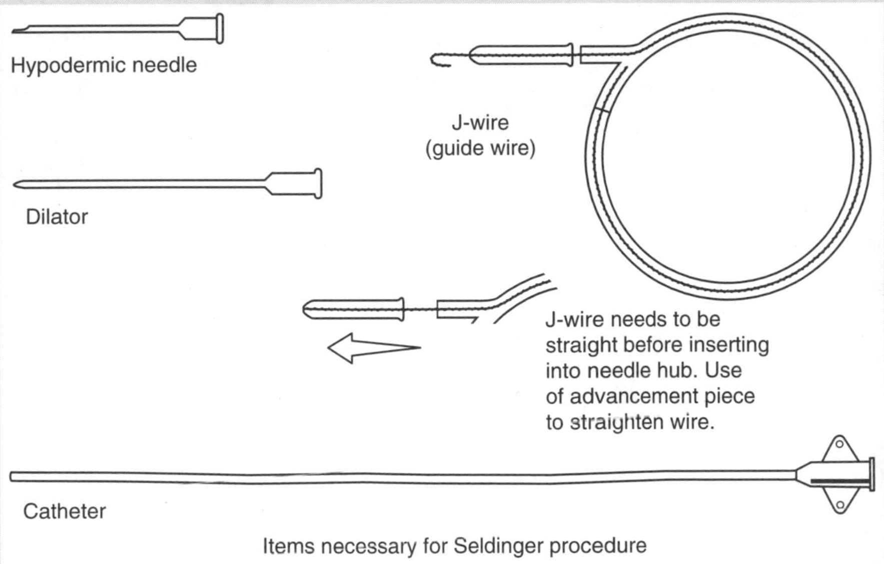

Items necessary for Seldinger procedure

Shave and surgically prep site. Drape around site. Sterile surgical gloves must be worn. Maintain sterility throughout procedure.

Continued

Box 3-2 Technical Tip: *Guidewire (Seldinger) Technique–cont'd*

1. Insert needle into vessel.

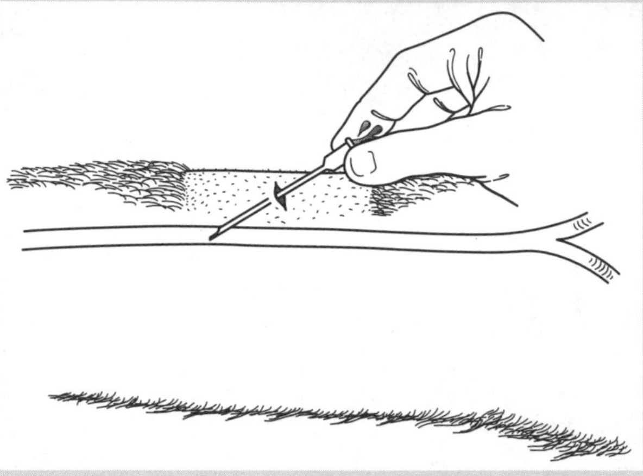

2. Place guidewire into vessel through needle. For smaller animals, cats, and dehydrated patients, insert straight end first.

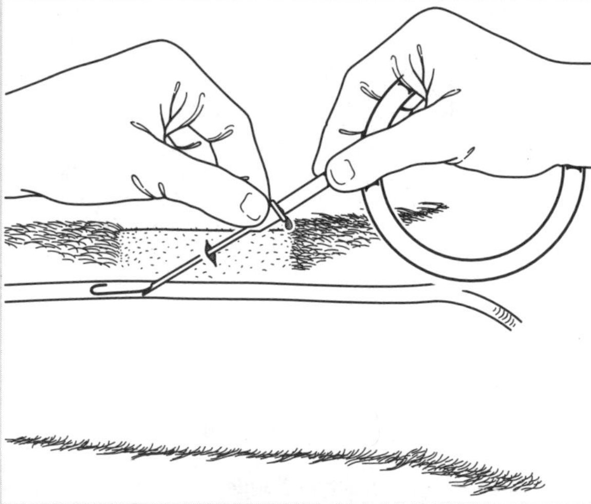

Box 3-2 Technical Tip: *Guidewire (Seldinger) Technique—cont'd*

3. Remove needle from vessel and off of wire.

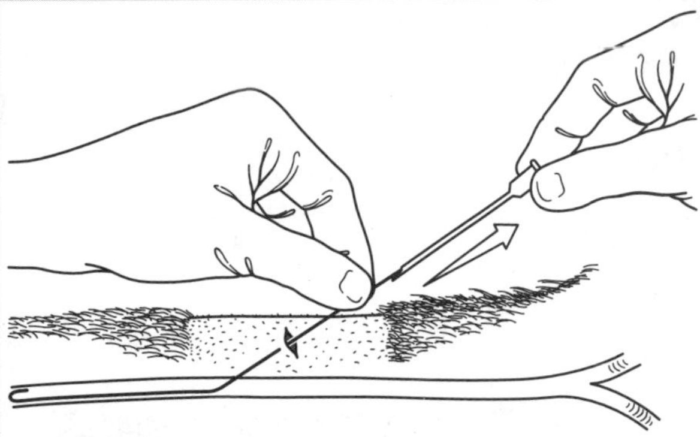

4. Place dilator over the wire into initial insertion point. Rotate back and forth to facilitate insertion. Insert about 50% of dilator, then remove. If patient's status deteriorates suddenly, this dilator can be inserted all the way, wire can be removed, and fluid therapy can begin. After stabilization occurs, wire can be reinserted, dilator removed, and long-term catheter placed.

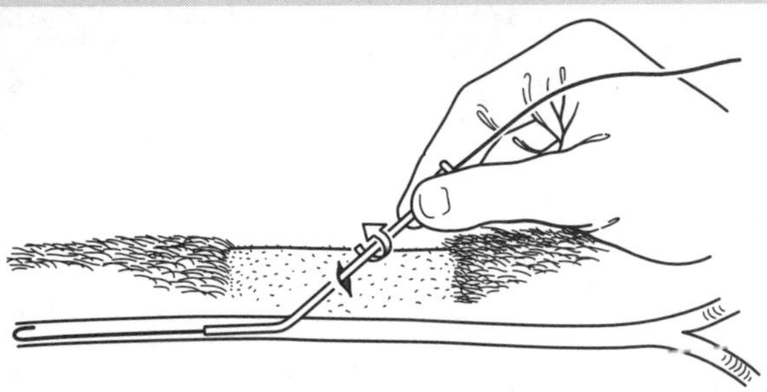

5. Place intravenous catheter over wire into vessel.

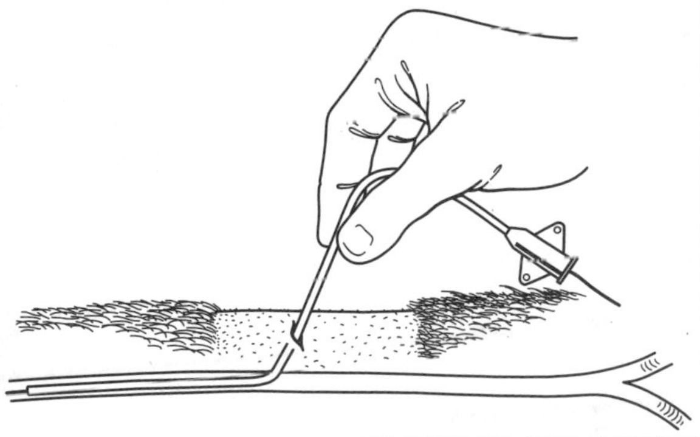

Continued

Box 3-2 Technical Tip: *Guidewire (Seldinger) Technique—cont'd*

6. Remove wire, cap, and flush with heparinized saline.

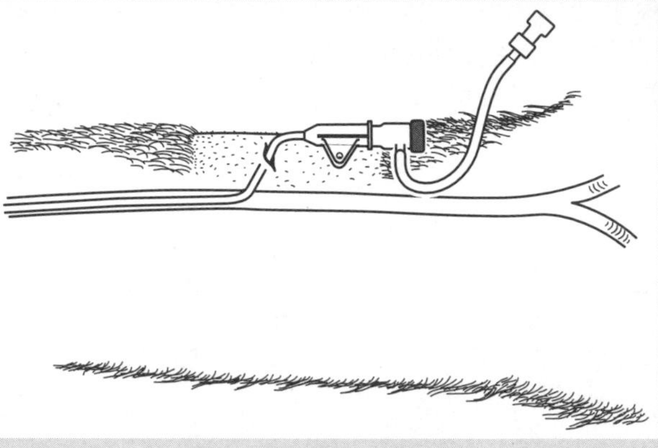

Box 3-3 Technical Tip: *Through-the-Needle Catheter Unit*

Items needed:

Through-the-needle catheter unit
Injection cap with extension line
Heparinized saline
Triple-antibiotic ointment
Materials for stabilization

1. Insert needle through the skin and into the vessel.

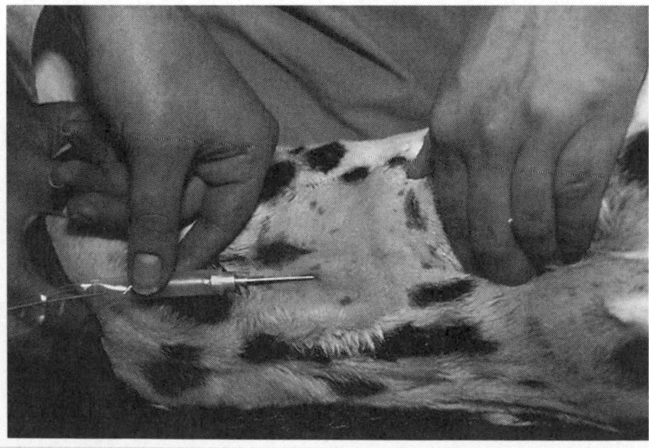

Box 3-3 Technical Tip: *Through-the-Needle Catheter Unit—cont'd*

2. Advance catheter into vessel and lock into needle hub.

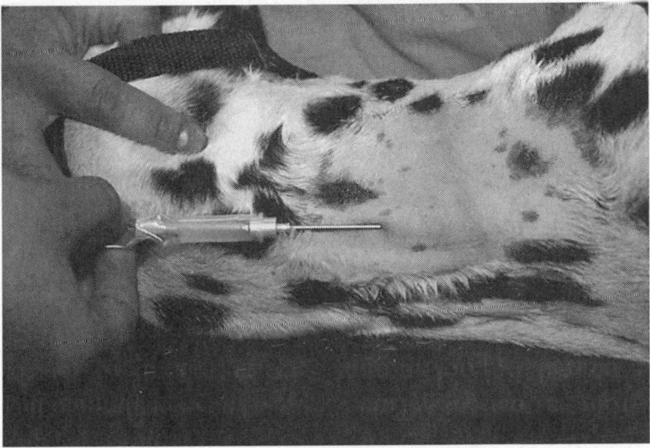

3. Remove needle from site.

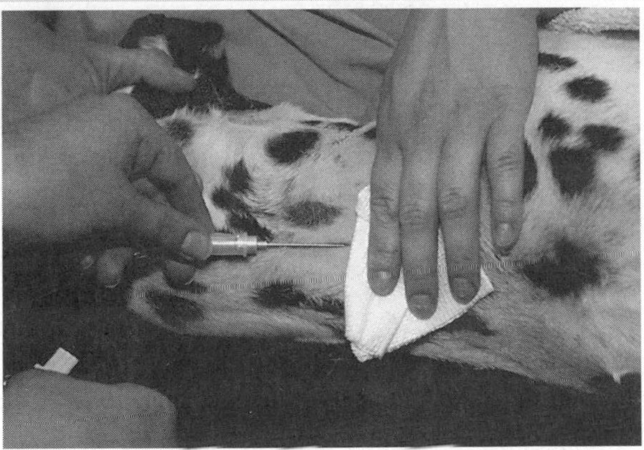

Continued

Box 3-3 Technical Tip: *Through-the-Needle Catheter Unit—cont'd*

4. Place needle guard over needle.

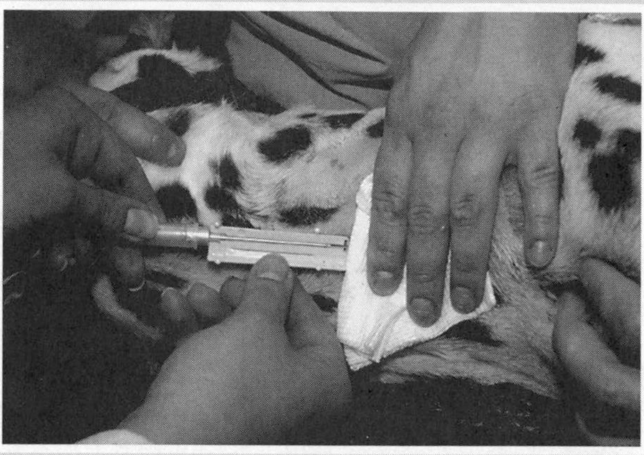

5. Apply pressure to insertion site and remove stylet.

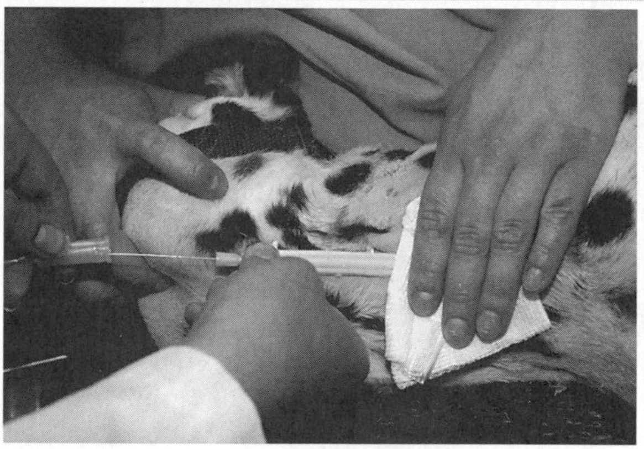

Box 3-3 Technical Tip: *Through-the-Needle Catheter Unit—cont'd*

6. Cap and flush.

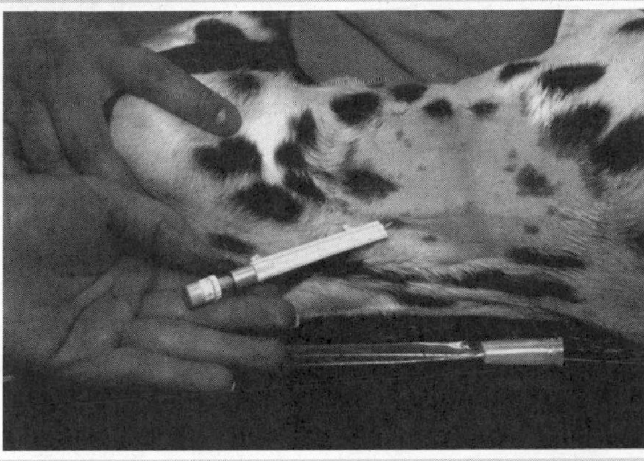

should remain uncovered so that it can be checked frequently throughout the treatment.

PERIPHERAL CATHETERS

Two ½-inch-wide pieces of tape, long enough to go around the leg, are used for initial stabilization. The first is placed at the base of the hub. Create tabs on either side of the hub and wrap firmly around the leg. The second piece is placed, adhesive up, under the catheter, with equal lengths of tape on either side. It is criss-crossed around the catheter and wrapped around the leg. Tissue glue can be used to further stabilize the catheter. A small drop on either side of the hub is sufficient. (Use tissue glue sparingly. Some animals may have a severe tissue reaction to the ingredients in the glue. When in doubt, use sutures instead of glue.) This technique is very useful for patients that are very active, especially fractious cats, or when quick stabilization is necessary.

A gauze pad with triple-antibiotic ointment is placed over the catheter insertion site. Cast padding is placed underneath the proximal portion of the hub to create padding between the leg and the catheter. It is wrapped around the leg to provide additional support.

Rolled gauze is used for additional support and for securing extended injection ports. Adhesive wrap (Vetwrap or Elastikon works well) can then be used to cover the entire bandage. Injection ports should always remain uncovered for quick venous access. Occasionally, it is necessary to extend the wrap to the toes to assist circulation. Cats usually need this extended wrap.

JUGULAR CATHETER

Three pieces of tape long enough to go around the patient's neck are needed for initial stabilization. The first piece is split 2 inches down the middle and placed so that the small strips go along either side of the catheter. It is wrapped around the neck, incorporating the small strips for the final connection. The other pieces are placed on either side of the catheter and wrapped around the neck. (For additional stabilization, a butterfly is placed at the base of the catheter or needle guard and a drop of tissue glue (or sutures) is put on each tab of the butterfly so that it adheres to the neck. This is done before the tape is placed.) Cast padding is placed over the tape to provide additional support. Rolled gauze is placed over the cast padding. Adhesive wrap is placed to secure the entire bandage to the

Box 3-4 Technical Tip: *Using an Over-the-Needle Catheter Unit and Feeding Tube for Jugular Catheter Placement*

Items needed:

- 14-gauge over-the-needle catheter with a 5-French feeding tube or 16-gauge over-the-needle catheter with a 3.5-French feeding tube
- Injection cap with heparinized saline
- Materials for stabilization

Before performing this technique, confirm that your materials are compatible. Some catheters are tapered differently on the distal end, and feeding tubes cannot pass through.

1. Shave and surgically prep the site.
2. Insert a 14-gauge over-the-needle catheter through the skin, into the vessel.
3. Advance the catheter off the stylet into the vessel.
4. Introduce a 5-French feeding tube through the catheter, into the vessel. A drop of 50% dextrose at the catheter hub may facilitate feeding tube introduction.
5. Cap and flush catheter with heparinized saline. Remove the over-the-needle catheter from vessel up to the initial insertion point. Loop and stabilize to patient.

For smaller patients, a 16-gauge over-the-needle catheter with a 3.5-French feeding tube can be used.

patient's neck. It is very important to check the tightness of the bandage around the neck after each layer is placed. If the patient shows any signs of discomfort or difficulty breathing, the bandage should be removed immediately and rewrapped more loosely, using less material. Leashes should be placed around the shoulder, or a harness can be used (Figure 3-2).

Through-the-needle catheters that are placed in the lateral saphenous veins of dogs can be secured using the following technique. The catheter is pulled out ½ inch and the needle guard placed pointing upward. A small piece of tape is placed on the catheter loop, with tabs on either side. The tabs are secured to the leg with tissue glue. This prevents the catheter from dislodging. Tape is used to secure the needle guard to the leg. A piece of cast padding is placed between the needle guard and the leg to provide a cushion. The entire needle guard and catheter site can then be wrapped. Rolled gauze is used for more stabilization. Then adhesive wrap is placed over the entire bandage.

Through-the-needle catheters placed in the medial saphenous veins of cats or small dogs can be secured using the following method. The patient remains in lateral recumbence for this step. The catheter is pulled out far enough to loop around the stifle. Two inches usually is sufficient. (When the catheter is looped out, expect bleeding to occur.) A piece of tape is placed around the catheter, with tabs on either side, and tissue glue is used for further stabilization. A gauze pad with triple-antibiotic ointment is placed at the insertion site, with tape to keep it in place. The patient is turned over carefully. The needle guard is placed along the lateral aspect of the patient's thigh and secured with tape. The catheter is secured using the same method and materials as mentioned previously.

Catheters placed in the medial aspect of the leg can also be wrapped without looping the catheter and leaving the needle guard on the medial side of the leg. The advantages of this method are less manipulation of the patient and a decreased risk of dislodging the catheter. The disadvantage (especially in cats) is the discomfort of the wrap. It extends to the toes, and a splint is needed, making it difficult for the patient to ambulate. It also must be changed frequently during the day because it is soiled easily.

CHALLENGES

SPECIFIC BREEDS

Placing catheters in basset hounds and dachshunds is very challenging because their limb structure and loose skin make it difficult to place and stabilize intravenous catheters. Other breeds with loose skin can also be a challenge.

Visualizing and palpating the vessel is easier for the person placing the catheter when the skin is stretched and rotated upward by the restrainer. Be very cautious about the degree of rotation.

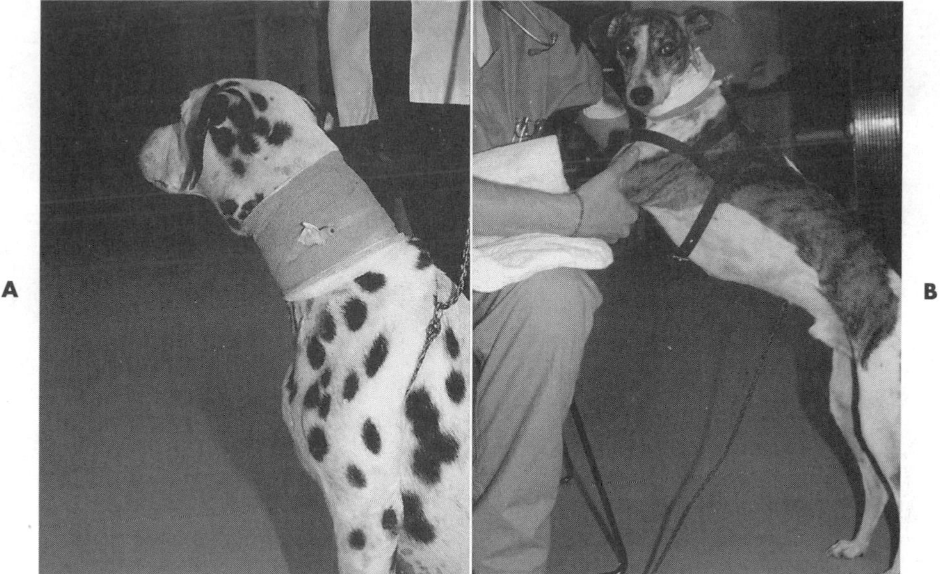

Figure 3-2

A, Place leash around shoulder to avoid additional stress to jugular catheter site. **B,** A harness can be used.

When the skin folds are released, the catheter port should be easy to access.

A small nick incision facilitates a smoother introduction of the catheter unit into the vessel. The catheter should be made of a rigid material such as Teflon. It is less likely to kink while being advanced and it will not migrate out of the vessel if stabilized properly.

Basset hounds have the advantage of long ears that contain accessible vessels. An 18-gauge, 2-inch catheter can be placed in an ear vein and can be maintained for up to 3 days (Figure 3-3).

Elastikon works well in stabilizing catheters in animals with loose skin folds. It is strong enough to hold the layers of skin back in most cases.

Neonates

Restraint is very important in facilitating a successful venopuncture in these animals. The jugular vessel is the most accessible vein.

Cradle the neonate in the palm of your hands, using their arms as a support for the body. Place the neonate on its back, head toward your fingers. Forelimbs must be held firmly to the chest. (Wrapping them in a towel sometimes works but can limit your ability to monitor the animal during this procedure.) The person placing the catheter extends the head back and rotates it slightly until the vessel can be visualized. Using the other hand, introduce the over-the-needle catheter into the jugular vessel. The animal should be held in an upright position when securing the catheter (Figure 3-4).

Fractious Feline and Cantankerous Canine

The restraining tools and the restrainer are the keys to successful intravenous catheter placement in aggressive animals. Do not take risks with animals that show any signs of aggression. Use the supplies available for protection. Restraining tools include muzzles, cat bags, rolling towels, catch poles, and sedation. Taking these precautionary measures will prevent injury to the animal and the staff.

It is important to use a catheter that will act as a multipurpose unit and that has a long indwelling

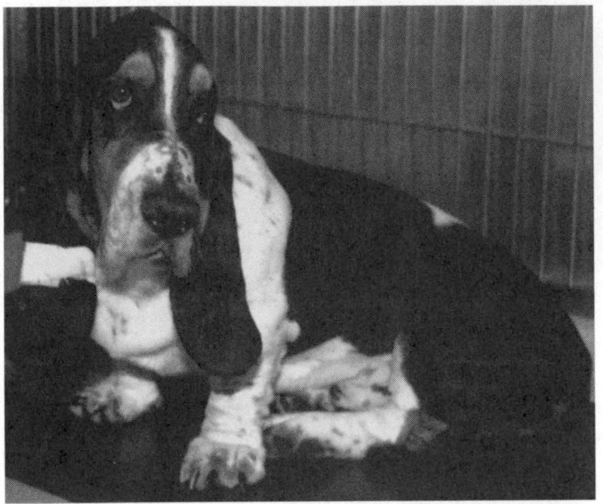

Figure 3-3

An 18-gauge, 2-inch over-the-needle catheter can be maintained in the ear vein of some dogs.

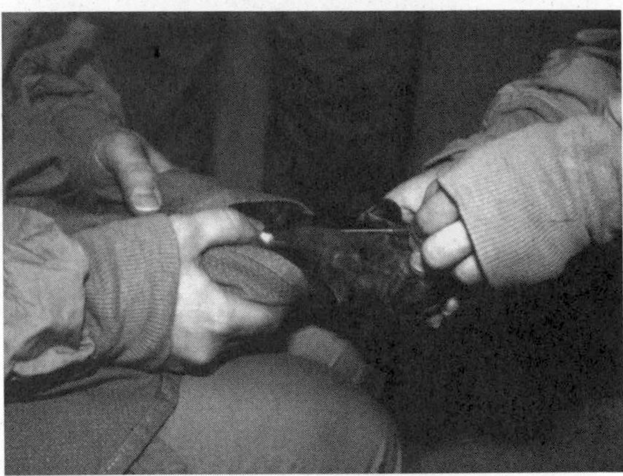

Figure 3-4

Restraining the neonate.

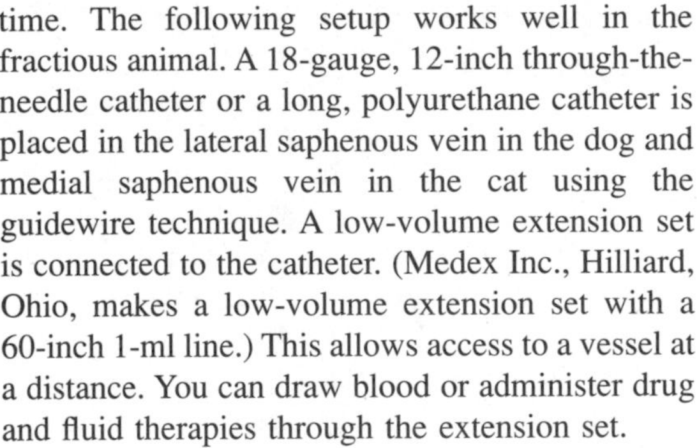

time. The following setup works well in the fractious animal. A 18-gauge, 12-inch through-the-needle catheter or a long, polyurethane catheter is placed in the lateral saphenous vein in the dog and medial saphenous vein in the cat using the guidewire technique. A low-volume extension set is connected to the catheter. (Medex Inc., Hilliard, Ohio, makes a low-volume extension set with a 60-inch 1-ml line.) This allows access to a vessel at a distance. You can draw blood or administer drug and fluid therapies through the extension set.

Putting an Elizabethan collar on these animals blocks their vision and makes it more difficult for them to bite. A leash is left around the animal's neck and the end placed outside the cage.

Collapsed Vascular System

A mini cutdown should be performed if an intravenous catheter cannot be placed quickly in an emergency situation. A hypodermic needle is used instead of a blade. Hold a 20-gauge hypodermic needle like a pencil and using the cutting edge of the bevel, make an incision through the skin, horizontally across the leg, to expose the vessel. Begin distally. If the catheter placement is not successful, incisions can be made parallel to the vessel, up the leg, until placement is successful.

Intraosseous cannulization also can be performed in an emergency. Intraosseous needles are available for this procedure. The most common sites include the medullary canal of the femur or humerus. Once the area is prepped with a local anesthetic, the needle is inserted into the greater tubercle of the humerus or the greater trochanteric fossa of the femur. Aspiration of bone marrow confirms the proper placement, or a radiograph can be taken.

MAINTENANCE

Proper placement technique, catheter choice, and site maintenance all play an important role in determining the indwelling time of an intravenous catheter. The intravenous catheter site should be assessed continually. Visual checks and palpation of the area above the catheter are done during treatment and throughout the day. Bandages should be changed every 24 hours or if they are wet or soiled. Intravenous catheters must be flushed with heparinized saline every 6 to 8 hours if a continuous intravenous drip is not being administered.

Once the bandage is removed, the site is evaluated for signs of redness or swelling. Phlebitis is one complication that can occur with an indwelling intravenous catheter. It is the inflammation of the vessel that results from an infection. The animal may show signs of discomfort when the catheter is flushed or palpated. The site may be hot and swollen. The catheter must be removed and the leg hot-packed every 4 hours until the swelling subsides if this is observed. Culturing the catheter tips will assist in determining the cause and type of infection.

Flush the catheter to check for any leakage around the site. The catheter is rewrapped and triple-antibiotic ointment replaced once it has been determined that the catheter will be used for another day.

The Centers for Disease Control and Prevention do not recommend routine application of antimicrobial ointment to venous catheter insertion sites because it macerates the site in humans. Chlorhexidine patches are used as an alternative. The patch slowly releases chlorhexidine, which is the only solution known to maintain its bactericidal effects in the presence of bodily fluids over a 7-day period.

If the catheter must be replaced, leave the old one in place (if still functional) until a new line has been established. It is important to maintain venous access at all times in the critically ill small animal. All fluid administration sets and fluid bags are changed along with the intravenous catheter.

The intravenous catheter is the patient's lifeline in many situations. The veterinary team must work together to place and maintain intravenous catheters properly. The entire staff must understand intravenous catheter placement, stabilization, and maintenance protocols to provide optimal patient care.

BIBLIOGRAPHY

Hanson B: Technical aspects of fluid therapy. In DiBartola SP: *Fluid therapy in the small animal practice,* Philadelphia, 1992, WB Saunders.

Manchon R, Raffe M, Robinson E: Central venous pressure measurements in the caudal vena cava of sedated cats, *Journal of Veterinary Emergency and Critical Care* 5(2):121, 1995.

Mathews K, Brooks M, Valliant A: A prospective study of intravenous catheter contamination, *Journal of Veterinary Emergency and Critical Care* 6(1):33, 1996.

Chapter 4

Fluid Therapy

Fluid therapy can play a vital role in the stabilization and recovery of emergency and critical care patients. The technician must begin with a basic understanding of the physiological requirements, available replacement solutions, fluid dosing and delivery systems, and patient monitoring. Fluid therapy in clinical medicine is used to replace hydration deficits, maintain normal hydration, replace lost blood volume, replace essential electrolytes and nutrients, and serve as a vehicle for infusing certain intravenous medications.

BODY FLUID AND DISTRIBUTION

The emergency or critical care patient may have an abnormal body weight. There may not be a normal baseline for the technician to use for calculation purposes. The first priority is to restore the blood volume, then to address the total body water and electrolyte needs. Average blood volume ranges from 50 to 55 ml/kg in cats and 89 to 90 ml/kg in dogs.

Total body water (TBW) accounts for approximately 60% of the patient's body weight. This fluid is further broken down to intracellular fluid (ICF) and extracellular fluid (ECF). The ICF can be measured as 40% of body weight or two thirds of TBW. ECF (20% of body weight or one third of TBW) is further divided into interstitial (15% of body weight or 75% of extracellular fluid) and intravascular (5% of body weight or 25% of extracellular fluid) (Table 4-1).

ELECTROLYTES

Understanding electrolyte concentrations in body compartments will aid the technician in administering fluid therapy. Whereas sodium and chloride exist in high concentrations in serum (ECF), potassium and phosphorus exist in high concentrations within the cells (ICF). Depending on the patient's condition, one area may be affected more than another. Fluid therapy is intended to maintain these areas in equilibrium. The body compartment's protein and sodium contents determine the fluid distribution (Figure 4-1).

FLUID TYPES

DEXTROSE SOLUTIONS

Solutions containing dextrose (an old chemical name for D-glucose, a sugar) are metabolized rapidly to carbon dioxide and water. Therefore administering dextrose physiologically becomes equivalent to administering distilled water. The technician should be particularly mindful of aseptic technique when handling these products because conditions in the solution are ideal for bacterial growth (Table 4-2).

Pros

- Dextrose can be used to provide free water to replace insensible losses or to correct hypernatremia resulting from a water deficit.
- When added to a crystalloid, it can be useful in providing an intracellular carbohydrate source in patients with sepsis.

TABLE 4-1 Distribution of Body Water

Intracellular Fluid	Extracellular Fluid: Interstitial (¾)	Extracellular Fluid: Plasma (¼)
40% of body weight is intracellular water.	15% of body weight is interstitial water.	5% of body weight is plasma water.
⅔ body water	⅓ body water	

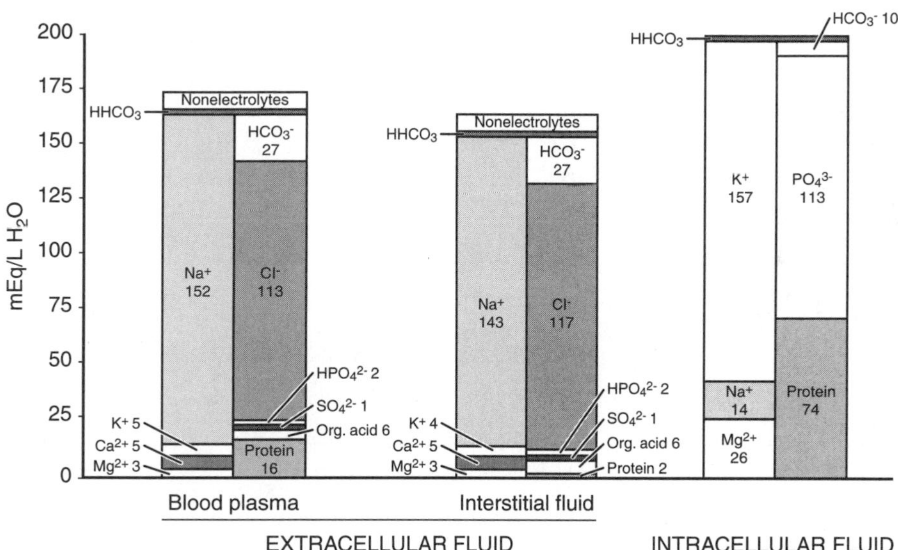

Figure 4-1

Electrolyte composition of human body fluids. Note that the values are in mEq/L of water, not of body fluid. (From Leaf A, Newburgh LH: *Significance of the body fluids in clinical medicine,* ed 2, 1955. Courtesy of Charles C Thomas, Publisher, Ltd., Springfield, Illinois.)

Cons

- Water redistributes quickly to the ICF and ECF. This can create edema.
- Dextrose should not be used as a replacement fluid in shock. The water will not stay in the intravascular space to provide needed expansion, but it will move to the ICF.
- Subcutaneous administration may cause electrolyte movement into these tissues, leading to a decreased circulating blood volume and shock.

Formulating Dextrose Solutions Using 50% Dextrose

5% dextrose solution = 1 ml 50% dextrose to 9 ml fluid

10% dextrose solution = 2 ml 50% dextrose to 8 ml fluid

CRYSTALLOIDS

These solutions contain sodium as their major osmotically active particle. They may or may not contain other electrolytes and buffers. Crystalloids are broken down into further categories based on their tonicity.

Hypotonic. Most of the fluids in this category are prepared as isotonic solutions. They contain dextrose, which results in a hypotonic solution when metabolized. An example

TABLE 4-2 Comparison of Commonly Used Parenteral Fluids in the Dog and Cat

	Electrolyte Content (mEq/L)									
Solution	**Na^+**	**K^+**	**Ca^{++}**	**Cl^-**	**Lactate**	**Acetate**	**Glucose (g/L)**	**Calories (kcal/L)**	**Tonicity**	**Osmolality (mOsm/L)**
Lactated Ringer's	130	4	3	109	28				Isotonic	273
Acetated Ringer's	131	4	3	109		28			Isotonic	275
Ringer's	147	4	4	155					Isotonic	309
Sodium chloride 0.45%	77			77					Hypotonic	155
Sodium chloride 0.9%	154			154					Isotonic	310
Dextrose 2.5%							25	85	Hypotonic	126
Dextrose 5%							50	170	Hypotonic	253
Dextrose 10%							100	340	Hypertonic	505
Dextrose 50%							500	1700	Hypertonic	2525
Dextrose 2.5% in half-strength lactated Ringer's	65	2	1	55	14		25	85	Isotonic	265
Dextrose 5% in lactated Ringer's	130	4	3	111	28		50	170	Hypertonic	525
Dextrose 2.5% with 0.45% sodium chloride	77			77			25	85	Isotonic	280
Dextrose 5% with 0.45% sodium chloride	77			77			50	170	Hypertonic	405
Dextrose 5% with 0.9% sodium chloride	154			154			50	170	Hypertonic	560

Data from Covington TR, Dipalma JR, Hussar DA et al, eds: *Drug facts and comparisons,* 1985 edition, Philadelphia, 1984, JB Lippincott.

of this type of fluid is 0.45% NaCl/2.5% dextrose.

Pros

- Hypotonic solutions are excellent fluid for maintenance when supplemented with KCl (potassium chloride).
- They are the fluid of choice in patients that are predisposed to sodium retention, such as those with congestive heart failure or liver disease.

Cons

- Hypotonic solutions are not to be used in shock because water will redistribute rapidly.

Isotonic. These fluids have an osmolality similar to that found in serum. Examples are 9% NaCl, lactated Ringer's solution, and Normosol-R. These solutions distribute evenly in the extracellular space when administered intravascularly. Only 25% of the administered crystalloid fluid remains in the intravascular space of the ECF compartment after 1 hour.

Pros

- Isotonic solutions are inexpensive and readily available.
- They are good replacement fluids for dehydration.
- They are good resuscitative fluids for small animals who need rapid volume expansion.

Cons

- Fluid redistributes rapidly, so infusion must be continued to maintain volume expansion.
- Isotonic solutions are not used for maintenance because of their high sodium and chloride content, osmolality, and inadequate potassium.

TABLE 4-3 Solutions for Fluid Therapy

	Electrolyte Concentration mEq/L					Buffer (mEq/L)	pH	Osmolality (mOsm/L)	Caloric Value (kcal/L)
	Na^+	K^+	Ca^{2+}	Mg^{2-}	Cl^-				
Colloidal solutions									
Hetastarch 6% in 0.9% saline	154	—	—	—	154		5.5		
Dextran 70 6% w/v in 0.9% saline	154	—	—	—	154		4.5-7	300-303	
Plasma (average values, dog)	145	4.2	5	2.5	108	20	7.4	290	
Electrolyte solutions									
Replacement solutions									
Lactated Ringer's	130	4	3	—	109	Lactate 25	6.5	273	9
Ringer's solution	147	4	5	—	156	—	5.8	310	—
Normal saline	154	—	—	—	154	—	5.4	308	—
Normosol-R	140	5	—	3	98	Acetate 27 Gluconate 23	6.2	295	18
Maintenance solutions									
2½% dextrose/0.45% saline	77	—	—	—	77	—	4.8	280	85
2½% dextrose/½ strength lactated Ringer's	65	2	1	—	54	Lactate 14	5.0	263	89
Normosol-M	40	13	—	3	40	Acetate 16	6.0	112	0
Normosol-M in 5% dextrose	40	13	—	3	40	Acetate 16	5.2	363	175
Other solutions									
5% dextrose in water	—	—	—	—	—	—	5.0	252	170

From Senior D: Fluid therapy, electrolyte, and acid base control. In *Ettinger textbook of veterinary internal medicine* (ed. 4). Philadelphia, WB Saunders.

HYPERTONIC

These solutions are highly osmolar and are meant for rapid resuscitation. An example of this type of solution is 7% NaCl (osmolality of 2400 mOsm).

Pros

- Hypertonic solutions are used for rapid volume expansion.
- Small volumes can be used to enlarge the intravascular space (i.e., when dealing with larger patients).

Cons

- The effect is transient. These solutions often are combined with a colloidal solution.
- They may cause hypernatremia, hyperosmolality, and increased bleeding.
- They are more expensive than other crystalloids (Table 4-3).

SYNTHETIC COLLOIDS

The term *colloid* refers to high-molecular-weight substances that do not pass readily across capillary membranes. These macromolecules are negatively charged, and their presence in the vasculature pulls additional water from the interstitium. Whereas large volumes of crystalloids will decrease the colloidal oncotic pressure, colloids actually increase oncotic pressure. Fluid will remain in the intravascular space as long as the colloidal pressure is greater than in the tissue. Normally, albumin provides this oncotic pressure. Albumin blood levels can be decreased dramatically in diseases associated with vomiting, diarrhea, fever, or excessive urination. Administering colloids along with crystalloid therapy during resuscitation and maintenance fluid therapy restores and maintains intravascular oncotic pressure.

The molecular weight of albumin is 69,000 Da,

and under normal circumstances albumin cannot cross vascular membranes. The colloidal solutions available vary in molecular weight and effective time for maintaining oncotic pressure.

Hydroxyethyl Starch. The most common products are pentastarch and hetastarch. The molecules are derived from a waxy species of maise or sorghum. These molecules resemble glycogen (a large polysaccharide that is the chief storage form of carbohydrates in the body). Pentastarch (PES) has an average molecular weight of 264,000 Da and hetastarch has an average molecular weight of 450,000 Da. The metabolism of these products depends on their absorption by tissues (liver and spleen). The half-life of concentration in the blood is about 2.5 hours for pentastarch and 25.5 hours for hetastarch.

Dextrans. Dextrans are high-molecular-weight polysaccharides composed of glucose residues but less highly branched than hydroxyethyl starch (HES). They are produced by the enzyme dextran sucrase during growth of various strains of bacterium *Leuconostroc* in media containing sucrose. The most commonly used are dextran 40, with an average molecular weight of 40,000 Da, and dextran 70, with an average molecular weight of 70,000 Da. Dextran is broken down completely to CO_2 and H_2O by dextranase present in the spleen, liver, lung, kidney, brain, and muscle. The half-life of dextran 40 is about 2.5 hours, and the half-life of dextran 70 is about 25.5 hours.

Gelatins. Modified fluid gelatins are available in veterinary medicine. An example of this type of fluid is Vetaplasm. It is produced from cattle-bone gelatin, prepared by a gradual controlled heating and chemical hydrolysis of raw material. Very few published clinical studies are available. The average molecular weight of the molecules is 30,000 Da. The duration of oncotic effect is about 4 to 6 hours. Little is known about the overall degradation of gelatins in blood.

Synthetic Colloid Pros

- They have a long effect on colloidal oncotic pressure. They are useful as both resuscitative and replacement fluids, and they can be given as boluses if the animal has poor perfusion because of hypovolemia.
- Colloids can be used safely to increase intravascular volume in animals with congestive heart failure. Underlying heart disease must be addressed and afterload reduced.
- Fewer incidences of peripheral edema result than when crystalloids are used.
- The need for positive inotropes or vasopressors (i.e., dopamine infusion) for blood pressure support is rare.
- They can reduce volume of crystalloid used by 40% to 60% when used concurrently with colloids.

Synthetic Colloid Cons

- The cost of these products can nearly equal that of blood products.
- In disease processes in which albumin leakage is already a problem, products that are equal to or smaller than the molecular weight of albumin will also leak into the interstitial space. The larger molecules found in HES and PES must be used in these instances.
- Anaphylaxis has been reported in a very small percentage of cases.
- HES and PES raise serum amylase levels, but there is no change in pancreatic function.
- Dextrans have been associated with acute renal failure and bleeding diathesis. These products interfere with cross-matching. Blood glucose and bilirubin levels may be falsely increased.

OXYGEN-CARRYING FLUID

Oxyglobin (hemoglobin glutamer-200 [bovine]) is an ultrapurified polymerized hemoglobin solution of bovine origin in a modified lactated Ringer's solution. It is used as an alternative to blood for animals with hemolytic anemia, blood loss caused by trauma or surgery, hypovolemia and other causes of shock, or other conditions involving poor tissue perfusion. It is contraindicated in animals with advanced cardiac disease (e.g., congestive heart failure).

The oxygen delivery system of Oxyglobin differs from the oxygen delivery system of blood. Hemoglobin, the protein that is encapsulated in the red blood cell, carries the oxygen from the lungs to the tissues through microcirculation. When an animal is anemic, there are not enough red blood cells to oxygenate the tissues adequately. Oxyglobin's polymerized hemoglobin molecules provide the animal with the substitute oxygen transporting system by circulating in the plasma and transporting oxygen from the lungs to the tissues.

The recommended dosage of Oxyglobin is 30 ml/kg of body weight at a rate of 10 ml/kg/hour. Oxyglobin has been used in cats, but an approved dosage has not been calculated. Rapid administration may result in circulatory overload. The animal's central venous pressure (CVP) should be monitored during the administration and immediately after administration. Oxyglobin can be stored for 24 months at room temperature or refrigerated. It cannot be frozen. Once the overwrap is removed, it must be used within 24 hours.

FLUID THERAPY FOR SPECIFIC DISEASES

Shock

Shock is a clinical syndrome in which the peripheral blood flow is inadequate to return sufficient blood to the heart for normal function, particularly for transporting oxygen to all organs and tissues. Shock may be caused by a variety of conditions, including hemorrhage, infection, drug reaction, trauma, poisoning, myocardial disease, and dehydration. Every injury is accompanied by some degree of shock and should be treated appropriately. Fluid therapy is the primary method of treating all types of shock. The main goal of the therapy is to increase the intravascular volume.

All of the types of fluids mentioned here could be used to treat shock. Typically, the mainstay of shock therapy fluids in the hospital is the use of crystalloids. As mentioned earlier, although crystalloids have their inadequacies (including limited intravascular time before redistribution), their easy availability and low cost make them hard to replace. With this said, it should be remembered that in large dogs and patients whose conditions will cause the state of shock to be protracted, colloids and hypertonic saline solutions may provide more effective shock management. When crystalloids are combined with the use of colloids, the crystalloid dosage should be reduced by 60% (Table 4-4).

Blood Loss

With blood loss, all components of the intravascular space are decreased along with the overall volume of the intravascular space. The type of fluid therapy used depends on the degree of blood loss encountered. Initial treatment with crystalloids and colloids will help increase the intravascular space, but the packed cell volume (PCV) and protein levels should be monitored closely. If PCV levels drop below 20% in cases of blood loss or destruction, packed cells or whole blood should be administered.

Dehydration and Prevention

Dehydration is often a sequela to a number of disease processes, especially those associated with vomiting and fevers. Hydration levels of every patient should be assessed. By evaluating clinical dehydration signs and laboratory data, the technician can initiate the proper fluid therapy. Dehydration is best corrected using the appropriate crystalloid solution because water from all of the spaces is decreased and must be replaced.

If the patient is about to be exposed to any situation (e.g., surgery) in which an extended period of time without water intake is to be expected both before and afterward, then maintenance crystalloid fluids should be started in advance. As mentioned earlier, several commercial fluid replacement solutions are available, or 0.45%

TABLE 4-4 Comparison of Fluid Therapies in Shock

Fluid Type	IV Dosage	Indications for Use	Benefits	Potential Complications	Miscellaneous Data
Isotonic crystalloids Lactated Ringer's Normal saline solution	Initial dog: 40-90 ml/kg Initial cat: 20-60 ml/kg	Intravascular volume expansion	Readily available Inexpensive Easy to use Help correct electrolyte imbalances	Dilutional anemia Hypoproteinemia Pulmonary and peripheral edema Stay in intravascular space only a short time	Lactate in lactated Ringer's does not potentiate lactic acidemia
Hypertonic crystalloids Hypertonic saline (3%, 7%)	3%: 5-20 ml/kg 7%: 4-8 ml/kg Infusion: 1 ml/kg/min	Intravascular volume expansion	Small volume needed Rapid improvement of cardiovascular function Positive inotropic effect	Reflex bradycardia, hypotension Potential hypokalemia, hypernatremia	Contraindicated in hyperosmolar or hypernatremic states, heart failure, dehydration
Colloids Dextrans 40, 70	10-20 ml/kg/day Infusion: 2 ml/kg/hr	Intravascular volume expansion Promotion of peripheral blood flow	Small volume needed Osmotically active Holds fluid in vascular space Remains in vascular space longer than crystalloids Volume expansion may persist for 4-8 hr Protentiates microcirculatory blood flow; coats endothelial surfaces Reduces incidence of thromboembolism	May decrease platelet function Renal failure possible if animal is oliguric and hypovolemia not corrected because of renal tubular obstruction Anaphylaxis (rare) Osmotic diuresis May interfere with cross-matching of blood May temporarily decrease immune competence Expensive	Contraindicated in thrombocytopenia, oliguric or anuric renal failure, heart failure
Dextran 70 + hypertonic saline (3%, 7%)	4 ml/kg over 5-10 min	Intravascular volume expansion in hypovolemic and septic shock	Longer dwell time in intravascular space than hypertonic saline alone Other benefits as listed above	As above for hypertonic saline, dextrans	As above for hypertonic saline, dextrans
Hydroxyethyl starch (Hetastarch)	20 ml/kg/day	Intravascular volume expansion	Small volume needed Remains in intravascular space longer than crystalloids Osmotically active	Expensive Rarely: anaphylaxis Rarely: coagulopathy at high dosages (>20 ml/kg/day) Pulmonary edema if volume overload occurs	Increases serum amylase but does not alter pancreatic function

TABLE 4-4 Comparison of Fluid Therapies in Shock—cont'd

Fluid Type	IV Dosage	Indications for Use	Benefits	Potential Complications	Miscellaneous Data
VetaPlasma (Marshalton Veterinary Group)	5 ml/kg every 4-6 hr as needed Infusion: 2-4 ml/min	Intravascular volume expansion Hypoproteinemia	Remains in vascular space longer than crystalloids Less coating of platelets than dextrans Can be repeated frequently	Expensive Not for use in dehydrated animals	Approved for use in dog and cat
Blood products				Osmotic diuresis	

NaCl/2.5% dextrose with 20 mEq KCl/L can be used for maintenance fluids.

SYSTEMIC DISEASE

Besides dehydration, a number of systemic diseases adversely affect the body's ability to stay in equilibrium. In these situations fluids are used to maintain hydration status, provide adequate perfusion to all tissues, diurese both endotoxins and exotoxins, restore normal serum osmolality, and help prevent shock secondary to sepsis. Many of these diseases also adversely affect electrolyte and protein levels. Careful monitoring of these parameters helps to determine the appropriate fluid therapy.

SUPPORTIVE TREATMENT

Fluid therapy can also be used to help support the cardiovascular system when procedures are performed that will decrease circulating blood volume and pressure, such as anesthesia or blood donation. Anesthetic agents, in general, decrease cardiovascular output, and in many surgical procedures a certain amount of blood volume is lost. In very young, very old, and critically ill patients, additional cardiovascular support can reduce the morbidity rate of the anesthesia.

DIURESIS

Fluid therapy can be used to increase urine production, assisting the body in eliminating substances that can be excreted by the kidneys. Instances in which diuresis is used include renal failure, liver failure, diabetes, electrolyte imbalances, and poisonings. Fluid rates for diuresis can be adjusted from 1.5 times maintenance to 3 times maintenance depending on the age of the animal, the nature of the disease, and health of the kidneys and heart. Depending on the laboratory values, the fluids to use for diuresis usually are the isotonic to hypotonic crystalloid and dextrose solutions (Table 4-5).

FLUID DOSING

The fluid dosing regimens presented in this section are guidelines for the veterinary technician for the purpose of understanding and preparing for emergencies. The veterinary practitioner must prescribe the final patient orders. It is best to review and learn your veterinarian's written protocols.

DAILY MAINTENANCE REQUIREMENTS

Maintenance volume is the amount of fluid and amount of electrolyte normally needed in a 24-hour period by a well-hydrated patient. This volume consists of two subcomponents.

- Insensible loss, not readily measured losses from respiratory evaporation, passage of normal feces, and sweat (which is negligible in dogs and cats). This loss can be estimated at 22 ml/kg/day (10 ml/lb/day) but can

TABLE 4-5 Selection of Fluids for Certain Diseases

	Serum					
Condition	**Na^+**	**Cl**	**K^+**	**HCO_3**	**Volume**	**Fluid of Choice**
Diarrhea	D	D	D	D	D	Lactated Ringer's + KCl, Normosol-R
Pyloric obstruction	D	D	D	I	D	0.9% NaCl
Dehydration	I	I	N	N/D	D	Lactated Ringer's 0.9% NaCl, 5% dextrose Normosol-R
Congestive heart failure	N/D	N/D	N	N	I	0.45% NaCl + 2.5% dextrose 5% dextrose
End-stage liver disease	N/I	N/I	D	D	I	0.45% NaCl + 2.5% dextrose + KCl
Acute renal failure						
Oliguria	I	I	I	D	I	0.9% NaCl
Polyuria	D	D	N/D	D	D	Lactated Ringer's + KCl, Normosol-R
Chronic renal failure	N/D	N/D	N	D	N/D	Lactated Ringer's solution, 0.9% NaCl
Adrenocortical insufficiency	D	D	I	N/D	D	0.9% NaCl
Diabetic ketoacidosis	D	D	N/D	D	D	0.9% NaCl (±KCl)

D, Decreased; *I*, increased; *N*, normal.

increase during febrile states, panting, and high environmental temperatures.

- Sensible losses, readily measured as urine production, approximately 22 to 44 ml/kg/day (10 to 20 ml/lb/day) in normal animals.

Normal maintenance volume for a dog or cat with normal urine output is approximately 50 to 60 ml/kg (25 to 30 ml/lb) of body weight per day. The normal animal loses approximately 65 to 75 mEq/L sodium and 15 to 20 mEq/L of potassium in the urine. Using these values, maintenance fluids should nearly equal the expected losses (Table 4-6 and Figure 4-2).

DEHYDRATION

Before a fluid therapy regimen is initiated, hydration status must be evaluated. Dehydration may be subtle or obvious, depending on the duration and severity of the disease affecting the patient. Patients with a history of vomiting or diarrhea but no abnormalities on physical examination may be estimated to be less than 5% dehydrated. The changes associated with dehydration are progressive, with each range including the signs previously noted:

5% to 6%: dry oral mucous membranes
6% to 8%: mild to moderate decrease in skin turgor, dry oral mucous membranes
10% to 12%: marked decrease in skin turgor, dry mucous membranes, weak and rapid pulse, slow capillary refill time, moderate to marked mental depression

The volume needed to correct dehydration is calculated as follows:

Volume (ml) of fluid needed = % Dehydration × Body weight (lb) × 500

Volume (ml) of fluid needed = % Dehydration × Body weight (kg) × 1000

This volume is then added to the maintenance volume.

TABLE 4-6 Daily Water Requirements for Dogs

Body Weight (kg)	Total Water/Day (ml)	Milliliters per kg
1	140	140
2	232	116
3	312	104
4	385	96
5	453	91
6	518	86
7	580	83
8	639	80
9	696	77
10	752	75
11	806	73
12	859	71
13	911	70
14	961	68
15	1011	67
16	1060	66
17	1108	65
18	1155	64
19	1201	63
20	1247	62
25	1468	59
30	1677	56
35	1876	54
40	2068	52
45	2254	50
50	2434	49
60	2781	46
70	3112	44
80	3431	43
90	3739	41
100	4038	40

From Ross L: Fluld therapy for acute and chronic renal failure, *Vet Clin North Am* 19:343, 1989.

Dehydration usually can be corrected in the first 24 hours of fluid therapy. Some practitioners order enough fluids to be administered during the first 4 to 8 hours to correct for dehydration. This is called front-end loading. In most cases, deficit replacement of 75% to 80% on the first day and the remaining 25% the second day is recommended. This approach may be advantageous physiologically because it allows more time for adequate equilibration of water and electrolytes between body compartments.

FEBRILE STATES

Fever increases an animal's metabolic rate. An increase in temperature of 1.8° F (1° C) will increase the metabolic rate by 13.8%. It is hard to quantify precisely what this means in water consumption, but in general, maintenance fluid rates should be increased by 10% for each 1.8° F rise in body temperature.

SUPPORTIVE TREATMENT

Anesthesia. Anesthetized patients undergo an obligatory water loss of about 1.5 to 3.0 ml/kg/hr. This amount should be replaced in addition to that lost from surgical wounds. General supportive therapy for anesthetized patients is 20 ml/kg fluid in the first hour, then 10 ml/kg each additional hour for dogs, and 10 ml/kg/hr fluid for cats.

SHOCK DOSES

Isotonic Crystalloids

Initial Rapid Infusion

Dogs: 20 to 40 ml/kg intravenously for the first 15 minutes, then 70 to 90 ml/kg over 1 hour

Cats: 10 to 20 ml/kg intravenously for the first 15 minutes, then 35 to 50 ml/kg over 1 hour

Maintenance Fluids

Dogs: 10 to 12 ml/kg/hr

Cats: 5 to 6 ml/kg/hr

Hypertonic Crystalloids

7.5% Sodium Chloride

4 ml/kg over 2 minutes

Response is seen in 1 to 2 minutes

Duration of response is 1 to 2 hours

Colloids. In cases of poor perfusion, dextran or hetastarch may be given as a rapid intravenous bolus (10 to 20 ml/kg for dogs, 5 ml/kg increments for cats).

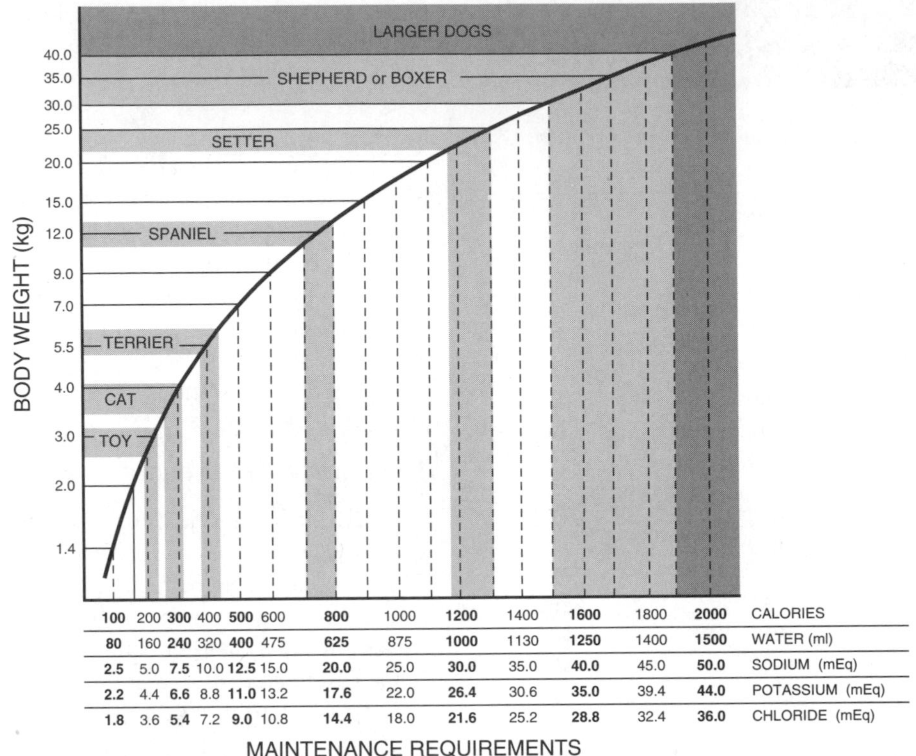

Figure 4-2

Maintenance fluid and electrolyte requirements of caged normal dogs and cats. (From Finco, after Harrison JB: *J Am Anim Hosp Assoc* 8:179, 1972.)

Be cautious when bolusing colloids to cats. Rapid infusion has been associated with vomiting, hypotension, and collapse. Titrate the colloids to effect. If the underlying disorder is trauma (without ongoing disease), a single colloid bolus usually is sufficient to bring blood pressure up rapidly while preserving the interstitium of the brain and lungs.

Cases of sudden inflammatory response syndrome (SIRS) take days to resolve. In these septic conditions, a constant-rate infusion of large-molecule colloids (HES or PES) may be necessary. After the initial intravenous bolus, the daily recommended dosage is divided over a 24-hour period and administered with crystalloids.

Daily Recommended Dosage

Dogs: 20 ml/kg/day

Cats: 10 to 15 ml/kg/day

Hypoproteinemia

Colloids and Plasma. If total protein levels are below 3.5 g/dl, then the use of colloids may help maintain normal oncotic pressure. If albumin levels are below 2.0 g/dl, then it is best to use plasma to bring the albumin level up to this point. Plasma usually is administered at a dosage of 5 ml/kg. The plasma used to treat hypoproteinemia may be either fresh frozen plasma or frozen plasma.

Once albumin volume has been improved, a colloid can be administered. As mentioned earlier, the type of colloid depends on whether ongoing losses of albumin are caused by capillary leakage. If albumin is low because of lack of production, the dextrans may be used at a rate no greater than 40 ml/kg/day. Hetastarch can be administered in volumes of up to 30 ml/kg/day.

DELIVERY SYSTEMS

Once the fluid prescription has been determined, the administration of therapy begins. Choices for therapy routes include oral, subcutaneous, intravenous (peripheral or central veins), intraperitoneal, or intramedullary. Oral fluid administration may be the easiest route, but it is contraindicated in life-threatening fluid imbalances. Subcutaneous fluid administration may be appropriate for some conditions. Fluids should be warmed to body temperature and must be isotonic (osmotic pressure equal to that of extracellular fluid). However, severe fluid deficits that warrant rapid replacement are best addressed via the intravenous or intramedullary routes. Intraperitoneal fluid administration generally is not recommended because of complications of peritonitis, intraabdominal abscessation, and low rate of absorption (Table 4-7 and Figure 4-3).

SETTING UP THE INTRAVENOUS LINE

There are many brands of intravenous fluid lines. The major manufacturers are Baxter/Travenol, McGaw, and Abbott. It is important to remember that if infusion pumps are to be used, the brand of infusion set must be compatible with the equipment. Extension sets should be matched with infusion sets; most brands are compatible with others. Aseptic technique should be maintained when dealing with intravenous lines. The fluid lines should be replaced after 48 hours of use.

The label on the administration set typically identifies the number of drops per milliliter that the set provides. For small animals, administration sets are available with an attached burette that can be filled with fluid from a primary container. Filtered administration sets also are available for infusing blood products.

Typically, administration sets can be found that deliver 10, 15, and 60 drops per milliliter. The drops normally are observed passing through a small drip chamber. This information is important when calculating fluid drip rates for gravity feed systems. With this information, drops per minute can be calculated. Buretrols are chambers that hold 150 ml fluid. The markers divide the buretrol by milliliters, allowing very accurate measurement of fluid administration in smaller animals. Buretrols can also be used for mixing different concentrations of solutions or drug therapies that must be given over a period of time (Figure 4-4). For small patients, fewer drops per milliliter allows for more accurate fluid dosing. In exceptionally small patients, the buretrol systems, with their attached burettes, offer accurate control of fluid dosages. Medications to be infused with these fluids can be added directly to the burette.

REGULATING FLUID RATES

To calculate the fluid rate, first the total volume to be given in a period of time must be determined.

Rate (drops/min) = Drops/ml calibrated
÷ 60 min/hr × Total volume to be
administered ÷ Total hr of infusion

The rate calibrated should be indicated on the packaging of the infusion set you are using. The veterinarian will prescribe a total volume dosage and the time frame in which the dosage is to be delivered, or you can calculate the total dosage by multiplying the patient's body weight by the percentage of dehydration.

Fluid Rate Monitoring. Although it is a common practice, while administering fluids by gravity flow it can be difficult to maintain regulated flow rates. Using a fluid pump can eliminate many of these complications. In a gravity feed system, fluids are kept in an elevated position above the patient. Gravity forces the fluids into the body. The drip rate is adjusted manually using the regulator on the fluid line. A timing measure should be affixed to the container so that dosing accuracy can be ascertained. Gravity feed systems depend on patient positioning and thus must be monitored very closely.

Several types of fluid pumps are used in veterinary practice. Fluid pumps help to regulate the flow of the solution to the patient. Two basic types of fluid pumps are available. Volumetric pumps can be programmed to deliver any quantity

TABLE 4-7 Routes of Fluid Administration for Dogs and Cats

Route	Indications and Advantages	Technique	Complications and Contraindications
Oral	For anorectic patients with short-term illnesses More appropriate for small animals (<20 kg) Very appropriate for neonates	Can use a stomach tube, pharyngostomy tube, small dosing syringe, or a small baby bottle and nipple, depending on the animal's size and underlying illness. Warm fluids to body temperature.	Aspiration pneumonia. Not useful for hypovolemic shock. Should not be used in vomiting animals. Avoid air administration.
Subcutaneous	For correcting mild to moderate dehydration For maintenance in patients that are not too severely ill Not appropriate for animals weighing >10 kg	Use isotonic fluid. Best to administer by gravity flow through an 18- to 20-gauge needle (for an adult-sized cat; use smaller needle for pediatric patients). Do not deposit more than 10-12 ml/kg per injection site. Fluid should be deposited dorsally along the area bordered by the scapulae anteriorly and the iliac crests posteriorly. The average 5- to 6-kg cat can receive 150-200 ml once or twice daily.	Avoid using hypertonic and hypotonic fluids. Do not deposit fluids under infected or devitalized skin. Not useful for hypovolemic shock. Do not use irritating solutions.
Intraperitoneal	When intravenous access is unavailable Provides a vehicle for delivering ample volumes of fluid over a short time period Rapid absorption	Use isotonic fluids. Use needle gauges 16-20, depending on the patient's size. Prepare a sterile injection site just lateral to the midline and midway between the umbilicus and the pelvic brim.	Hypertonic fluids worsen the dehydration. Do not use if patient has abdominal sepsis, ascites, or peritonitis. Do not use with pending abdominal surgery.
Intravenous	Preferred route for severely dehydrated and hypovolemic patients Best route for correcting hypotension Provides rapid delivery at the most precise dosage Most effective for medium and large dogs	Prepare a sterile site for needle or cannula intravenous insertion. Amount and rate of fluid delivery depend on patient's status. Use isotonic fluids for volume repletion. Maintain sterile intravenous cannula and infusion system.	Avoid intravenous overload caused by excess fluid delivery. Avoid catheter sepsis and phlebitis. Avoid catheter displacement and the inadvertent extravascular placement of the fluid infusion.

Modified from Schaer M: General principles of fluid therapy, *Vet Clin North Am [Small Anim Pract]* 19:203, 1989.

Table 4-7 Routes of Fluid Administration for Dogs and Cats—cont'd

Route	Indications and Advantages	Technique	Complications and Contraindications
Intraosseous	When intravenous access is unavailable Particularly useful in small animals Provides direct access to the vascular space	Prepare a sterile site 1 cm distal to tibial tuberosity, proximal medial tibia, or trochanteric fossa of the femur. Make a small nick skin incision. Insert an 18- to 20-gauge hypodermic needle, a spinal needle, or a small bone marrow needle. Secure with tape and bandage.	Avoid growth plates. Use needle proportional to bone size to avoid trauma. Bone infection is rare.

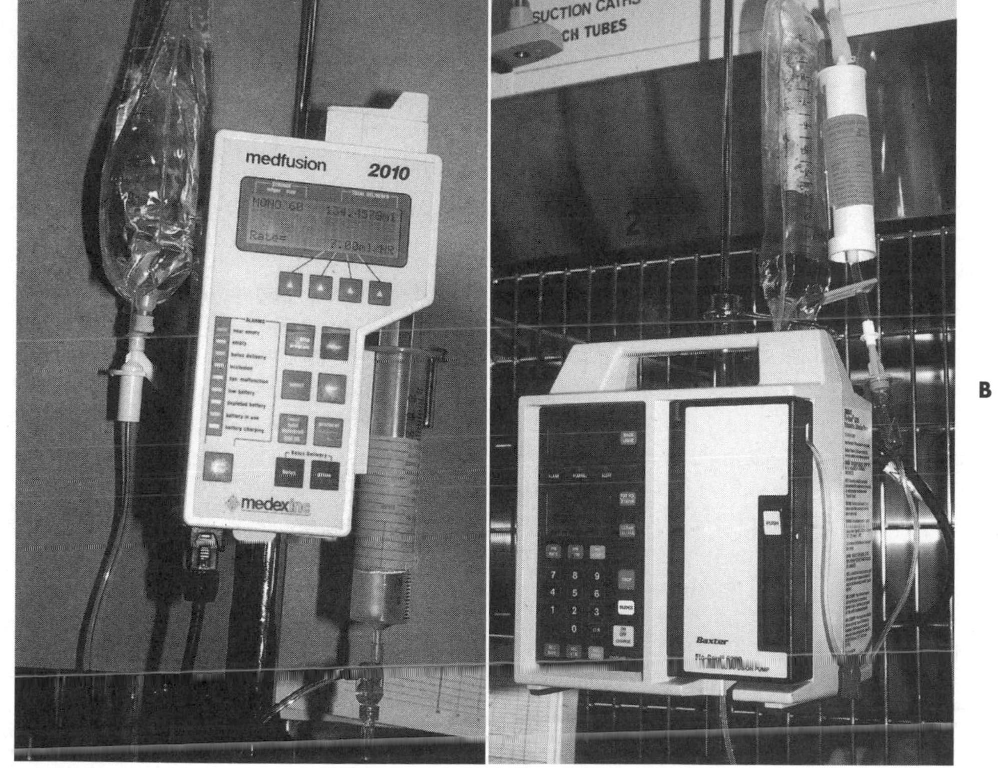

Figure 4-3

A, Syringe pump. **B,** Fluid pump. (In Allen DG, Kruth S, eds: *Small animal cardiopulmonary medicine.* Philadelphia, 1988, BC Decker, p. 142.)

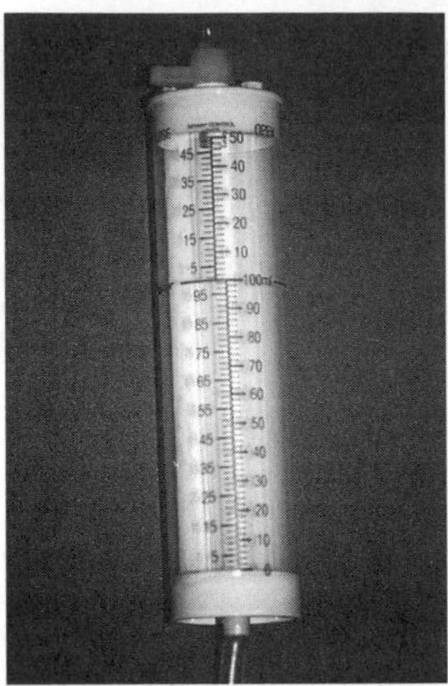

Figure 4-4
Buretrol.

of fluids over a determined period of time. These systems work based on the calculated volume (diameter) of the administration set; the pumps work independently of the drip size.

Other pumps use a photoelectric eye to count the drops as they are being administered. These pumps are adjusted on a drops per minute basis. The sensor is placed on the drip chamber. Calculations must be made to determine the appropriate drop rate to obtain the proper fluid dosage over time. Syringe pumps are mechanical devices that use a syringe with a measured volume of solution to administer a fluid. These are used most often on very small animals or when administering blood products. Settings for these devices allow accurate administration of small volumes over a long period of time. They are usually adjusted at milliliter per hour rates.

Most of these models are reconditioned and refurbished human units. The three most common types are produced by Baxter/Travenol, Sigma (McGaw), and IVAC. These electronic units are battery operated, and the most common complication is user error in regard to battery charging.

These brands often are species specific to the intravenous fluid lines produced by the same manufacturers. For example, the Baxter/Travenol 6100 should be used with Baxter/Travenol intravenous infusion sets. When reconditioned or refurbished units are purchased, the owner's manual must be reviewed for compatibility with the brands of intravenous lines. The veterinary technician must read and follow the operating instructions. Even when using a mechanical pump, it is still useful to label the fluid container with the expected volume goals over time. Mechanical pump administration can be hindered by occlusions in the catheter system. Careful monitoring of fluid administration by the technician is still essential to safe therapy (Technical Tip Box 4-1).

MONITORING RESPONSE TO TREATMENT

Although fluid therapy is critical to successful treatment, misuse of fluids, especially the overuse of fluids, can be life threatening. Careful monitoring of the patient's condition can alert the veterinarian and technician that problems may be about to develop.

PHYSICAL EXAMINATION

A physical examination should be performed several times daily during the initial fluid management to document rehydration, prevent overhydration, and detect ongoing fluid losses such as vomiting, diarrhea, and polyuria. Body weight should be noted at admission and then checked at least daily to document adequate hydration. Knowledge of the patient's baseline body weight can be used as a quantitative guide. An acute gain in body weight of 1 pound equals 500 ml in body water. However, in an anorexic animal, weight can be lost at a rate of 0.1 to 0.3 kg/day/1000 calories of the daily requirement.

Hydration status can be evaluated by a number of parameters. These factors include skin turgor, capillary refill time, mucous membrane color and moisture, pulse strength, and alertness (Table 4-8).

Box 4-1 Technical Tip: *Regulating Fluid Rates*

The following equations can be used to calculate drip rates for accurate fluid administration. These rates are also calculated to ensure proper functioning of fluid rate monitors and pumps.

Choosing the Fluid Delivery Set for Accurate Fluid Administration

Animals receiving 60 ml/hr or less need a buretrol and mini-drip set (60 drops/ml). Animals receiving more than 60 ml/hr need a regular drip set (10 drops/ml)

Types of Sets Available

Mini-drip set (60 drops/ml)*

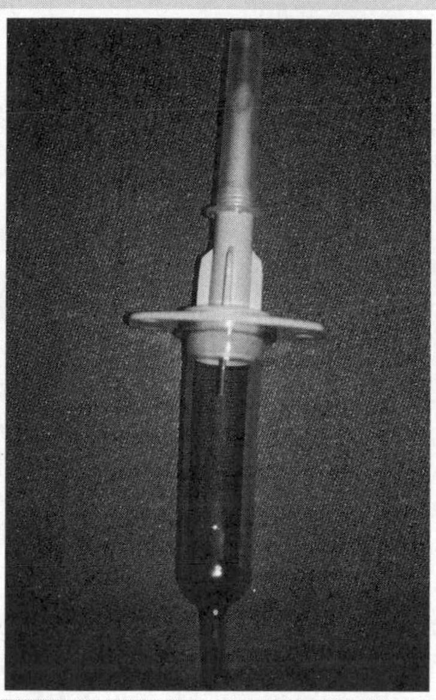

Regular drip set (10 drops/ml)*

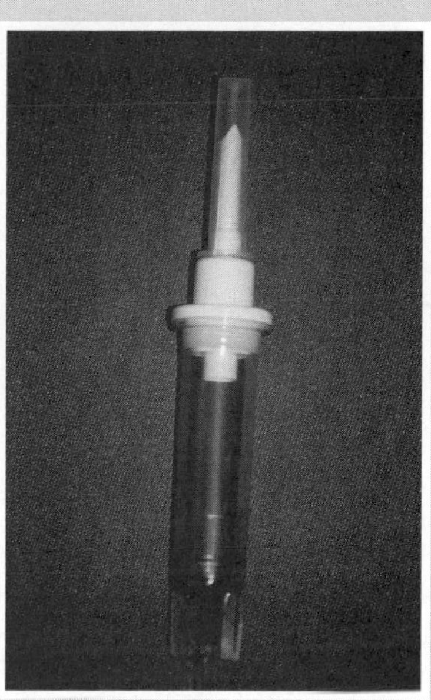

Calculating the Rate with Total Volume to Be Administered over a Specific Number of Hours

Rate (drops/min) = Drops/ml calibrated* ÷ 60 (minutes/hour) × Total volume to be administered ÷ Total hour of infusion

Seconds/drop = 60 ÷ Rate

Example: 400 ml is needed over a 6-hour period of time

$(10 \div 60) \times (400 \div 6) = 11$ drops/min $\quad 60 \div 11 = 5$ seconds/drop

Calculating the Rate with ml/hr to Be Administered

Rate (drops/minute) = ml/hr × drops/ml calibrated* ÷ 60 (minutes/hour)

Seconds/drop = 60 ÷ Rate

Example: 40 ml/hr to be administered

$40 \times 60 \div 60 = 40$ drops/min $\quad 60 \div 40 = 1.5$ seconds/drop

*Drops per milliliter are calibrated for each individual set. This information is on the package of the fluid administration sets.

TABLE 4-8 Clinical Signs of Extracellular Fluid Volume Depletion and Overload

Depletion	Overload
Pale, dry mucous membranes	Serous nasal discharge
Poor skin elasticity	Subcutaneous edema
Reduced urine output	Increased urine output with normal kidney
Microcardia on thoracic radiographs	Ascites
Sunken orbits	Chemosis
Cool distal extremities	Exophthalmos
Slow capillary refill time	Restlessness, coughing
Weak rapid pulse	Increased respiration rate
Increased temperature	Vomiting

URINE PRODUCTION

The normal animal produces 22 to 44 ml/kg (10 to 20 ml/lb) of urine in a 24-hour period, or 1 to 2 ml/kg/hr. Urine production should be monitored closely, especially in patients undergoing diuresis. In such patients, urine production should nearly equal fluid input. Indirect measurement of urine output can be performed by free catch of urine in a bowl, use of a disposable diaper placed underneath a recumbent patient (weighed before and after urination), or weighing the litter pan before and after urination. One milliliter of urine is equivalent to 1 mg increase in weight when using this method. However, the most accurate measurement of urine production entails bladder catheterization and a closed collection system.

The urinary collection system must be sterile and introduced asceptically. Use a red rubber or polyvinyl chloride feeding tube for male dog catheterization or a Foley catheter for female dogs. Cats are catheterized with an open-ended tomcat or 3.5-French red rubber feeding tube. The catheters are lubricated with sterile jelly and slowly advanced through the urethra to the neck of the urinary bladder. Extreme care should be taken with this procedure so as not to kink the catheter or cause iatrogenic trauma to the urethra or bladder. The catheter should be sutured, glued or stapled in place, and connected to a sterile, closed urinary collection system. An empty sterile fluid bag or a commercial urine collection bag can be used, connected to an intravenous line. The collection bag should be placed below the level of the catheter but off the floor.

Once the system is in place, the bladder should be emptied and the time recorded on the patient's chart. Urine output should be measured and the collection bag drained every 2 hours. The urine sediment should be evaluated daily for signs of infection. Catheter care should be performed every 8 hours and includes cleaning the prepuce or vulva (betadine scrub and water rinse). Flush the surrounding area with a 1:10 solution of betadine and water. Inspect the urinary catheter for kinks or clots by flushing the system with sterile saline.

BLOOD VALUES

Before any fluid regimen is begun, a baseline set of blood data should be evaluated. These baseline data not only help in choosing the fluid and blood volume replacements to be administered but also act as a reference point to determine any changes in the therapy.

Packed Cell Volume or Hematocrit. The PCV should be followed closely during fluid administration, whether treating for shock or dehydration or administering supportive care. If the PCV drops abruptly below 20%, then a blood transfusion should be administered.

Total Protein. Total protein (TP) relates to the relative serum oncotic pressure. If the serum oncotic pressure falls, then more fluid will enter the interstitium. This edema can create life-threatening disease. TP (and more importantly albumin) levels can decrease rapidly in disease and rehydration. TP levels should be maintained above 3.5 g/dl and albumin levels should be maintained above 2.0 g/dl. Plasma is the best source of TP replacement therapy in the patient. Alternatively, colloids can be used to help maintain serum oncotic pressure.

Electrolytes. Serum electrolyte levels should be evaluated to determine the need for replacement therapy. Serum sodium levels normally are between 140 and 155 mEq/L. Serum potassium levels normally are between 3.6 and 5.5 mEq/L.

Other. Other parameters should be monitored depending on the disease being treated. Examples include renal disease, diabetes, and hepatic disease. Monitoring these blood chemistry values allows the technician to assess the patient's status and evaluate the success of diuresis and rehydration.

Assessing Perfusion

Mucous Membranes. Normal nonpigmented mucous membranes are pink. Variations may be found with disease states (white for shock, anemia, or blood loss; blue for hypoxia; red for sepsis; yellow for liver disease). Mucous membrane color depends on peripheral capillary blood flow, hemoglobin concentration, and tissue oxygenation. The gums are the most commonly evaluated tissue, but the vulva, penis, or conjunctiva of the eye also may be used.

Capillary Refill Time

Peripheral perfusion is evaluated by capillary refill time (CRT). Digital pressure applied to the mucous membranes reduces the capillary blood flow, resulting in a blanching of the tissue. The period of time for blood flow to return to the area normally is 1 to 2 seconds and depends on vascular tone and cardiac output. Prolonged CRT may be an indicator of late stages of shock, heart failure, severe vasodilation or vasoconstriction, or pericardial effusion. Capillary refill time of less than 1 second may be an indicator of compensatory shock, fever, pain, or anxiety.

If a patient demonstrates abnormal CRT, the veterinarian should be notified and appropriate therapy initiated. When fluid therapy is indicated to replace blood volume, perfusion should improve, the mucous membranes should moisten, the color should improve to a pink, and the capillary refill time should be less than 2 seconds.

Skin Turgor

Hydration status may be approximated by skin turgor, defined as fullness, which in this case would be fluid. Subjective evaluation of skin turgor may be performed by pinching a fold of skin and assessing the time for the skin to return to its normal position. Skin that has a slight delay in return to normal may be approximated as 5% to 6% dehydrated. A pronounced tenting effect resulting from the skin fold pinch may be approximated as 10% to 12% dehydration.

Skin turgor can be misleading in the obese animal because adipose tissue replaces subcutaneous interstitial water and maintains elasticity despite a negative water balance. Older, cachectic patients lose skin resiliency and may give a false impression of marked dehydration.

Auscultation

It is important for the veterinary technician to become proficient in lung sound auscultation. Common terms used to describe lung sounds, such as *rales* or *rhonchi,* are nonspecific. Sounds may better be described by frequency (low or high), intensity (loud or soft), quality or complexity, and duration (long or short). Sounds are produced by tissue vibration and the movement of air through the structures. Normal lung sounds may be bronchial (larger airways), vesicular (peripheral airways), or bronchovesicular (between bronchial and vesicular). Bronchial sounds usually are louder and vesicular normally are quieter. The intensity may be increased by panting breaths, lung consolidation, thin chest walls (underweight or young patients), or airway inflammation (bacterial pneumonia). Decreased intensity (silent lung) may be caused by obesity, pleural effusion, pneumothorax, diaphragmatic hernia, or lobar consolidation.

Abnormal lung sounds should be identified by the same parameters as normal sounds but should include the time when the sounds were heard (inspiratory-expiratory cycles) and the quantity of sounds noted. Crackles are sounds that can result from the opening of airways and can be described as low- or high-pitched, depending on the length of the sound. They are explosive sounds that are nonmusical. Pleural friction rub is heard as an abnormally loud but focal sound that is low pitched and noted during both inspiration and expiration. This "creaking leather" sound may be present in patients with a history of pleural effusion or pleuritis. Wheezes are continuous, nonexplosive musical sounds of air passing at a high velocity through a narrowed airway. The airway may be decreased from constriction or filling and may cause a monophonic wheeze (single-site obstruction) or a polyphonic wheeze (widespread airway narrowing). Stridor is an abnormally intense monophonic wheeze that is heard continuously, often without the aid of a stethoscope. When stridor is heard it is often associated with an upper airway obstruction.

Pulse Quality

The emergency patient should be evaluated for pulse quality or pressure. Hypovolemic shock may be observed as a weak (hypokinetic) pulse pressure. Increased pulse pressure is noted when the clinical signs of shock begin to resolve. Early compensatory stages of shock may be indicated by a bounding (hyperkinetic) pulse pressure. The pulse also is valuable for assessing cardiovascular status. The femoral artery is the most common location for pulse palpation, although the palmar aspect of the carpus also can be used. The heart should be auscultated between the left fourth and sixth intercostal spaces while the pulse is taken. If the pulse is less than the heart rate (pulse deficit), there may be a cardiac dysrhythmia. If both the heart rate and the pulse increase and decrease, respectively, during inspiration and expiration, the patient may have a sinus arrhythmia (considered a normal variation). Normal pulse rate ranges are similar to heart rates (cats, 160 to 240/minute; dogs, 60 to 160/minute); puppies and small breed dogs may have higher rates.

Central Venous Pressure

In patients that are prone to developing hypertension, particularly those with renal or heart failure, the CVP should be monitored. This must be done through a central line (jugular) catheter, the tip of which is level with the right atrium. The catheter is connected by an extension set to a three-way stopcock. The intravenous line and fluids are connected opposite from the extension set and a water manometer is connected to the upright opening of the stopcock. While the patient is receiving fluids, the stopcock is turned off from the manometer. To measure CVP, fluids are turned off to the patient and the manometer is filled with fluid. The incoming fluids are then turned off, and the extension set to the patient is opened. The fluid level in the manometer (which is placed level with the sternum) will equilibrate. The measured level will fluctuate within a few millimeters during respiration or heartbeat. A minimum of three readings should be performed to ensure consistency and an accurate CVP.

The normal CVP range is 0 to 10 cm H_2O. Patients with values less than 5 cm H_2O may have insufficient blood volume. Those with CVP values greater than 14 cm H_2O may have a significant volume overload or right heart failure. The optimal range is between 5 and 8 cm H_2O. When high CVP measurements are seen or there is an absence of respiratory fluctuation in the manometer level, the veterinary technician should examine the catheter for a possible blood clot or occlusion. It is important to note that serial CVP measurements should be performed, with attention given to resulting trends (Figure 4-5).

Pulse Oximetry

Arterial oxygen saturation (Sao_2) is measured noninvasively with pulse oximetry. Veterinary models are available as well as reconditioned and

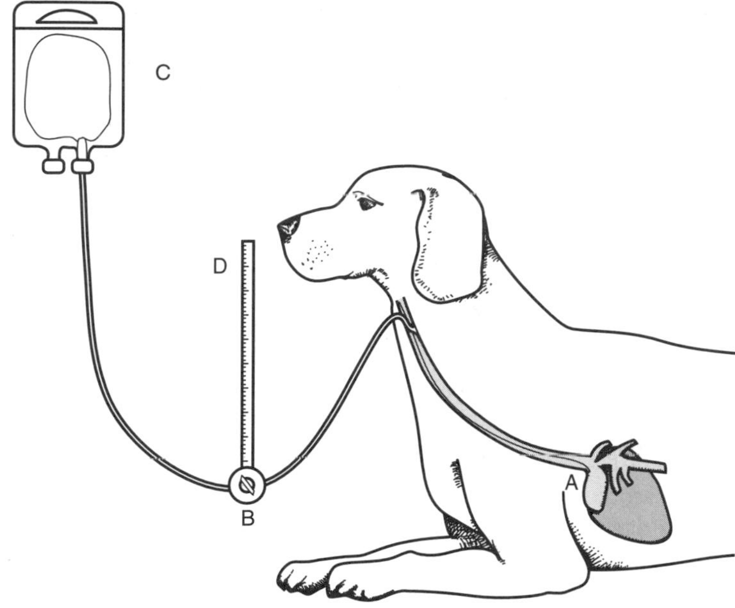

Figure 4-5

Central venous pressure measurement. With the patient in sternal recumbency, a jugular venous catheter is advanced to the level of the right atrium *(A)* and connected to a stopcock *(B)*. The stopcock is connected to an intravenous delivery system *(C)* and a manometer *(D)*. (Allen DG: Ancillary aids to cardiopulmonary medicine. In Allen DG, Kruth SA, eds: *Small animal cardiopulmonary medicine,* Philadelphia, 1988, BC Decker, p 142.)

refurbished human units. Light wavelengths are passed through body tissue (red and infrared) to a photodetector. The strength of the signal that is measured is reported as the SaO_2 level. The clamp style probe is placed on the tongue or on nonpigmented skin. Rectal probes are available with some models. Probe placement, tissue color, and thickness can affect the accuracy of the SaO_2 reading. The pulse oximeter is a valuable monitoring device for patients with SaO_2 levels between 90% and 95%. Normal SaO_2 level is 98%. Patients with values less than 90% should be monitored closely and may need oxygen therapy. Cardiopulmonary function should be assessed if there is a sudden drop in SaO_2. Patients undergoing blood volume replacement therapy can be evaluated further with pulse oximetry.

CONCLUSION

Fluid therapy, when used appropriately, can be crucial in the successful care of any patient. Careless use of fluids can endanger the patient. Technicians involved in administering fluids must understand the basic principles of fluid therapy, including the contents of the fluids and the proposed goal of the fluid treatment. By monitoring the parameters described, the technician plays a key role in patient care.

BIBLIOGRAPHY

Bell F, Osborne C: Maintenance fluid therapy. In Kirk RW, ed: *Current veterinary therapy X,* Philadelphia, 1989, WB Saunders.

Fagella AM: Introduction to critical care. In Morgan RV, ed: *Handbook of small animal practice,* ed 3, Philadelphia, 1997, WB Saunders.

within 6 hours. After 24-hour storage, platelet function is lost and the concentration of labile coagulation factors decreases. The product is then defined as stored whole blood (SWB), which provides RBCs and plasma proteins. The length of time whole blood can be stored under refrigeration depends on the anticoagulant preservative solution used in collection. Because of the well-documented advantages of using blood components and the greater availability of these products, using whole blood is no longer considered the treatment of choice. However, SWB can be used in patients that need intravascular volume expansion and oxygen-carrying support.

Using whole blood, fresh or stored, is not recommended in severe chronic anemia. Chronically anemic patients may have a reduced RBC mass but have compensated over time by increasing their plasma volume to meet their total blood volume needs. Administering whole blood may carry the risk of volume overload, especially in patients with preexisting cardiac disease or renal compromise.

Packed Red Blood Cells

Packed red blood cells (pRBCs) are the component of choice for increasing red cell mass in patients who need oxygen-carrying support. Decreased RBC mass may be caused by decreased bone marrow production, increased destruction, or surgical or traumatic bleeding. Although it seems logical to use whole blood, most blood loss is treated adequately by replacing blood volume with pRBCs and crystalloid or colloid solutions. This therapy is adequate for the majority of acutely bleeding patients. In human medicine, more than 80% of all transfusions incorporate pRBCs. With recent advances in veterinary medicine and an increase in the understanding of component therapy in animals, the rate of pRBC use in veterinary transfusions soon may equal that in human medicine.

pRBC transfusion is not recommended in patients whose anemia is well compensated (e.g., those with chronic renal failure). The decision to perform red cell transfusion should never be based solely on hematocrit or hemoglobin levels. Patients should be evaluated properly and pRBC administration based primarily on clinical status (e.g., tachycardia, poor pulse quality, respiratory distress, or lethargy).

Platelet-Rich Plasma and Platelet Concentrates

Platelet-rich plasma (PRP) is harvested from a unit of FWB that is less than 8 hours old and has not been cooled below 20° C. Refrigerated platelets do not maintain function or viability as well as platelets stored at room temperature. The PRP may be administered just after harvesting, or the

surably in larger dogs. In some patients, however, bleeding ceases after platelet transfusion without a measurable increase in platelet number. Because of the impracticality of producing this component in the volume needed for significant impact, its specific storage requirements, and its short shelf life, veterinarians routinely treat thrombocytopenia or thrombocytopathia with active bleeding with FWB, from which the patient receives both platelets and RBC support. In situations of platelet destruction, such as idiopathic thrombocytopenia purpura, the survival of transfused platelets is a matter of minutes rather than days. If the patient is must be administered in large volumes to have a measurable impact on the acute effects of hypoproteinemia (e.g., pulmonary edema and pleural effusion). In this case, synthetic colloid solutions should be considered. They are more effective in increasing oncotic pressure and are more readily available. Like FFP, FP and LP are not recommended for use as blood volume expanders.

CRYOPRECIPITATE

Cryoprecipitate (CRYO) is the cold-insoluble portion of plasma that precipitates after FFP has been thawed slowly at 1° to 6° C. The precipitated material contains concentrated amounts of von Willebrand factor (vWF), factor VIII:C, fibrinogen, and fibronectin. After production, CRYO can be frozen at −18° C or colder and has a shelf life of 1 year from the original date of whole blood collection. CRYO can be used in patients with suspected or diagnosed von Willebrand disease, hemophilia A, or fibrinogen deficiency. Each unit of CRYO contains approximately 25 to 50 ml liquid plasma, so many units can be administered without the risk of volume overload (Table 5-1).

BLOOD SOURCES

Historically, veterinarians have relied on donor dogs living in the hospital facility as a source of blood for transfusion purposes. Blood was collected for immediate use, and little emphasis was placed on quality control. These few in-house donors could not meet the growing need for transfusion. During the past few years, university-based blood donor programs and several commercial animal blood banks have been established to help meet blood transfusion needs. These facilities supply safe and high-quality blood products that are processed according to the standards of the American Association of Blood Banks (AABB). Blood banking staff also share expertise in transfusion medicine through newsletters and individual case consultation requests. Purchasing products from these blood banks and maintaining an

TABLE 5-1 Blood Components

Component	Contents	Indication
Fresh whole blood (FWB)	RBCs: plasma proteins; all coagulation factors; WBCs; platelets (approx. Hct 40%)	Acute active hemorrhage; hypovolemic shock; thrombocytopenia with active bleeding
Stored whole blood (SWB)	RBCs, plasma proteins (approx. Hct 40%)	Anemia with hypoproteinemia; hypovolemic shock
Packed red blood cells (pRBCs)	RBCs (approx. Hct 80%; reduced plasma	Increase red cell mass in symptomatic anemia
pRBCs, adenine-saline added	RBCs (approx. Hct 60%); reduced plasma; 100 ml additive solution	Increase red cell mass in symptomatic anemia
Platelet-rich plasma/platelet concentrate	Platelets; few RBCs and WBCs; some plasma	Bleeding due to thrombocytopenia or thrombocytopathy
Fresh frozen plasma	Plasma, albumin; all coagulation factors	Treatment of coagulation disorders/factor deficiencies; liver disease; DIC; anticoagulant rodenticide toxicity
Frozen plasma	Plasma; albumin; stable coagulation factors	Treatment of stable coagulation factor deficiencies
Cryoprecipitate	Factor VIII; vWF; fibrinogen; fibronectin	Hemophilia; von Willebrand disease; hypofibrinogenemia

Hct, Hematocrit; *RBCs,* red blood cells; *WBCs,* white blood cells; *vWF,* von Willebrand factor.

Shelf Life	Preparation	Comments
Less than 8 hr after initial collection	Use immediately following collection (refrigeration compromises platelet and certain coagulation factor function)	Restores blood volume and oxygen-carrying capacity, may help control some microvascular bleeding
Greater than 8 hr old and up to 35 days (dependent on anticoagulant-preservative solution used); refrigerate at 1°-6° C	Allow to come to room temperature (temperatures exceeding 37° C will result in hemolysis and bacterial proliferation)	Restores blood volume and oxygen-carrying capacity (WBCs, and platelets not functional; factor V & VIII diminished); not recommended for chronic anemia
Dependent on anticoagulant-preservative solution used; refrigerate at 1°-6° C	Allow to come to room temperature (temperatures exceeding 37° C will result in hemolysis and bacterial proliferation); may reconstitute with 0.9% NaCl prior to administration	Same oxygen-carrying capacity as whole blood, but less volume
37 days; refrigerate at 1°-6° C	Allow to come to room temperature (temperatures exceeding 37° C will result in hemolysis and bacterial proliferation)	Additive solution extends shelf life and reduces viscosity for infusion
5 days at 22° C; intermittent agitation required	Should administer immediately following collection and preparation	Do not refrigerate; usually require multiple units
12 mo frozen at −18° C or below	Thaw in 37° C water bath (temperatures exceeding 37° C will result in protein denaturation and bacterial proliferation)	Frozen within 8 hr after collection; no platelets; can be relabeled as frozen plasma after 1 yr for additional 4 yr; administer as soon as thawed
5 yr frozen at −20° C or below	Thaw in 37° C warm water bath (temperatures exceeding 37° C will result in protein denaturation and bacterial proliferation)	Frozen after more than 8 hr following collection; no platelets; can be used to treat some cases of acute hypoproteinemia; administer as soon as thawed
12 mo frozen at −20° C or below	Thaw in 37° C warm water bath (temperatures exceeding 37° C will result in protein denaturation and bacterial proliferation)	Administer as soon as thawed

Canine donors must
- weigh at least 25 kg
- Healthy
- Vaccs against - distemper
hepatitis, parainfluenza,
parvovirus and rabies
- not on any meds

Do Not sedate for sampling.

…e

S…

te…

do…

cha…

pred…

Altho…

optima… …al excellent

care in… …vironment.

Othe… …anks have established volunteer donor programs to meet veterinary transfusion needs. Donors are recruited from among employees' pets, healthy client-owned animals, breeders, and dog clubs. Client education about the importance of blood product availability and the need for blood donors is instrumental in establishing a large donor pool. Informed pet owners are a valuable asset to this type of program. Most are willing to volunteer their animals for periodic blood donation (i.e., three or four times yearly) once they understand the need for blood products and the elements of the donation process. The program involves owners and heightens their awareness of transfusion medicine.

One could argue that the people attracted to this type of program are those who care about animal welfare and provide very good health care to their pets. Like human blood donors, these people are motivated by altruism. Nevertheless, potential donors may carry illnesses that could affect the safety of the donation process or the safety and quality of the blood products. For this reason, it is important to verify donor health status through a brief history, physical examination, and appropriate laboratory testing, all of which are performed on the day of the donation. The staff must be well trained and proficient. To attract volunteer donors initially and to encourage their continuing support, conditions surrounding the blood donation should be as pleasant and safe as possible.

Canine donors must meet specific requirements before being accepted into the program. Donors must be at least 1 year old and weigh at least 25 kg to allow the collection of a full unit (i.e., 450 ml ± 10%). They should be healthy; have a current vaccination status for distemper, hepatitis, parainfluenza, parvovirus, and rabies; and not be on medication at the time of donation (excluding heartworm and flea preventive medications). Because canine donors are not sedated for blood collection, good temperament is needed for successful donation. A complete blood cell count, chemistry profile, and testing for geographically specific infectious agents (e.g., *Ehrlichia canis, Babesia canis, Dirofilariasis immitis*) should be performed annually. The hematocrit or hemoglobin concentration should be at least 40% or 13.5 g/dl, respectively, before each donation. Donors can be screened for vWF antigen levels to identify those that have the highest plasma concentration of this platelet adhesion protein and reserve their blood for use in patients with von Willebrand disease.

Thirteen specific antigens, or blood types, have been identified on the surface of canine erythrocytes. The current nomenclature is listed as dog erythrocyte antigen (DEA) 1.1, 1.2, and 3 through 13. Because of the limited donor availability and the inadequacies of typing reagents, limited work has been done to determine the incidence of all blood types or their significance in transfusion.

Blood donor dogs should be typed for DEA 1.1 and possibly others (DEA 1.2 and 7). The most severe antigen-antibody reaction is seen with these antigens, most specifically DEA 1.1. Dogs that are negative for DEA 1.1 are considered universal donors. Significant naturally occurring alloantibodies are not seen in the dog, so antigen-antibody reactions are not likely to occur on initial transfusion. However, dogs that are DEA 1.1, 1.2, and 7 negative can develop alloantibodies to DEA 1.1, 1.2, and 7 from a mismatched transfusion. This can occur within 4 to 14 days from initial transfusion. These antibodies can destroy the donor's red blood

Canine.
- Blood donors should be typed DEA 1.1
(other possibly DEA 1.2 + 7)
- Negative blood can be given to a negative or positive type
- Positive blood only to positive type.

performed using a small amou... blood, is based on the agglutination reaction that occurs within 2 minutes when erythrocytes that are DEA 1.1 positive interact with a murine monoclonal antibody specific to DEA 1.1. Because of the strong antigenicity of DEA 1.1, typing of donors and recipients for DEA 1.1 is strongly recommended. DEA 1.1 negative blood can be given to DEA 1.1 negative and DEA 1.1 positive patients. Dogs positive for the DEA 1.1 antigen can be accepted into the donor pool as long as recipients are typed before administration, with DEA 1.1 positive blood being given only to patients positive for DEA 1.1. If typing is unavailable, or in an emergency, recipients should be cross-matched with universal donors before transfusion to avoid sensitization.

The approach to feline donors is much more complicated. At present, there are few commercial feline blood banks. In addition, volunteer programs for cats hold many risks. Although dogs donate blood voluntarily, most cats must be sedated for blood donation purposes. The legal risk associated with sedating personal pets solely for blood donation is far too great. Another concern is that cats can harbor infectious agents more readily than dogs. For this reason, indoor-only cats should be used.

Feline blood donors should be young, good-natured adults. They should be large and lean, weighing at least 4 kg. Blood collection is easiest in cats with short hair, which facilitates vascular

Feline donors should be young, good natured adults
- indoor cats only
- weigh at least 4kg.
- Good health
- Vaccs - rhinotracheitis, calicivirus panleukopenia and rabies.

Blood types
A + B + AB

on the surface of the red blood cell. Nearly all domestic shorthair (DSH) and domestic longhair (DLH) cats have type A blood, the most common. Many purebred cats (and some DSHs) have type B blood (Table 5-2 and Figure 5-1). The proportion of A and B type varies not only among the different breeds but also nationally and internationally. Cats differ from dogs in that they have significant,

TABLE 5-2 Incidence of Blood Type B in Purebred Cats in the United States*

Type B Incidence (%)	Breeds
0	Siamese and related breeds, Burmese, Tonkinese, Russian blue
1-10	Maine coon, Norwegian forest, DSH/DLH
11-20	Abyssinian, Birman, Persian, Somali, Sphinx, Scottish Fold, Himalayan
25-50	Exotic and British Shorthair cats, Cornish and Devon Rex

*Type AB occurs rarely (<1%).

< 1% type B 1-2% type B 2-3% type B 4-6% type B

Fig
Ge
in tl

natu
bloc
stro
whe ... weak anti-B alloantibod-
ies. These alloantibodies can cause two serious problems:

- Transfusion reactions. Cats with rare type B blood can experience potentially fatal reactions if they are given a transfusion with the common type A blood. Mismatched transfusions have short half-lives and are ineffective.
- Neonatal isoerythrolysis. If a queen with type B blood is bred to a type A tom and produces kittens with type A blood, the antibodies in the colostrum of the queen will destroy RBCs in the kittens.

When type B blood is administered to a type A cat, there may be no obvious clinical reaction, but the transfused RBCs have a half-life of approximately 2 days. If type A blood is administered to a type B cat, RBC survival can be minutes to hours, with severe clinical signs, sometimes fatal. Administering a small amount of blood to test for incompatibility is no longer an acceptable procedure. Life-threatening acute hemolytic transfusion reactions can be observed with administration of as little as 1 ml of AB-incompatible blood. These reactions can be prevented by typing and cross-matching donors and patients. Blood typing cards similar to those used in dogs are commercially available, yielding accurate results in minutes (DMS Laboratories, Inc., 2 Darts Mill Road, Flemington, New Jersey 08822, [800] 567-4367).

Because of the presence of naturally occurring alloantibodies, there is no universal blood type in the cat. All feline blood donors and recipients must be blood typed, and only typed, matched blood should be administered. The extremely rare blood type AB cat can be transfused safely with type A blood.

BLOOD COLLECTION

Blood Collection Systems

Quality should be the primary goal in collecting, processing, storing, and administering all blood products. At each step, it is critical to prevent or delay adverse changes in blood constituents and minimize bacterial contamination and proliferation. Many improvements in the preparation of components from whole blood have been

e
d
ie
al
in
od
eet
een

col-
lect whole ... d as
whole blood. It consists of a main collection bag,

containing anticoagulant preservative solution, and integral tubing with a 16-gauge needle attached.

Vacuum glass bottles containing acid-citrate dextrose (ACD) anticoagulant-preservative are easier to use but is an open collection system and foam caused during collection can cause hemolysis

* High rapid blood flow containers are not recommended

collection is easier with this system, there are many limitations and disadvantages: this is considered an open collection system, the glass activates platelets and certain clotting factors, the foam created during collection disrupts the red cell surface and causes hemolysis, and component preparation is not possible. For these reasons, vacuum glass bottles are not recommended. Vacuum chambers that allow more rapid blood collection are available.

Feline Blood Collection

The recommended collection s
ily accessible jugular vein. Du
size and increased blood flow,
trauma is minimized during colle
should be performed with a
rupted single venipuncture to av
and excessive activation of coa
Strict aseptic technique and th
equipment minimize the possibi
contamination.

Although commercially produ
tion bags are suitable for collecti
the size of these systems prohibit

Feline Blood collection.
1 unit of blood = 40-50ml of whole blood.
14-gauge needle.

Altenatively blood can be collected with a 19/21 gauge butterfly catheter or 20 gauge needle attached to a 3way stopcock

Currently, smaller closed collection systems are not available. In addition, blood component preparation is difficult due to the small volume of blood with which to work. Recommendations have been made to utilize the 450-ml CPDA-1 whole blood collection system used in dogs. The majority of anticoagulant is expressed from the main collection pack into a satellite container via integral tubing. The remainder of anticoagulant-preservative solution in the collection tubing will be appropriate for one unit of blood, defined as approximately 40 to 50 ml of whole blood. This maintains the system as "closed." Because of the size of the collection bag and its attached 14-gauge needle, this approach is less than optimal.

Because of the lack of commercially prepared closed blood collection systems for cats, the difficulty in preparing blood components from small whole blood units, and the limited storage life of blood collected with an "open" system, cats in need of transfusion support have most often received fresh whole blood. By modifying current blood collection protocols, a closed collection system that allows component preparation and storage of small blood volumes (35 to 45 ml) was developed using commercially available blood collection products. Connections were established and sterility was maintained by using a tube-welding instrument (Terumo Sterile Tubing Welder
a vacuum chamber,
litated by establish-
ssful collection de-
., animal restraint,
amount of vacuum
n, the whole blood
y, stored as whole
ponents and stored
banking procedures.
n may serve as a
nanufactured closed
ats. Until then, this
of processing and
ts.
collected utilizing
9/21-gauge butterfly

catheter or 20-gauge needle attached to a three-way stopcock and sterile 10- to 30-ml syringes containing anticoagulant may be used. During collection, the syringes should be gently inverted to allow for mixing of blood and anticoagulant, thus preventing clot formation. Blood collection utilizing this technique is effective but considered an "open" system. Following collection, blood can be transferred from the syringes into an empty sterile bag, or transfer pack, making delivery more efficient. Blood products collected via syringe are not suitable for storage.

Anticoagulant Preservative Solutions

Several anticoagulants, anticoagulant preservatives, and additive solutions are available for collecting blood for transfusion purposes. The primary goal of preservative solutions is to maintain red cell viability during storage and to lengthen the survival of red cells after transfusion. According to AABB standards, 75% of transfused RBCs must survive for 24 hours after infusion for the transfusion to be considered acceptable and successful. The longer cells are stored, the more viability decreases. Predetermined storage times are based on studies that have investigated adverse biochemical changes that take place during red cell storage. These changes, called the storage lesion, include a decrease in ATP, pH, and 2,3-DPG (increasing hemoglobin-oxygen affinity) and an increase in lactic acid. All of these ultimately lead to a loss of red cell function and viability. Storage time varies with the anticoagulant preservative solution used:

- Citrate-phosphate-dextrose-adenine (CPDA-1)
  - RBC 2,3 DPG, and ATP are better maintained.
  - Best anticoagulant preservative solution; canine and feline whole blood can be stored for 35 days, canine pRBCs can be stored for 21 days.
  - Used at ratio of 1 ml CPDA-1 to 7-9 ml blood.
- Citrate-phosphate-dextrose (CPD)
  - pRBCs can be stored for 21 days.
  - Used at ratio of 1 ml CPD to 7 ml blood.
- Acid-citrate-dextrose (ACD)
  - pRBCs can be stored for 21 days in dogs, 28 days in cats.
  - Used at ratio of 1 ml ACD to 7 ml blood.
- Heparin
  -Not recommended for transfusion purposes.
- Additive solutions (e.g., Adsol, Fenwal Laboratories, Baxter Healthcare Corp., Deerfield, Illinois; Nutricel, Miles, Pharmaceutical Division, West Haven, Connecticut; Optisol, Terumo Medical Corporation, Somerset, New Jersey)
  - Protein-free solution added to red cells after plasma removal from unit of whole blood.
  - Canine pRBCs can be stored for approximately 37 days.

PROCESSING AND STORAGE

The centrifuge rotor size, speed, and duration of spin are the critical variables in preparing components by centrifugation. Each centrifuge must be calibrated for optimal speed and specific time of spin for each component. pRBCs can be harvested from whole blood (fresh or stored) by centrifuging the unit at 5000 *g* and 4° C for 5 minutes. If a refrigerated centrifuge is not available, the red blood cells can be allowed to separate from refrigerated whole blood by sedimentation over a period of time. Unfortunately, natural sedimentation decreases the volume of plasma that can be removed and increases the chance of red cell contamination of the final product. After separation has occurred, plasma is removed, ideally with a plasma extractor, leaving enough in the unit to maintain a hematocrit that does not exceed 80%. Removing more plasma than recommended results in insufficient preservative solution to support storage. Ideally, pRBCs should be reconstituted with a nutrient solution before storage to maintain the cells in a healthier environment. Using additive solutions allows increased plasma yield (approximately 50 ml) and extended storage time. In addition, reconstituting the cells reduces viscosity during administration. pRBCs can be refrigerated at 1° to 6° C, with storage time defined by the anticoagulant preservative or additive solution used in collection and processing. If the RBCs were separated in a system that was open at any time, the product must be used within 24 hours. If a nutrient solution is not used in processing, pRBCs can be reconstituted with approximately 100 ml 0.9% NaCl before administration to reduce viscosity. Only isotonic saline should be used to dilute blood components because other intravenous solutions may cause red cell damage (e.g., D_5W) or initiate blood coagulation (e.g., lactated Ringer's solution).

Fresh plasma contains plasma proteins and coagulation factors. It does not contain viable platelets. The same value is retained for up to 1 year if fresh plasma is frozen at a minimum of −18° C within 8 hours of collection. If the natural separation method is used to prepare plasma, clotting factor efficacy will be compromised. FFP has a shelf life of 1 year from the original collection date. If not used within this time, it can be relabeled as FP, providing plasma protein only, for an additional 4 years.

CRYO is harvested from a unit of FFP that has been allowed to thaw slowly at 1° to 6° C for approximately 12 to 18 hours. The slurried plasma is centrifuged at 5000 *g* and 4° C for 6 minutes. The supernatant plasma is expressed using a plasma extractor, leaving behind a white, foamy precipitate (mostly adhered to the bag) in 25 to 50 ml liquid plasma. Units of CRYO can be pooled before storage or administration. If CRYO is to be pooled prior to freezing, it should be pooled immediately after preparation. If it is thawed and then pooled, the product must be administered within 4 hours.

PRP is harvested from FWB that has been centrifuged at 1000 *g* and 20° to 24° C for 4 minutes, a much slower speed and warmer temperature than used for routine plasma harvesting. The FWB should not be cooled below 20° C before the PRP is removed, and the separation must occur within 8 hours after collection. After centrifugation, the bag is allowed to sit undisturbed for 30 minutes and PRP is removed. This product can be stored at room temperature for approximately 3 days with intermittent agitation. Refrigerated platelets do not maintain function or viability as well as platelets stored at room temperature; therefore, this component should be prepared and administered as quickly as possible after collection.

BLOOD ADMINISTRATION

Blood Cross-Match

Ideally, patients should be blood-typed and cross-matched before blood transfusion. If blood typing reagents or cards are not available, at the very least a blood cross-match (BCM) test should be done. Blood typing determines the blood group antigens on the surface of the RBC. A BCM test detects any serum (plasma) incompatibility between donor and recipient.

The BCM test is used to identify antibodies in donor or recipient plasma against recipient or donor RBCs. The major portion of the BCM detects the presence of alloantibodies in the recipient's plasma against donor RBCs, whereas the minor BCM test looks for alloantibodies in the donor plasma against recipient RBCs. If there is evidence of macroscopic agglutination of the patient's blood (rarely seen in cats) or severe hemolysis of the patient's blood sample, a BCM test cannot be performed.

Dogs being transfused for the first time (non-sensitized) can have a compatible cross-match despite differing blood types because they often do not have significant naturally occurring allo-antibody. Even if type-specific blood components are used for the first transfusion, cross-matching is still advised because all RBC antigen groups have not been characterized fully. Although the BCM detects many incompatibilities, it does not guarantee against future sensitization. A BCM should always be performed in a dog that was previously transfused. In dogs, if neither cross-matching nor typing is available, or it is an emergency with no time for cross-matching, universal donor blood (DEA 1.1 negative) should

Box 5-1 Technical Tip: *Blood Cross-Matching*

Materials

Anticoagulated blood from donor and recipient
- Centrifuge
- Test tubes
- 0.9% Sodium chloride
- Microscope slides

Procedure

1. Collect 2 ml ethylenediaminetetraacetic acid anticoagulated blood from donor and recipient.
2. Centrifuge the blood samples for 1 minute at 3000 *g*. Remove the plasma to prelabeled tubes.
3. Make a 2% RBC suspension by mixing 0.1 ml RBCs and 5 ml 0.9% saline solution. Mix the suspension.
4. Centrifuge the suspension for 1 minute. Discard the supernatant. Resuspend the RBCs in another 5 ml 0.9% saline, centrifuge, etc. This washing procedure is performed three times.
5. Place two drops of the recipient's plasma and two drops of the donor's RBC suspension in a 3-ml test tube. This is the major part of the cross-match. Then place two drops of the recipient's RBCs and two drops of the donor's plasma in another 3-ml test tube. This is the minor part of the cross-match. Mix well and incubate the tubes for 30 minutes at room temperature.*
6. For controls, use the donor's and recipient's own cells and plasma, following the procedure just described. Centrifuge for 1 minute at 3000 *g*. You now have a total of four tubes.
7. Reading the crossmatch: Check for agglutination, check for hemolysis, and place a drop on a slide and examine microscopically at 40× for agglutination.

*For optimal results, incubate at 4° C, room temperature, and 37° C.

be given. All cats with unknown blood type should be cross-matched. It is possible to predict the blood type of a cat based on the BCM test results because of the presence of naturally occurring alloantibodies (excluding the rare blood type AB) (Technical Tip Box 5-1).

COMPONENT PREPARATION

Refrigerated blood can be warmed gently by sitting at room temperature for approximately 30 minutes. Properly administered cold blood will not increase the chance of a transfusion reaction, but large amounts of cold blood given at a rapid rate can induce hypothermia and cardiac arrhythmias. Routine warming of red cell products is not recommended except in neonates or hypothermic patients and with massive transfusion. Several types of blood warmers are available commercially. In an emergency, the tubing of the administration set can be placed in a warm water bath, not to exceed 37° C, so that warming can occur as blood passes through the tubing. The entire unit should not be immersed in the bath. Frozen products should also be thawed in a 37° C warm water bath. No blood product should be exposed to temperatures exceeding 42° C because this damages RBCs and denatures blood proteins. Warming RBC products or thawing plasma products in a microwave oven is not recommended unless it is an AABB-approved microwave.

ADMINISTRATION VOLUME

The aim of transfusion in the anemic patient is not to return the packed cell volume (PCV) to normal values but to correct the clinical signs. One generally aims to raise the PCV by approximately 10%. The following equations are used to determine the plasma volume needed.

$$\text{Weight (lb)} \times \frac{40\ \text{(dog)}}{30\ \text{(cat)}} \times \frac{\text{Desired PCV} - \text{Actual PCV}}{\text{Donor PCV}} = \text{Whole blood needed (ml)}$$

$$\text{PCV rise (\%)} \times \text{Weight (lb)} = \text{Whole blood needed (ml)}$$

Six to ten ml/kg of plasma can be given up to four times daily; transfusions are repeated depending on disease process and patient status.

Administration Routes

Blood and blood components can be administered via many routes. Intravenous administration is the most effective route because the infused RBCs or plasma products are immediately available to the general circulation. The intraosseous route is used in puppies or kittens when vascular access is difficult or unsuccessful. When blood products are delivered intraosseously, infused cells and proteins are available to the general circulation within minutes. The most common sites for intraosseous catheter placement are the trochanteric fossa of the femur, the wing of the ilium, and the shaft of the humerus. These catheters must be placed carefully to minimize the risk of osteomyelitis. Intraperitoneal infusion of blood products is not recommended. This delivery route can be painful and carries a risk of peritonitis. Absorption will occur, but it is delayed because only approximately 50% of the infused RBCs and proteins reach the circulation within 24 hours.

Administration Rates

Administration rates are variable. For example, a patient with massive hemorrhage may need a more rapid transfusion than a normovolemic patient with a chronic anemia. Blood should not be administered at a rate greater than 22 ml/kg/hr. However, the administration rate is less critical in a hypovolemic animal than in a normovolemic animal, where circulatory overload is a potential problem. Cardiovascularly compromised animals cannot tolerate infusion rates greater than 4 ml/kg/hr.

For all patients, blood components should be infused slowly (e.g., 1 ml/kg) for the first 10 to 15 minutes and the patient observed closely for signs of an acute transfusion reaction. The blood product should then be infused as quickly as tolerated, but it should not take longer than 4 hours. Before infusion, baseline values of attitude, rectal temperature, pulse rate and quality, respiratory rate and character, mucous membrane color, capillary refill time, hematocrit, total plasma protein, and plasma and urine color should be monitored. These parameters should be checked every 30 minutes during transfusion and evaluated routinely after transfusion to ensure that the desired effect has been achieved.

TRANSFUSION REACTIONS

Animals should be monitored carefully for any adverse reactions during and for several weeks after transfusion. Transfusion reactions can be classified as immune mediated or non–immune mediated.

Immune-mediated transfusion reactions can be hemolytic, with either acute (caused by preexisting isoantibodies or prior sensitization) or delayed (can be exhibited 2 to 21 days after transfusion) presentation. Hemolytic transfusion reactions are the most serious but the most rare. In acute situations, intravascular hemolysis is caused by preexisting antibodies, as seen in the mismatched transfusion of feline type A blood to a cat with type B blood or in previously sensitized DEA 1.1 negative dogs receiving DEA 1.1 positive blood. Clinical signs include fever, tachycardia, weakness, muscle tremors, vomiting, collapse, hemoglobinemia, and hemoglobinuria. Hemolytic transfusion reactions can lead to renal failure as a result of damage caused by clearance of antibody-coated RBC stroma. The most common hemolytic transfusion reaction is delayed in presentation. Sensitization can result from a mismatched transfusion, resulting in hemolysis. This phenomenon can occur for up to 21 days as antibodies are produced.

Nonhemolytic transfusion reactions are a result of antibodies to white blood cells, platelets, or plasma proteins. These reactions most often are transient and are not life threatening. Clinical signs include anaphylaxis, urticaria, pruritus, pyrexia, and neurologic signs. Vomiting can be noted with any type of transfusion reaction. In humans, transfusion therapy is reported to promote nausea.

Patients receiving blood products should fast before administration to avoid this potential complication.

A variety of factors is associated with non–immune-mediated transfusion reactions. Any type of trauma to the red blood cells can cause hemolysis. Overheating blood products causes protein denaturation and may increase bacterial growth during infusion. Mixing RBC products with nonisotonic solutions may cause cellular damage. Freezing RBC products, warming and then rechilling, and collecting or infusing blood through small needles or catheters also can cause hemolysis.

Bacterial pyrogens and sepsis can be complications of improper blood collection and storage. Dark brown to black supernatant plasma in stored blood indicates digested hemoglobin from bacterial growth. Any blood with discolored supernatant should be discarded immediately. Patients experiencing this most often mount a febrile response 15 to 20 minutes from start of infusion, which usually subsides within 2 to 4 hours of transfusion completion.

Citrate intoxication may occur when the citrate to blood volume ratio is disproportionate or in massively transfused patients, particularly in patients with liver dysfunction. Common clinical signs include involuntary muscle tremors, cardiac arrhythmias, and decreased cardiac output. This compromised state can be confirmed by obtaining an ionized serum calcium. If citrate toxicity is in question, blood administration should be discontinued and calcium gluconate administered.

The appropriate volume of blood must be administered to each patient. One should use only the blood component necessary to treat the specific disorder, and cardiovascular status always should be assessed before the infusion volume and administration rate are determined. Because blood is a colloid solution, vascular overload is a potential complication. Clinical signs include coughing (as a result of pulmonary edema), dyspnea, cyanosis, tachycardia, and vomiting. If volume overload is of concern, blood administration should be discontinued at least temporarily and supportive care instituted.

All blood products should be filtered to help prevent thromboembolic complications. Standard blood infusion sets have in-line filters with a pore size of approximately 170 to 260 μm. A filter of this size will trap cells, cellular debris, and coagulated protein. Infusion sets can be used for several units of blood products or for a maximum time of 4 hours. Trapped debris at room temperature may promote proliferation of bacteria. Pulmonary microembolism can occur with massive transfusion as a result of microaggregates of platelets, leukocytes, and fibrin strands that form in blood after several days of storage. This is prevented by using a microaggregate filter system with a pore size of 20 to 40 μm. It is not necessary to use microaggregate filters for routine low-volume transfusion.

CONCLUSION

Many positive changes have taken place in veterinary transfusion medicine in the last two decades that have improved the quality of medicine practiced. This evolution will continue as it has in human medicine. The Society of Veterinary Hematology and Transfusion Medicine will help develop standards in veterinary blood banking and investigate some exciting future trends in blood banking and transfusion medicine. These will include improved red cell availability and storage, autologous donation, and the use of blood substitutes.

One of the most significant discoveries in human blood banking is the ability to freeze RBCs. Depending on the preservative solution used, the process can prolong shelf life to more than 10 years. This simple procedure involves adding a cryoprotective agent (e.g., glycerol) to the RBCs and freezing them rapidly at −65° C. Before transfusion, the thawed product must be deglycerolized to prevent hemolysis. The expense and expertise involved in freezing RBCs may be prohibitive in veterinary medicine.

The appearance of the acquired immunodeficiency virus in human medicine and the discovery that it could be transmitted through blood transfusion sparked development of the autologous and directed donation path. In many respects, there is no safer transfusion than an autologous one. It eliminates the risk of infectious disease transmission and alloimmunization to cellular and plasma protein antigens. Human autologous donation programs can include four procedures: presurgical deposit, acute normovolemic hemodilution, intraoperative blood salvage, and postoperative blood salvage. These alternatives may have a role in veterinary medicine.

Some of the risks associated with homologous blood transfusion, combined with the practicality issues we face in veterinary medicine, have led us to focus research efforts on blood substitutes. Many products have been tested extensively and their clinical application confirmed (e.g., synthetic colloid solutions, desmopressin, erythropoietin). Other promising blood substitutes have been approved recently for use in veterinary medicine (e.g., synthetic hemoglobin solutions).

BIBLIOGRAPHY

Cutter SM, ed: *Comparative transfusion medicine. Advances in veterinary science and comparative medicine,* Vol 36, San Diego, Calif, 1991, Academic Press.

Hohenhaus AE, ed: *Transfusion medicine, problems in veterinary medicine,* Philadelphia, 1992, JB Lippincott.

Kristensen AT, Feldman BF, eds: The Veterinary Clinics of North America: *Small animal practice: canine and feline transfusion medicine,* Philadelphia, 1995, WB Saunders.

Walker RH, ed: *Technical manual of the American Association of Blood Banks,* ed 12, Arlington, Va, 1996, American Association of Blood Banks.

Chapter 6

Nutrition for the Critically Ill Hospitalized Patient

Nutrition historically has been used as a secondary tool in veterinary medicine to promote healing in critically ill patients. Over the past several years, however, it has been recognized as one of the most important factors in restoring animals' health, whether they are short-term, stable patients or long-term, critically ill patients.

Almost all hospitalized veterinary patients experience some form of malnourishment because of anorexia and a decrease in the total amount of food ingested. The major consequences of malnutrition, particularly in critically ill or injured patients, are a depressed immune system, decreased tissue synthesis and repair, altered intermediary drug metabolism, and change in organ function. Therefore preventing and treating malnutrition and providing early nutritional support play important roles in the recovery of the critically ill patient, affecting almost every body function and optimizing the effects of medical treatment.

The old belief that patients will eat when they feel better has gradually been replaced with the knowledge that they will feel better when they eat as our understanding of nutritional support and its benefits increases. This chapter describes how to assess a patient's nutritional needs, calculate daily caloric requirements, choose the appropriate route of administration if nutritional support is needed, and manage those complications associated with nutritional support.

NUTRITIONAL ASSESSMENT

Nutritional assessment is a must for every hospitalized patient. This assessment should include a thorough history, current body weight, patient age, normal activity level (working versus sedentary), physical examination, body condition score, normal diet at home (brand name and daily amount fed), and laboratory and other tests.

BODY CONDITION SCORING

Body condition scoring (BCS), a tool used to evaluate body composition in the cat and dog, is part of patient assessment. This includes evaluating four general regions of the body: the abdomen, ribs, pelvic bony prominences, and tailhead. Palpating these regions is essential because the appearance of fur can be very deceiving. One must consider the patient's age and history when evaluating body condition. For example, a swollen abdomen in a puppy or kitten may be a sign of parasite infestation rather than obesity. Conversely, a swollen abdomen in an older animal may indicate ascites or other medical conditions rather than obesity. Several BCS systems are available, with the number of categories ranging from five to nine. Category descriptors include *emaciated, ideal, underweight,* and *obese*. Table 6-1 is a list of compa-

TABLE 6-1 Product Information and Body Condition Scoring Resources

Company	Information and Products Available
Hill's Pet Nutrition, Inc. 1-800-892-4621 www.hillspet.com	BCS and nutritional supplies
Waltham Veterinary Diets (England) www.waltham.com	Nutritional supplies
Iams Co. 1-800-535-8387 www.iams.com	BCS and nutritional supplies
Ralston Purina Co. 1-800-222-8387 www.purina.com	BCS and nutritional supplies
Ross Laboratories 1-800-551-5838 www.rossmn.com	Human liquid diets, feeding tubes, and setups
Cook Veterinary Products P.O. Box 2327 Bloomington, IN 47402 1-800-826-2380 (fax) 812-332-1359	Intravenous catheters, feeding tubes, and other medical supplies
Abbott Laboratories, Animal Health North Chicago, IL 1-847-935-4849	Veterinary liquid nutritional products (feline and canine)
Becton Dickinson Sandy, UT 84070	Intracaths

BCS, Body condition scoring.

nies that supply body condition scoring information and other resources.

CALCULATING DAILY CALORIC REQUIREMENTS

Once a thorough history, current body weight, and body condition score have been obtained, the patient's nutritional requirements can be determined. Although daily caloric requirements previously were calculated using a basal energy requirement (BER) multiplied by some stress factor, this method now is thought to be inaccurate for hospitalized patients. The BER is defined as the amount of energy a healthy animal metabolizes 12 hours after ingesting a meal while lying quietly in a warm, stress-free environment. Although some critically ill patients may be completely inactive (i.e., those that are comatose or recumbent), most of them are somewhat active and eating and therefore need more energy than BER. Resting energy requirement (RER) is used to calculate a patient's daily caloric requirements. RER is approximately 10% to 20% higher than BER to compensate for the greater caloric needs of alert patients.

The belief that critically ill patients (postoperative patients and those with trauma, debilitating disease, cancer, or fever) have higher caloric needs than healthy animals may be inaccurate. New information is currently being published that the caloric needs of critically ill patients are not greater than those of healthy animals. Some veterinarians still use a stress factor to compensate for what they believe to be the increased caloric need caused by a specific illness or injury. However, using a stress factor often results in overfeeding the patient. Energy requirements per pound decrease as body weight increases. Therefore larger animals need fewer calories per kilogram or pound than smaller animals.

Daily Resting Requirements (RER)	
Cats	40 kcal/kg/day
Dogs	30 kcal/kg/day
Animals <2 kg	50 kcal/kg/day

To calculate RER in kilocalories per day, use one of the following equations:

$$\text{Animals} <2\text{ kg: RER} = 70 \times (\text{Body weight in kg})^{0.75}$$

or

$$70 \times \sqrt[4]{(\text{Body weight in kg})^3}$$

$$\text{Animals} >2\text{ kg: RER} = (30 \times \text{Body weight in kg}) + 70$$

Examples

A 40-kg dog had abdominal exploratory surgery for a foreign body that perforated his intestine and may be septic. What is this patient's daily caloric requirement?

$$\text{RER} = (30 \times 40\text{ kg}) + 70 = 1270\text{ kcal/day}$$

A 1.5-kg kitten was caught in a fire and fell five stories, sustaining multiple fractures. What is this patient's daily caloric requirement?

$$\text{RER} = 70 \times (1.5\text{ kg})^{0.75} = 95\text{ kcal/day}$$

ENTERAL AND PARENTERAL NUTRITION

Once the patient's daily caloric requirements have been calculated, we then determine the most beneficial route for the patient to receive nutritional support. A patient can receive nutrition by two main routes: enteral, or via the gastrointestinal tract, and parenteral, or via nongastrointestinal administration (e.g., intravenously). Whenever possible, animals should receive nutrition enterally because it is the most physiologic method with the lowest complication rate. The health of the intestinal mucosa and normal peristalsis of the intestine are of utmost importance. Because the intestine normally receives bolus feedings of solid food intermittently, any change in caloric intake, type of food, and frequency of feeding in conjunction with disease or injury can lead to the destruction of the lining of the intestine, ultimately affecting nutritional absorption and peristalsis of the intestinal tract. Maintaining intestinal mucosal integrity (i.e., structure and function) and thereby minimizing bacterial translocation is important in preventing secondary infections. For this reason, enteral feeding is the route of first choice. The optimal method of enteral nutritional support depends on the length of time nutritional support is needed, the patient's temperament and neurologic status, the function of the patient's gastrointestinal (GI) tract, the presence of other diseases such as pancreatitis and hepatic lipidosis, the equipment available, the veterinarian's experience, and the availability of supportive care. As a rule use the easiest, least expensive, least invasive method first if there are no contraindications. The easiest and most natural way to supply patients with nutrition is to offer food orally. When not contraindicated, the technician must first determine the patient's voluntary food intake over a 24-hour period. This 24-hour period allows the patient's body to reap the benefits of intravenous fluids and perhaps antibiotics, which may help the patient feel better, and the animal may start eating on its own. Once the patient's voluntary food intake is equal to the calculated RER, enteral feeding can continue, and no other form of nutritional support may be needed. However, if voluntary consumption does not meet RER, another route of administration is needed.

ENTERAL NUTRITION

Choosing the Right Diet

Oral feeding is the easiest and least expensive way to provide nutrition, and choosing the right type of food is very important. Many disease-specific types of food are available from several companies, including Hill's, Purina, Iams, and Waltham Veterinary Diets. When choosing the patient's diet, consider the animal's history, current condition (disease or injury), weight, and age.

Geriatric and Juvenile

Although in healthy animals age is very important in determining the correct diet to offer, it is less important in critically ill patients; age becomes secondary to the patient's diagnosis and laboratory values. For example, most healthy older animals are overweight, so a well-balanced, low-calorie, low-fat, high-fiber diet with adequate protein is appropriate. Fiber is thought to increase bulk and reduce hunger, helping the animal feel full after each meal. A good example is Hill's Prescription Diet r/d, which is low in fat and calories and high in fiber. However, if an older animal experiences massive protein losses (as in patients with severe burns, open abdomens, or severe inflammatory bowel disease), this patient needs enough protein to compensate for its ongoing losses. A puppy diet such as Hill's Prescription Diet p/d, which is high in protein, would be a more appropriate choice for this patient until protein losses are minimized.

In the same context, juvenile patients may also have special age-related needs, but diagnosis and laboratory results are of primary importance and age is secondary. Until about 6 months of age, the energy needs of healthy puppies and kittens are almost twice those of adults of the same size. They need more nutrients and energy to help build the new tissue that occurs with growth. Because puppies and kittens have higher energy needs but consume smaller volumes of food than adults, they need a more concentrated diet. Keeping these special nutritional needs in mind, a diet formulated for growth, with higher levels of all nutrients, in a highly digestible form, is appropriate for healthy growing animals (e.g., Hill's Prescription Diet p/d). However, in critically ill patients such a diet may not be appropriate. For example, a 4-month-old puppy with congenital renal failure or a portal systemic shunt should not consume liberal amounts of protein. The liver and kidneys must metabolize excess protein, and these organs may not be able to handle additional protein if already compromised by disease. Therefore, although we would feed this puppy at its RER, we would do so with a lower-protein diet than that normally fed to growing pups. A renal diet, such as Hill's Prescription Diet k/d, with protein levels at actual requirements, would be an appropriate choice.

Gestation and Lactation

Another category of patients with special nutritional needs includes lactating or gestating animals. These patients must be fed above RER because of their increased nutritional needs, regardless of the disease or injury present. For example, a lactating bitch must be fed at 25% above her RER for every puppy she is nursing, regardless of her disease or injury. If she cannot eat the necessary amount because of her injuries or disease-related problems, a decision must be made to wean the puppies or supply added nutrition via other routes, whether enteral or parenteral. In the same context, a gestating patient must be fed approximately 10% above RER to meet her increased nutritional needs, regardless of the presenting injury or disease. In both cases, a well-balanced diet formulated for growth with increased nutrient density, such as Hill's Prescription Diet p/d, should be offered frequently and in proper quantities to help these patients maintain their physiologic states of lactation or gestation. In such cases, the patients' bodies often respond by aborting the fetuses or ceasing lactation in response to a lack of nutrition or the animal's disease or injury.

Many factors are involved in choosing the correct diet for patients. Although age may still play a role in choosing nutrition for hospitalized patients, the diagnosis and most recent laboratory work results are of primary importance, as is the patient's ability and desire to ingest food voluntarily and tolerate the nutrition offered. Because all these factors can change from day to day, a daily nutritional assessment should be performed for each patient. As long as the patient is fed at RER and is offered a complete and well-balanced diet, it is likely that its nutritional needs will be met, and separate calculations for each nutrient requirement are not necessary. Thus diagnosis and test results, as well as voluntary food intake, food tolerance, age, current body weight, and body condition, all are used in deciding what type of nutritional support the patient needs.

Megaesophagus

Although many patients need special nutritional support, ranging from hand feeding to monitoring of feeding tubes, few diseases or injuries necessitate the specific and specialized feeding techniques that megaesophagus does. This can be a very frustrating condition in which technician time, knowledge, and effort can mean the difference between life or death for the patient.

Megaesophagus, which is most common in dogs, is a generalized dilation of the esophagus, with a lack of or decrease in motor function. Food is not pushed down toward the stomach but stays in the esophagus, often causing the patient to regurgitate. Frequent regurgitation in these patients causes many to develop aspiration pneumonia, the most common cause of death in these patients. For this reason, technicians must understand this disease and the dietary management necessary to help these patients survive.

Treatment of megaesophagus depends on the underlying cause. Most patients with megaesophagus are treated with dietary management rather than surgery. Because of the lack of esophageal peristalsis, gravity is used to help move the food down the esophagus and into the stomach. These patients must be fed from a level above the neck. Several positions are possible. The technician can hold the bowl above the patient's neck level while it eats from a sitting position, the bowl can be placed on a high stool and the patient allowed to eat on its own from a standing or sitting position, or the patient can be taught to eat on stairs or a countertop, with its front paws on the countertop or a stool. After eating, the patient's head must remain elevated for at least 15 minutes, although this is often difficult with active patients and time constraints. Keeping the patient's head elevated prevents the food from pooling in the esophagus, which often causes regurgitation and aspiration pneumonia. This can be achieved by holding the patient, pointing its nose to the ceiling while it is in a sitting position, or keeping its upper body elevated by having it stand with its front paws up on a stool or countertop. Monitoring for food pooling is also an important step. If a lump in the throat is visible, it is likely that pooling has occurred, and the patient should be kept with its upper body elevated for more than 20 minutes. Massaging the lump gently may also help the food move down into the stomach. If these techniques do not work, the patient probably will regurgitate some or all of the food. All patients with megaesophagus should be monitored closely for aspiration pneumonia, which includes monitoring mucous membrane color, respiratory rate, and respiratory effort. If aspiration pneumonia is present, usually the patient shows signs of a moist cough and possible nasal discharge. The veterinarian should be notified and the patient may be started on antibiotics, nebulization, or coupage.

Once the technician understands the feeding techniques that must be used in these patients, a choice of nutrition can be made. The type and consistency of food must be decided on a patient-by-patient basis, often through trial and error. One patient may do well with gruel, whereas another patient may not tolerate gruel and may need canned food. When starting a feeding program, a semiliquid gruel is a good first choice because it will flow quickly down the patient's esophagus. However, there is an increased possibility of aspiration pneumonia with liquid diets. The consistency of the food must be adjusted according to the patient's response, as should the number of feedings per day. When a patient is started on a new feeding program, the patient's daily caloric requirements should be divided into three to four equal feedings per day because smaller meals help prevent regurgitation and reflux. If a liquid or gruel diet is used, it is best to use a high-calorie diet because liquid and gruel forms usually contain a large amount of water. If reaching a patient's daily caloric requirements becomes difficult, especially with gruel, a commercial liquid diet can be added to the gruel instead of water to add nutrients and energy. Once the patient is tolerating the new feeding regimen, it can be started gradually on more normal, solid food. As with any new feeding regimen, changes in diet should be made gradually, and the patient should be allowed up to a week to adjust to the new diet.

Because patients with megaesophagus usually are malnourished, cachexic, and anorexic and suffer from chronic bouts of regurgitation, a gastrostomy tube is another option for nutritional support. This allows the patient to receive maximum nutrition but bypasses the esophagus, decreasing the chances of aspiration pneumonia, although the possibility of regurgitation from the stomach still remains. However, gastrostomy or percutaneous endoscopic gastrostomy (PEG) tube placement entails anesthesia and a minor surgical procedure, which can place any critically ill patient at risk. This choice must be made on a patient-by-patient basis. In some cases, a gastrostomy/PEG tube may make the difference between getting the patient home and euthanizing it.

Although with any diagnosis of megaesophagus, regardless of the type, the prognosis is almost always guarded or poor, technician skill and care can mean the difference between life or death for these patients. Thorough knowledge of this disease, the important role of gravity in feeding these patients, and the signs of aspiration pneumonia is critical in treating patients. Knowing patients and their personalities can help the technician and veterinarian develop a recovery and feeding plan that best suits the patient not only in the hospital but also at home. Many of these animals are hospitalized frequently because of repeated episodes of aspiration pneumonia. However, with quick owner recognition and prompt treatment, these animals can be treated with antibiotics, nebulization, and coupage and sent home, sometimes within a couple of days. Team effort and communication between the veterinarian, the technician, and the owner can help these patients survive this disease for up to several years.

Anorexia

Although oral feeding is the easiest, least expensive, and most natural way to provide nutrition, anorexia is common in hospitalized animals. Almost every critically ill patient suffers from some form of anorexia while hospitalized, whether caused by stress, pain, or nausea. General knowledge of the patient's eating habits is helpful in tempting the patient to eat. A nutritional assessment of the patient upon admission is very useful. What type of food does the patient normally eat at home? Is it used to dry food, canned food, or table scraps? When does the patient normally eat at home: several times a day, free choice throughout the day, or once a day? Many animals are so accustomed to their home routine that they will eat only at their normal mealtimes, even when hospitalized, and they are more apt to eat the food they usually eat at home. Many hospitalized animals will not eat for strangers but will eat happily for their owners. For this reason it is helpful to encourage owners to visit during visiting hours and ask them to bring in their animal's normal diet to tempt them to eat while they are present. Each patient should be given the chance to ingest food voluntarily over a 24-hour period. If voluntary food intake does not equal RER, then we must try to tempt these patients to eat.

Cats and Dogs

To tempt animals to eat, the technician must understand the species-specific differences between patients and their normal eating habits. Cats are very particular about their food, sometimes nibbling at it up to 20 times in a 24-hour period. They can be erratic eaters, at times eating only small amounts for several days and then eating large amounts the next day. Dogs almost never pass up food when it is offered, often gorging themselves. In cats, anorexia often is secondary to stress, whereas in dogs anorexia usually is a complication of illness or injury, although dogs also can be affected by stress.

In a hospital setting, many environmental factors can play a part in anorexia in both cats and dogs, but cats are particularly sensitive to environmental changes. These changes can include noise level, the number of people milling around, the amount of lighting, the size and shape of the food container, and even the type of cleaner used on the food container. Disposable containers are the best option, if financially feasible, to avoid contamination and foreign odors. For most cats, a flat, wide, shallow dish is much more inviting then a small, deep bowl. If lighting or other elements are disturbing the patient and no other rooms or cages are available, try covering the cat's cage one half to two thirds of the way with a mat or towel. This will enable you to monitor the patient while allowing it to calm down in a dark, quiet place. Another alternative is to give the cat a rolled-up cage mat to tuck itself into or a paper diaper to hide under, giving the cat a sense of security by allowing it to hide. Unless extremely fearful, most dogs are not as sensitive to environmental stress, but each animal should be dealt with individually.

Both dogs and cats have a keen sense of smell and use this in selecting their food. Therefore any injury or illness that affects an animal's sense of smell will also affect its appetite. Trauma and radiation can decrease the function of taste buds and sensory receptors, drastically reducing the patient's desire to eat. Many patients' nasal passages are blocked by discharge or bleeding, and these passages must be cleaned gently and kept open to optimize the animal's ability to smell. Patients with fractured jaws who experience pain but still have good swallowing and gag reflexes can be enticed to eat a warm, blended gruel diet fed by syringe. Often these patients are hungry, but with the dried blood in their mouths and perhaps clogged nasal passages, they will not try to eat on their own until tempted.

Increasing Food Palatability

The type of food the patient prefers also can be species specific. A cat may strongly prefer dry or moist food, whereas dogs have a tendency to prefer canned food, perhaps because it contains more fat and protein. A cat or dog can be tempted with a highly odorous diet, and the food can be warmed to maximize odors and increase palatability. In addition, caressing the animal while encouraging it to eat may be all it takes to get it started on a few mouthfuls of food. If all else fails, a diet high in fat and protein can be used because these ingredients usually increase palatability. A dog can be tempted with cat food or a cat with kitten food. Human food also can be used, but any change in a patient's normal diet can cause stress diarrhea. These diets should only be used to entice the anorexic patient to start eating again and then should be decreased slowly as the patient's normal diet is reintroduced and increased gradually.

Foreign Physical Obstructions

Technicians must also be aware of the stress new apparatuses, bandages, and Elizabethan collars (E-collars) put on patients and how these can affect their appetites. E-collars can act as obstructions, preventing the patient from reaching its food. Cats especially hate these collars, often refusing to eat with them on. If time allows, remove the E-collar and give the cat an opportunity to eat without this obstruction. On the other hand, dogs usually do not refuse food simply because they are wearing an E-collar. Strange new bandages and wraps, casts, and KE apparatus can also cause added stress, especially if they affect the patient's movement or ability to reach food and water. Although patients usually adjust quickly to these foreign objects, they may need some help getting to their food and water until they have adapted to moving with these objects on.

Other obstacles that can affect patients' appetites include vitamin B_{12} deficiencies, low serum zinc levels, hypokalemia, and the effects of certain medications. These levels must be monitored throughout a patient's recovery.

Drug-Induced Stimulation

If the aforementioned techniques have failed, certain medications can be administered as appetite stimulants. Cyproheptadine hydrochloride can be used in both dogs and cats at a dosage of 1 mg/kg orally every 8 to 12 hours for dogs or 2 to 4 mg (total) orally every 8 to 24 hours for cats. Usually this drug is given about 30 minutes before feeding and can be used for several days. Benzodiazepines such as diazepam 0.05 to 0.4 mg/kg (i.e., a usual dosage in cats would be 1 mg intravenously twice a day or 2 mg orally) or oxazepam 2.5 mg (total) are two other alternatives, but they should not be used in cats with liver problems and do not have good results in dogs. Both of these medications have a rapid response, and a sufficient amount of food should be available as soon as the drug is given because its effect can be rapid but short term. Oxazepam and diazepam usually are used for only 1 or 2 days, and if the desired effect does not occur, they should be discontinued because their repeated use can reduce their effect on the patient's appetite.

Anabolic steroids such as stanozolol at a dosage of ¼ of a 10-mg tablet or 25 or 50 mg intramuscularly weekly or nandrolone decanoate at a dosage of 5 mg/kg maximum or 200 mg intramuscularly per week are used only in patients that have been ill for a long time and may be cachexic. These drugs increase muscle mass by decreasing tissue and protein breakdown, and in so doing they can increase caloric intake. How these drugs increase tissue growth is not known, and their use is controversial. The deciding factor is the veterinarian's experience with these drugs.

Although these drugs can work well in stimulating a patient's appetite, very rarely do they cause an anorexic patient to ingest enough food for it to reach its RER. Sometimes these medications can be used for a few days while the patient is recovering and can be stopped when the patient continues to eat on its own as it feels better. Other times, however, these drugs may not be enough and other alternatives for nutritional support must be used.

Force Feeding

If all other attempts to stimulate the patient to eat voluntarily have been unsuccessful, force feeding can be attempted. Force feeding usually is fairly easy in a critically ill, weakened patient but may meet with great resistance in a patient that is stronger and more apt to fight. Force feeding can be a long and tedious process, and a lot of patience and understanding are needed. A simple method of force feeding is to syringe feed the patient a liquid diet, keeping its head in a natural position. Whether a commercial liquid diet from a can or a homemade gruel diet is used, the nutrition offered during syringe feeding should be a high-calorie, easily digestible food. A high-calorie food can reduce the number of feedings needed. Although the old technique for force feeding involved holding the patient's head up while placing solid food via syringe in the pharyngeal area to stimulate swallowing, this position is unnatural for the patient and may predispose it to aspirating the food. Several complications, including vomiting and severe aspiration pneumonia, can result from force feeding. Most animals, but especially cats, hate being restrained, and the increased stress force feeding can cause may be more harmful then helpful, despite the benefits of the additional nutrition. If the patient is too ill and its level of consciousness decreased, its gag reflex and ability to swallow may be impaired, allowing the food to be drawn into the trachea and the lungs instead of the esophagus, resulting in severe aspiration pneumonia. Aspiration pneumonia also can occur if the patient is too strong to force feed and it puts up an intense fight. For these reasons, force feeding should be avoided if possible. Many other forms of enteral support are much easier and less stressful and still allow the patient to eat on its own. Furthermore, most force-fed patients do not ingest enough nutrition to reach their daily RERs. For this reason, other routes of enteral nutritional support are recommended.

Enteral Nutritional Support

Enteral feeding can be done orally or through various tubes that preclude oral feeding but still use the gastrointestinal tract for absorption. The appropriate route depends on the patient's injury or illness. Indications for enteral support via tube feeding include anorexia; persistent weight loss of more than 20% in less than 14 days; central nervous system disorders; disorders of the oral cavity, pharynx, or esophagus (including functional, traumatic, and radiation side effects); trauma and burns; and disease states including hepatic and renal disease and diabetes mellitus. Tube feeding almost always is less stressful and much quicker and can supply more nutrition to the patient than any amount of force feeding. If the patient continues to be anorexic or oral feeding is contraindicated for more than 24 hours, tube feeding should be started. Both dogs and cats can be tube fed via the orogastric, nasoesophageal, or nasogastric route or by pharyngostomy, esophagostomy, gastrostomy, PEG, or enterostomy (Table 6-2).

Orogastric Tube Feeding. Orogastric tube feeding can be used in patients that have fought force feeding or are too weak to be force fed. This is an appropriate choice if it can be done with little restraint and minimal stress on the patient. A red rubber urinary catheter is used as the tube (8 to 12 French for cats and small dogs and 12 to 24 French for larger dogs). The tube is measured from the nose to the ninth intercostal space and marked with a piece of tape or marker to aid in gastric placement. The tube can be lubricated with water or a tasteless lubricant to help it pass more easily. The patient's mouth should be opened only as wide as necessary to pass the tube through the mouth and over the tongue, with the head kept in a normal position. The patient should be swallowing during passage of the tube, a sign that it is in the esophagus, and not coughing, a sign that it may have gone into the trachea. Slow passage of the tube helps prevent damage to the pharyngeal and esophageal muscle. When the patient begins to swallow, the tube should be advanced down the esophagus to the premeasured mark. Once in place, 5 to 10 ml sterile water or sterile saline should be instilled into the tube before feeding to ensure that

TABLE 6-2 Enteral Tube Feeding

Tube Type	Location	Purpose	Product Type	Type Infusion
Nasoesophageal	Placed through the nose into the upper esophagus	Short-term nutritional support	Liquid only	Bolus or CRI
Nasogastric	Placed through the nose into the stomach	Short-term nutritional support	Liquid only	Bolus or CRI
Pharyngostomy	Placed surgically from the lateral pharyngeal wall into the upper esophagus	Short- and long-term nutritional support	Liquid only unless tube >18 French	Bolus or CRI
Esophagostomy	Placed surgically through a stab incision into the cranial esophagus and advanced into the distal end of the esophagus	Short- and long-term nutritional support	Liquid only unless tube >18 French	Bolus or CRI
Gastrotomy/PEG	Placed surgically via an abdominal laparotomy (gastrotomy tube) or endoscopically through the ventrolateral abdominal wall directly into the stomach (PEG tube)	Long-term nutritional support	Liquid or gruel	Bolus or CRI
Enterostomy (duodenostomy or jejunostomy)	Placed surgically via an abdominal laparotomy directly through the abdominal wall into the small intestine (in the duodenum or jejunum), bypassing the stomach	Long-term nutritional support	Liquid only (monomeric diet)	CRI only

PEG, Percutaneous endoscopic gastrostomy; *CRI,* constant-rate infusion.

the tube is not in the trachea. Complications from orogastric tube feeding can include stress on the patient, gastrointestinal tract trauma, and aspiration pneumonia. Because of these complications, some veterinarians recommend alternative routes of tube feeding but may use this technique for single doses of food or medication.

Nasoesophageal and Nasogastric Tube Feeding. Oral feedings often are supplemented with additional enteral support when a patient is eating but not consuming enough nutrition to meet its daily caloric needs because of stress, pain, or nausea. Two forms of tube feeding that can provide additional nutrition while allowing the patient to continue to eat and drink are the nasoesophageal (NE) tube and the nasogastric (NG) tube. Placing these tubes is easy and quick and causes minimal stress on the patient. Both dogs and cats tolerate these tubes well, and they can be kept in place from several days to several weeks.

Many different types of tubes can be used for NG intubation, including polyvinyl, polyurethane, and silicone tubes. Polyvinyl tubes function well and are less expensive, but if left in the stomach for more than 2 weeks they will harden. Therefore they must be changed weekly or be placed in the caudal esophagus rather than the stomach. Unlike polyvinyl tubes, polyurethane and silicone tubes can be used in the stomach without hardening because they are not susceptible to gastric acid, and silicone tubes are reusable, which may make them more feasible for practitioners with limited resources (Technical Tip Box 6-1).

Tube placement begins with choosing the appropriate size (3-French tubes for puppies and kittens, 5 French for cats and small dogs, and 8 French in medium to large dogs). If the tube is too small, even the most dilute solution may not pass through and the tube may clog (Figure 6-1).

As mentioned earlier, nasogastric and nasoesophageal tubes are indicated for short-term nutritional support. Whether the tube is placed in the esophagus or the stomach is determined by doctor preference and the patient's condition. Some veterinarians believe that when the tube is placed in the esophagus there is less chance of vomiting and therefore less chance of aspiration pneumonia because the tube is not penetrating the lower esophageal sphincter at the junction of the esophagus and the stomach. Some believe that this placement creates a small opening that can allow reflux to occur. Others believe that with placement of a nasoesophageal tube there is increased possibility of esophageal erosion by a constant-rate infusion (CRI) dripping nutrition into the esophagus at the same location. Complications with these tubes include not only those mentioned earlier (esophagitis, gastritis, and the most severe, aspiration pneumonia) but also vomiting, regurgitation with expulsion of the tube, and diarrhea. Because of these complications, NE and NG tubes are contraindicated in patients predisposed to aspiration, including comatose and recumbent patients, patients with esophageal dysfunction, and patients that are actively vomiting or have severe diarrhea. These tubes also are contraindicated in patients that have injuries to the head or neck or diseases or surgical procedures of the nasal cavity, pharynx, or esophagus.

Maintaining these tubes is fairly simple. Monitoring the tube to make sure it is not slipping out is the main concern. The patient with an NE or NG tube must be observed closely because if the patient vomits, it can expel the tube, bite it in half, and aspirate it into the trachea. Placing a mark on the tube with an indelible marker at the point of entry into the nares allows the technician to see even the smallest movement of the tube. These tubes often are more annoying to the patient than painful, so an E-collar must be used to prevent the patient from pawing out the tube. Flushing the tube with warm water or sterile saline before and after feeding helps verify its patency and prevent clogging. The opening at the top of the tube should be covered with a male plug at the tip to prevent air buildup in the stomach. Feeding protocols for these tubes are discussed later in this chapter.

For all other enteral nutritional support routes, tubes must be placed surgically whether with short-term anesthesia and simple surgical procedures (as for PEG tubes) or long-term anesthesia and major surgical procedures (as for gastrostomy and jejunostomy tubes). These risks are important factors in considering which enteral route to use in a critically ill patient.

Box 6-1 Technical Tip: *Nasogastric Tube Placement*

Items Needed

Tube
Ophthalmic topical anesthetic
2% Lidocaine jelly
Tape or tissue glue
Suture material

1. Instill a drop of ophthalmic topical anesthetic in nostril.

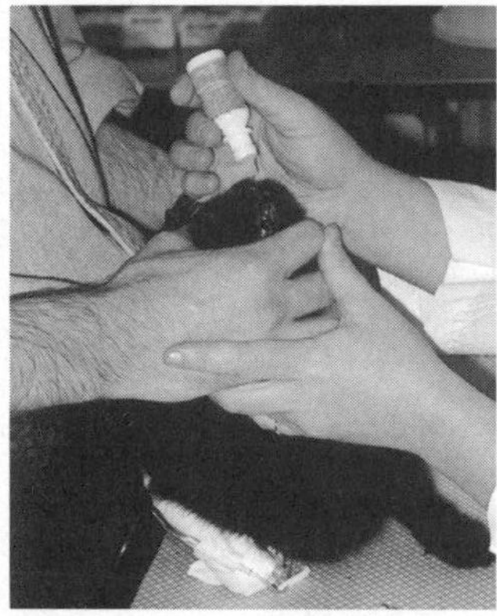

2. Measure the tube and mark it at the ninth intercostal space (or seventh intercostal space for esophageal placement).

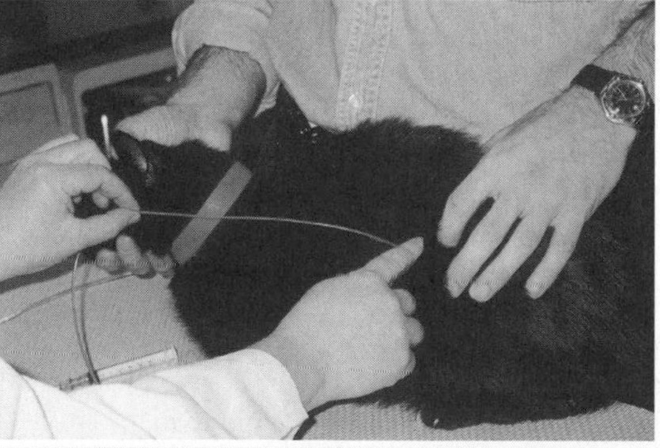

3. Instill another drop of ophthalmic topical anesthetic into same nostril.
4. Lubricate tube with 2% lidocaine jelly.

Box 6-1 Technical Tip: *Nasogastric Tube Placement—cont'd*

5. In dogs, direct tube ventromedially to the alar fold. In cats, tube can be directed ventromedially and passed through the ventral meatus, nasopharynx, pharynx, and esophagus to the premeasured mark. (Keeping the head at a normal angle while placing and advancing the tube while the patient swallows is critical in ensuring its placement into the esophagus and preventing tracheal intubation.)*

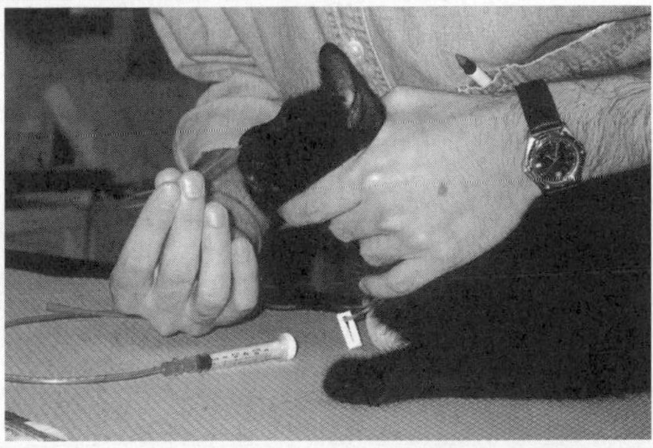

6. Once the tube is in place, oral examination and injection of air into the tube while ausculting for gurgling sounds can verify placement into the esophagus or stomach. Injecting water into the tube to stimulate a cough reflex if in the trachea is not a reliable method for determining correct placement. Not all patients cough if water is injected into the trachea. Some are too weak for the cough reflex to occur. Radiographs are taken if necessary.
7. The tube is sutured into place. The first suture is placed as close to the external nares as possible. The other suture is placed on the dorsum of the muzzle and a third on the forehead. Tissue glue can be used as an alternative but should be used sparingly and with caution. Some animals can have negative reactions to the glue. Avoid securing the tube near cat's whiskers to prevent irritation.

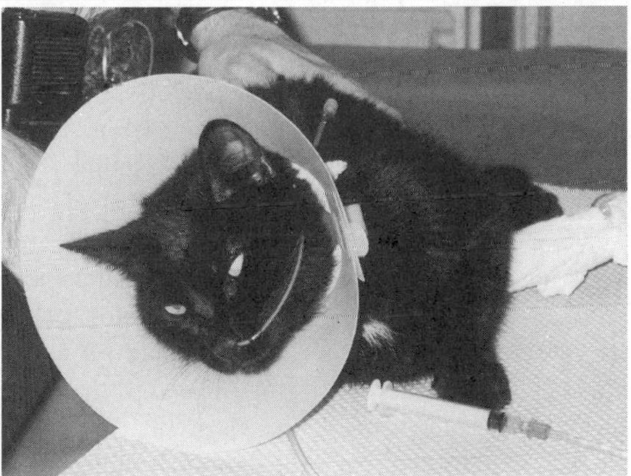

8. A mark is placed on the tube at the nares to indicate tube migration.
9. Place an Elizabethan collar around neck to keep patient from removing tube.

*If any resistance is encountered during placement, remove all but 1 to 2 cm of tube, then reintroduce. If sneezing occurs, stop advancing the tube until the sneezing stops, then continue advancement.

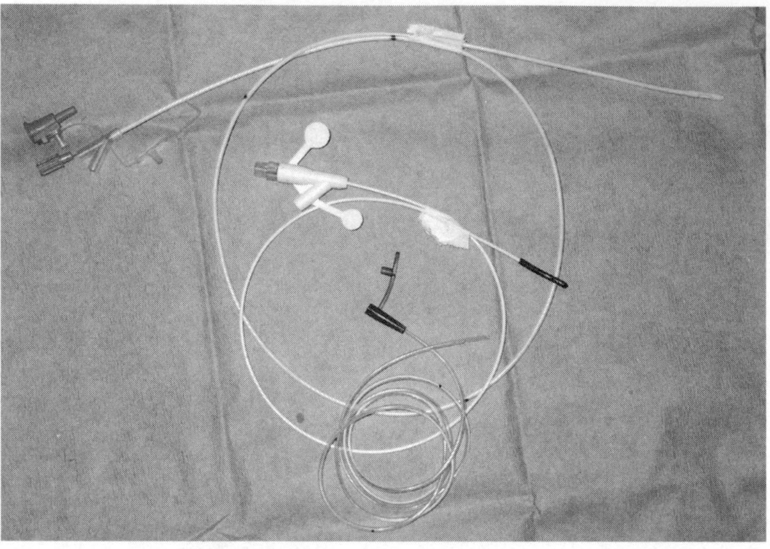

Figure 6-1

Several types of tubes are available for nasoesophageal or nasogastric placement.

Pharyngostomy Tube Feeding. Unlike NE and NG tubes, pharyngostomy tubes are placed surgically. If a large-bore feeding tube (12 French or larger) is placed, the patient can receive canned food gruel rather than only liquid diets, as would be necessary with NE or NG tubes. Pharyngostomy tubes are indicated in patients with prolonged anorexia that are not voluntarily ingesting enough nutrition to meet their daily caloric needs, such as those treated for disease or trauma; those who have undergone surgery of the maxillary, mandibular, or facial region; and those whose swallowing is impaired by neuromuscular disorders. However, pharyngostomy tubes can be left in place longer than NE or NG tubes and usually are considered for patients that may need prolonged nutritional support.

Pharyngostomy tube placement carries a risk of complications, and because problems can occur when this tube is placed through the piriform recess, a modified procedure has been recommended. A tube of the appropriate size is placed surgically by blunt introduction into the pharynx caudodorsally and directed as close to the esophageal entrance as possible. The tube is sutured in place and a bandage placed for added support and sterility.

The use of pharyngostomy tubes is controversial because of their potential complications. These can include upper airway obstruction, dysphasia, and aspiration pneumonia. Gastroesophageal reflux and vomiting also can occur, but the modified procedure of distal esophageal placement decreases these risks. The patient may vomit and expel the tube, or with constant tongue manipulation the patient can move the tube into the oral cavity and thus increase the possibility of aspiration pneumonia. Because of its close location to many nerves and the jugular vein, the tube also can damage vascular and nervous structures. Choice and placement of this tube depend on the veterinarian's experience with its use.

Daily maintenance includes changing the bandage to monitor for tube slippage and checking the insertion site for cleanliness, discharge, and swelling. The tightness of the bandage also should be monitored. Because of the tube's location, an E-collar should not be needed and patients appear to tolerate this tube well.

Esophagostomy Tube Feeding. The esophagostomy tube is similar to the pharyngostomy tube but can be used in both dogs and cats when a pharyngostomy tube is contraindicated, as in patients recovering from major surgery of the pharynx or those with disease involving the pharynx, or when placing a pharyngostomy tube would delay healing or interfere with normal pharyngeal function. Esophagostomy tube feeding was developed for cats because pharyngostomy tubes appear to cause more problems in cats than in dogs.

The advantage of pharyngostomy and esophagostomy tubes is that no endoscopic equipment is needed to place them. Esophagostomy tube placement involves brief anesthesia and a minimally invasive surgical procedure. This tube is inserted through a stab incision into the cranial esophagus. The tube is then advanced until the distal end of the tube is in the distal end of the esophagus. The tube is sutured in place and a bandage placed. The end of the tube should be capped with a male plug.

Most patients tolerate esophagostomy tubes well and do not need an E-collar. Maintenance of these tubes is exactly the same as for pharyngostomy tubes, including monitoring the surgical site with daily bandage changes. Complications of this type of tube are the same as those of pharyngostomy tubes, including aspiration pneumonia, vomiting, tube expulsion, and esophageal reflux. Therefore these tubes should not be used in patients with esophageal dysfunction; those that are actively vomiting, comatose, or recumbent; or those with disease or surgical procedures of the nasal cavity, pharynx, or esophagus.

Gastrostomy Tube and PEG Tube Feeding. Gastrostomy tube placement is indicated when the oral cavity, pharynx, or esophagus must be bypassed and nutritional support is needed for more than 3 days. This includes cases in which pharyngeal or laryngeal surgery has been performed and the tube's presence could interfere with normal function or healing, a mass is present in the pharynx or esophagus that would block the tube's passage into the stomach, or esophageal tears, lesions, or obstructions would prevent safe tube passage into the stomach. Gastrostomy tubes work well in both cats and dogs and do not interfere with their normal daily activity. For this reason, this tube is a good choice for long-term nutritional support. Patients can be sent home with this tube in place if the owner is able to perform the necessary feeding and monitoring tasks.

Gastrostomy tubes can be placed by two methods. The first method is percutaneous placement. Since PEG tubes were invented, gastrostomy tube placement has become much easier and is used much more often for nutritional support. Although the patient must be placed under general anesthesia, the procedure is fairly quick and easy and minimally invasive. The endoscopic equipment and specialized training needed may not be available to every practitioner, but PEG tube placement carries little risk of complications.

First the patient's stomach is inflated with air. A French Pezzar mushroom-tip catheter is used (18 French for cats and small dogs, and 22 French for medium and large dogs). An intravenous catheter is inserted through the skin into the dilated stomach, monitored visually with a fiberoptic gastroscope. A long piece of suture material inserted through the catheter is retrieved by the biopsy forceps of the gastroscope and pulled out of the stomach, through the esophagus, and out of the mouth. The gastrostomy tube is then pulled through the mouth, into the esophagus, and into the stomach by the suture. As the PEG tube is pulled down through the esophagus, the endoscope is used to monitor placement. Once the tube is in place, it is firmly pulled so that the mushroom tip is secured against the wall of the stomach. The tube is not sutured into place. A dry 4-inch by 4-inch gauze square with sterile betadine ointment is put over the exit site at the base of the tube. A full abdominal bandage is placed to secure the tube and protect it from infection and mutilation. In most dogs an E-collar should be placed to prevent chewing. However, most cats seem to tolerate the tube well and do not need the collar. Feeding should not start until 24 hours after the tube has been placed to ensure that a good seal forms between the visceral and parietal peritoneum. After 12 hours, start with a small bolus of water to assess the patient's comfort level and check for any complications, such as subcutaneous leakage. Twelve hours after tolerating water, the patient can be started on a slow bolus of gruel via the tube.

The second method of gastrostomy tube placement is via a formal laparotomy. Because it is a major surgical procedure, this method should be used only when surgical intervention for the underlying disease or injury is needed or when endoscopic equipment is not available. Laparotomy usually is performed in the left flank or on the midline. A double pursestring suture is placed in the left side of the stomach, and a Foley or dePezzar tube is advanced into the stomach via the left flank and through the center of the pursestring suture. If a Foley tube is used, it is then expanded with sterile saline and a small amount of air. At this point, a continuous suture pattern circling the gastrostomy tube is used to fix the stomach to the abdominal wall, where the tube enters the peritoneum. Suture styles similar to those used with esophagostomy and pharyngostomy tubes, such as pursestring sutures and Chinese finger-tie sutures, are used to fix the tube to the skin and external abdominal fascia. Once the abdominal incision is closed, a sterile dressing and bandage are placed to help secure the tube and protect it from infection and mutilation. Dogs should wear an E-collar to prevent chewing, but in most cats this is unnecessary.

Complications of gastrostomy tube placement include stomal infection, blockage, dislodgment, migration, or extraction of the tube, which can cause stomach contents or the instilled feeding formula to leak into the peritoneal cavity, causing peritonitis. Vomiting and diarrhea can result from poor choices in feeding practices, including type of nutrition and feeding frequency. Although complications can arise, both placement techniques are reliable, with few complications.

Gastrostomy tube maintenance includes daily bandage changes to observe for any discharge or irritation at the ostomy site. Tube migration can be monitored with daily bandage changes. When monitored properly, these tubes can be maintained from several weeks to several months without complications.

Enterostomy (Duodenostomy or Jejunostomy) Tube Feeding. Enterostomy tube feeding is indicated when the patient's stomach or duodenum must be bypassed because of disease, injury, or dysfunction. These cases include patients that have had surgery of the stomach, duodenum, and pancreas and those with chronic vomiting, stomach ulcers, and gastroparesis. The patient's small intestine must be functional.

Enterostomy tubes can be placed surgically (when an abdominal laparotomy is needed to intervene in the case of disease or injury) or through an existing gastrostomy tube. In an abdominal laparotomy, the enterostomy tube is placed directly into a functional segment of intestine, through a hole in the intestinal wall, and exits through the peritoneum and the abdominal wall. A duodenostomy tube is placed into the duodenum and a jejunostomy tube into the jejunum. Alternatively, an existing gastrostomy tube that was placed for gastric decompression can be used. The enterostomy tube is led through the gastrostomy tube to the desired placement in the intestine. A third procedure also involves placing an enterostomy tube via an abdominal laparotomy, but this time the tube is placed into the stomach and is advanced down into a functional segment of intestine. This type of tube is called a gastroduodenostomy tube if placed in the duodenum or a gastrojejunostomy tube if placed in the jejunum. However, most enterostomy tubes are placed with a traditional needle catheter jejunostomy procedure during an abdominal laparotomy. The disadvantage of traditional enterostomy tube placement is that the tube can back out of the intestine and end up in the abdomen. This can allow tube feeding solutions and bowel secretions to leak peritoneally or subcutaneously and cause peritonitis. However, an enterostomy tube placed through a gastrostomy tube, would not back out into the abdominal cavity but could end up in the stomach. In this procedure it is more difficult to place an enterostomy tube because it is hard to pass the tube through the pylorus.

For all enterostomy tube placement methods, complications include clogging and kinking of the tube, infection, diarrhea, and possible perforation of the small intestine by the catheter tip. As with gastrostomy tubes, vomiting and diarrhea can result from poor feeding practices.

As with other enteral feeding tubes, maintenance and care of the enterostomy tube should include daily bandage changes to monitor for infection, leakage, and migration, as well as placement of E-collars in dogs to prevent tube mutilation. Cats often do not need an E-collar. The enterostomy tube should be flushed several times throughout the day to prevent clogging of the tube and monitor its function. Advantages of enterostomy tube feeding include postoperative nutritional support. Although the stomach and colon may remain aperistaltic for up to 72 hours postoperatively, nutritional support through the enterostomy tube can be started shortly after surgery, promoting a quicker return of intestinal function than in patients not supported with enteral nutrition.

DIET CHOICES FOR TUBE FEEDING

Selecting the appropriate diet for the chosen feeding route is important. Two basic forms of liquid diets are used for feeding through tubes: homemade blenderized diets and canned commercial human and veterinary diets (Box 6-2 and Table 6-3). Blenderized diets tend to cause less diarrhea, are administered as bolus feedings (so fewer feedings are needed per day), and usually are less expensive than commercial liquid diets. However, commercial liquid diets are more convenient and less likely to block the tube, and the patient can be started on a CRI, which may be very beneficial in patients that have been anorexic for several days or longer.

Liquid commercial diets can be used with any form of enteral tube feeding. However, these diets usually are used with nasoesophageal, nasogastric, and jejunostomy tubes because only liquid formula, not gruel, can pass through these tubes (usually 8 French or smaller) without plugging them. Many forms of these commercial diets are available today, including Peptamen (produced by the Nestlé Corporation), CliniCare, CliniCare RF, Jevity, and Perative (all produced by Ross Abbott Laboratories). All of these diets are isoosmolar, meaning that their osmolality is approximately equal to that of blood, or about 300 mOsm/kg. Unlike hyperosmolar diets (those that have an osmolality greater than 400 mOsm/kg) they do not draw fluid in from the tissues and promote dehydration. Peptamen and Perative are human products that have been used successfully in animals and are monomeric, meaning that the nutrients in these liquid foods are in their simplest form and therefore are absorbed easily. Therefore Peptamen and Perative are good choices for patients that have abnormal gastrointestinal function, such as puppies with parvovirus. These puppies often slough their intestinal lining and suffer from severe bouts of diarrhea, and these patients cannot digest a complex diet. Peptamen and Perative also are appropriate choices for patients with jejunostomy tubes because these tubes bypass the stomach, pancreas, and liver and must supply nutrition that the jejunum can absorb easily without causing additional complications such as diarrhea (Figures 6-2 and 6-3).

The other forms of commercial diets mentioned (CliniCare, CliniCare RF, and Jevity) are polymeric diets, meaning that their nutrients are in high–molecular-weight forms that must be digested. These diets can be administered only to patients with nearly normal gastrointestinal function and can be given through nasoesophageal, nasogastric, pharyngostomy, esophagostomy, and gastrostomy tubes. Because they must be digested, these polymeric diets are contraindicated in patients with jejunostomy tubes. CliniCare is a nutritionally balanced veterinary liquid diet that is available in canine and feline forms. CliniCare RF also is a nutritionally balanced veterinary liquid diet available in canine or feline forms but is lower in protein and electrolytes. The *RF* stands for *renal*

Box 6-2 Homemade Gruel Recipes for Tube Feeding

2 Cans Hill's Prescription Diet a/d
50 ml H_2O
Blend until thoroughly mixed.
Caloric density = 1 kcal/ml
½ Can Hill's Prescription Diet Feline p/d
170 ml (⅔ cup) water
Blend at least 1 minute.
Sieve twice through a kitchen strainer.
Caloric density = 0.8 kcal/ml

TABLE 6-3 Commercial Liquid Diets for Tube Feeding

Product	Caloric Density (kcal/ml)	Osmolality (mOsm/kg H_2O)	Comments
CliniCare (canine and feline)	1	Canine, 230 Feline, 235	Veterinary product (polymeric solution)
CliniCare RF	1	165	Veterinary product for use in renal disease management (polymeric solution)
Peptamen*	1	380	Human product (monomeric solution)
Jevity*	1.06	310	Human product with added fiber to help control bowel function (polymeric solution)
Perative*	1.3	385	Human product (monomeric diet)

45 ml/kg is the maximum stomach capacity of any animal.
*These are human products that can be used in most adult dogs.

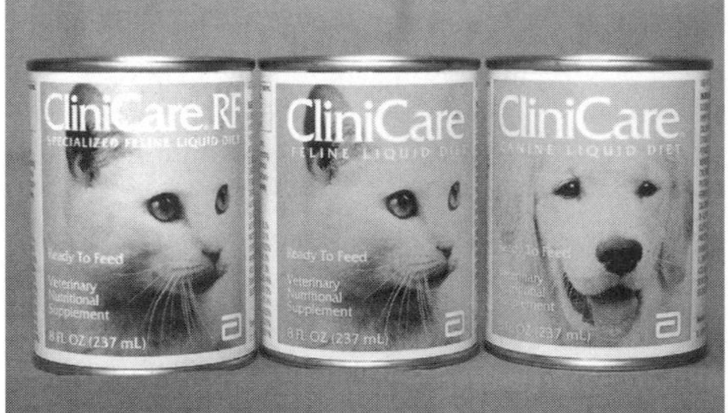

Figure 6-2
Veterinary liquid nutritional products.

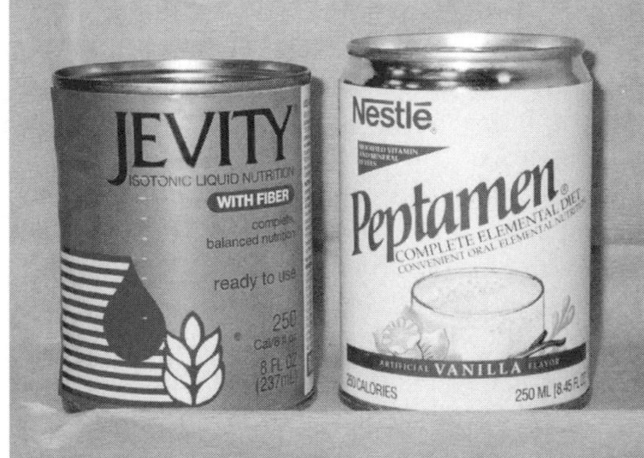

Figure 6-3
Two human liquid nutritional products found to work well in animals.

failure, and it is intended for patients with specific medical conditions such as azotemia, kidney disease, renal failure, and liver disease. Jevity, a human product, is a nutritionally balanced liquid diet that includes fiber, unlike the other products. This product can be used to stabilize bowel function in patients with diarrhea and constipation. The nutrient density of all these products is 1 kcal/ml, which makes daily caloric calculations easy.

Blenderized gruel can be administered only through large tubes (10 French and larger) with openings in their tips. Tubes with only side ports often plug with gruel. The standard recipe for blended gruel is half of a 15-oz can (225 g) of high-calorie cat food, such as Hill's Prescription

Diet Feline p/d, and ⅔ cup (170 ml) of water. This mixture must be blended at high speed for at least 1 minute. Once blended, it should be strained twice through a kitchen strainer. This produces approximately 360 ml gruel, which contains 0.8 kcal/ml of energy. Another recipe for a gruel with a smoother texture is to blend or mix well two cans of Hill's Prescription Diet a/d (canine or feline) with 50 ml water. This gruel has no particles that could plug a tube, so straining is unnecessary. Each milliliter of this recipe contains 1 kcal of energy. These gruels should be given only to patients with functional intestinal tracts because these are complex diets that must be digested. If the tube is large enough (size 10 French or larger), these gruels can be used with pharyngostomy, esophagostomy, and gastrostomy or PEG tubes.

Constant-Rate Infusion and Bolus Feedings

When starting tube feeding, one must decide whether to use a CRI or bolus feedings. CRI can be done only with liquid diets; many feeding pumps and setups are available that make CRIs convenient (see Table 6-1 for a list of suppliers). If the patient has been anorexic for more than 2 days, it may have decreased digestive function and some degree of gastric contraction. CRIs may allow the stomach and gastrointestinal tract to return to normal function in these patients, whereas bolus feeding may cause vomiting, diarrhea, and cramping. It was believed once that anorexic patients could not tolerate introduced feeding of their daily caloric requirements in the first day because of decreased digestive function and gastric contraction. However, if these patients are fed their daily RERs by CRI (preferred) or by many small, slow boluses throughout the day, they usually tolerate feedings. However, if vomiting does occur, the infusion or bolus feedings should be stopped for at least 2 hours; when infusion resumes, the CRI rate or bolus feedings should be decreased by 50%. Bolus or continuous-rate feeding can be used with nasoesophageal, nasogastric, pharyngostomy, esophagostomy, and gastrostomy or PEG tubes. Bolus feeding should not be used with jejunostomy tubes because it will cause abdominal cramping and result in diarrhea. To calculate the volume needed for bolus feeding, divide the patient's 24-hour RER by 4 and feed the patient equal doses every 6 hours. No more than 20 ml/kg should be fed at one time to prevent overfilling the stomach. Only very small amounts (5 to 15 ml) should be given until it is clear that the patient will tolerate the food. Food should be warmed; a warm water bath can be used to heat the food, and the food's temperature should be checked before feeding. Bolus feedings should be given over approximately 10 minutes to reduce nausea and avoid reflux. If the patient still shows sign of nausea (e.g., licking the lips, drooling, swallowing excessively), stop the feeding for several minutes to allow the patient to recover. When the feeding is resumed, proceed slowly and monitor for signs of nausea. All feeding tubes should be flushed before and after feedings with lukewarm water to ensure that the tubes are functional and to prevent clogging.

To calculate the hourly CRI rate, divide the patient's 24-hour RER by 24. CRI may be not be appropriate for every practice because it entails 24-hour monitoring. If the patient vomits up the tube or the pump stops infusing because the tube is kinked, someone must be available to correct these problems and maintain accurate infusion. A patient with a feeding tube in place should not be left alone.

Complications with Tube Feeding

Most complications associated with enteral tube feeding are either mechanical, gastrointestinal, or metabolic. Mechanical problems are associated with tube placement and maintenance. Proper tube placement should be verified with radiographs. Tube placement can also be verified before feeding by flushing the tube with lukewarm water. The correct food must be used or the tube may clog. Clogging can also occur when medications are crushed and pushed through the tube or food is not flushed out of the tube after bolus feeding. Once the tube is flushed, a male plug should be inserted into the hub of the tube. This will leave only water in the tube to keep it patent until its next use. Cranberry juice or carbonated beverages can be instilled to dissolve clogs.

Most gastrointestinal problems are the result of poor nutrition choices or overzealous feeding practices. Feeding a patient a type of nutrition it cannot digest properly can result in vomiting, cramps, and diarrhea; upset the fluid and electrolyte balances in the gut; and lead to cramping and abdominal distention. Choosing the correct nutrition and the correct rate of administration for each patient can prevent these complications. These complications can be alleviated by decreasing the rate of administration or decreasing the concentration of the solution. If these measures are not successful, choosing a diet that contains fiber or higher concentrations of fat may help by delaying gastric emptying.

Metabolic complications include hypokalemia and hypophosphatemia, which can be monitored through regular blood tests and treated. Now that more veterinary nutritional products are available, these problems have decreased because hospitals are using fewer human products, which can have inappropriate levels of fats, proteins, and electrolytes for veterinary patients' need (Table 6-4).

Terminating Enteral Tube Feeding

The decision to discontinue enteral tube feeding must be individualized. Depending on the type of tube placed, the patient's injury or illness, the expected time to recovery, and the patient's level of voluntary food intake, enteral feeding can continue for months. If the patient's voluntary food intake begins to increase, the enteral nutrition supplied via the tube can be decreased as long as the total nutrition equals that patient's RER. Once the patient is voluntarily eating enough on its own, the tube can be pulled. However, one must be certain that the patient can

Table 6-4 Enteral Tube Feeding Complications and Suggested Solutions

Complication	Solution
Vomiting	Stop feeding for 1-2 hr. Restart more slowly.
Diarrhea	Choose the correct nutritional product for the patient's needs. Check osmolality (should be 200-400 mOsm/kg). Check fiber to modulate water and motility. Ensure that the correct type of infusion has been chosen for the type of tube (e.g., CRI for a jejunostomy tube).
Tube ejection	Prevent vomiting. Prevent tube removal by placing an E-collar on the patient. If the tube has been ejected, remove it immediately.
Aspiration pneumonia	Ensure proper placement of the tube with radiographs or saline instillation. Suture the tube securely in place and monitor for migration or movement.
Clogging (blockage)	Flush the tube with water before and after each feeding to clean tube and verify function. Do not push crushed medications through the tube. Ensure that tube size and nutritional product are compatible. If blockage occurs, instill a carbonated beverage or cranberry juice to break down the plug.
Infection	Where applicable, change bandage regularly to monitor insertion sites for signs of infection including redness, swelling, and discharge.
Medication reactions	Check the manufacturer's directions for compatibility of medications with nutritional products. Some medications are not compatible.
Continued complications	If complications persist, replace the tube.

meet its daily RER on its own before pulling the tube. For this reason, the patient should be observed for several days of voluntary food intake to verify that it will sustain its daily nutritional needs. When this is accomplished, the tube can be pulled.

PARENTERAL NUTRITIONAL SUPPORT

When enteral nutritional support is contraindicated, parenteral nutritional (PN) support can be initiated. With PN support the nutrients are supplied intravenously, bypassing the gastrointestinal tract. This method is indicated in patients with complete mechanical intestinal obstruction, ileus or hypomotility, severe diarrhea, or chronic vomiting; those that are unconscious or have severe neurologic deficits (which increase the risk of aspiration); and those with acute pancreatitis or hepatitis. PN also can be used in conjunction with enteral nutrition when complete caloric requirements cannot be met by enteral support alone. PN is a very important tool in treating many critically ill patients. However, it is very expensive, demanding a lot of time and care from the medical staff. PN should not be administered until the patient has been rehydrated to normal levels and electrolyte and acid-base abnormalities have been corrected.

PN for veterinary patients is very different from PN for human patients. PN support can meet human patients' long-term nutritional requirements, but for veterinary patients, PN support is described as partial parenteral nutrition (PPN) because these solutions are nutritionally incomplete, meeting only the patient's most important and immediate nutritional needs, including energy, most amino acids, electrolytes, some B vitamins, and trace minerals. These solutions lack taurine and lesser important nutrients such as fatty acids, other vitamins, and trace minerals. Veterinary PN solutions also are not nutritionally balanced for long-term (more than 10 days) administration and are used only for short-term administration, usually no longer than 3 to 4 days.

Depending on the solution's final osmolarity, PPN may be administered through a central line or a peripheral line. Most veterinary PN solutions have a final osmolarity of 400 to 550 mOsm/L because most patients are receiving maintenance or greater fluid amounts. These PN solutions can be administered through a peripheral vein, depending on the type of catheter. However, in fluid-restricted patients, PN solutions could have a final osmolarity of more than 550 mOsm/L, and these solutions must be administered through a central vein because of their possible caustic effects. A central line can include a jugular or saphenous catheter. With both types of catheters, the tip must be advanced into the cranial vena cava for it to be used as a central line. The cranial vena cava has a large opening with increased blood flow and therefore tolerates the high osmolarity of the PN solutions better than a peripheral vein. Because these catheters must enter the cranial vena cava, saphenous catheters can be used only in cats and small dogs because they are not long enough to reach the vena cava in medium to large dogs. Thus jugular catheters must be substituted for saphenous catheters in larger breeds. However, jugular catheters can be used in any size animal.

Complications with PN Administration

Several complications can occur with PN administration, the most common of which is thrombophlebitis. This can be caused by many things, including poor catheter placement, inadequate catheter care, and use of the central line for blood drawing and drug administration as well as PN administration. Thrombophlebitis prevention includes aseptic catheter placement technique, daily bandage changes, close attention to catheter care, and use of the central line for PN administration only. The catheter should not be used to draw blood, administer medications, or measure central venous pressure.

Catheter occlusions can be prevented with proper catheter care and flushing with heparinized saline.

Sepsis is the most severe complication associated with PN administration. All PN solutions must be sterile. These solutions usually are made for 3 to 4 days of administration. Therefore, there are three or four different bags of PN solution, each representing one 24-hour period. Once PN is started, all extra bags must be refrigerated. After 24 hours, a new bag must be used, with fresh setups and intravenous lines. The new bag of PN solution should be taken out of the refrigerator ahead of time and allowed to warm to room temperature before administration. Bags and intravenous lines must be dated to indicate when bags and setups are to be changed (Figure 6-4).

Other complications of PN administration can include metabolic abnormalities such as hyperglycemia, but these can be monitored and controlled with blood tests and appropriate treatment.

PN is a very important tool in treating many critically ill patients. Its benefits far outweigh any complications that may occur, and it may be the only tool that enables certain patients to recover from an illness or injury.

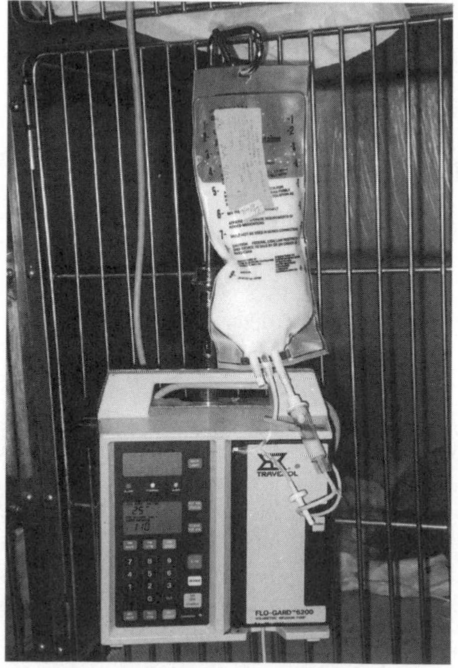

Figure 6-4

Partial parenteral nutrition should be administered via an infusion pump to maintain the proper infusion rate.

Technician Skills

Understanding patients' species-specific and individual differences allows technicians to optimize care for each hospitalized patient. Getting to know patients and their personalities usually is as important as understanding their diseases or injuries and their complications. From a very shy and frightened cat who will eat only when its cage is covered to a nauseated dog with a PEG tube who cannot tolerate cold gruel, attention to detail counts.

Such attention to detail, combined with common sense, improves patient care. Understanding certain techniques helps the technician prevent, reduce, or solve problems that arise. For example, if you are bolus feeding a patient through an enteral feeding tube and the patient begins to show signs of nausea (e.g., drooling, lip licking, restlessness, and ultimately vomiting), what should you do? First, stop the feeding until these signs disappear and the patient calms down. When restarting the feeding regimen, continue at a slower rate. If the patient is nauseated but you still must feed it a bolus through an enteral feeding tube, do all of its medical treatments first, while the patient's stomach is empty. Then start the feeding very slowly, and do not touch or move the patient during or after feeding; allowing the patient to lie still reduces the chances of nausea and vomiting. If vomiting persists, consider starting CRI. Warming nutritional solutions also makes bolus feeding more comfortable for the patient. Never feed a patient a cold nutritional solution. Warming the amount needed in a warm water bath is recommended, but you should always check the temperature of the solution and ensure that it is mixed well before administering it to the patient. Microwaving solutions is not recommended because they can become too hot, and may not warm evenly.

Because certain pain medications can cause nausea and sedation, the patient should be fed before such medications are administered. Similarly, many oral medications can have an awful taste, causing stomach upset. Whenever possible, feed your patients before giving them oral medications to decrease the chance of nausea. Patients may then start eating on their own or tolerate tube feedings better.

Enteral feeding tubes can become plugged, even with close monitoring. When this occurs, a carbonated beverage or cranberry juice can be flushed into the tube to break down the plug. However, some nutritional formulas are not compatible with these solutions, and they may be contraindicated by the location of the tube. Make sure these solutions are not contraindicated before you try them.

Clear and open communication between the technician, the veterinarian, and the owner of each patient is essential. Technicians must inform the veterinarian of any changes in the patient's behavior, physical status, or tolerance of medications or nutritional support. Knowing the patient, recognizing problems quickly, and notifying the veterinarian immediately can prevent small problems from becoming major complications. Likewise, the veterinarian should inform the technician of any changes in diagnosis or status or any foreseeable problems. Finally, good communication with clients enables them to make informed decisions. To help clients make realistic decisions, keep them informed about any home care the patient will need. This can include tube feeding and daily monitoring for infection. When the client cannot perform the necessary home care or afford suggested treatments, understanding the clients' physical and financial limitations can enable the technician and veterinarian to develop alternatives. Helping patients recover more quickly and return home takes a team effort.

CONCLUSION

Nutritional support is an important part of treating critically ill patients. Technicians must learn about the advantages of nutritional support, recognize complications and side effects of enteral and parenteral nutrition, and seek the solutions to these problems. With this knowledge, good communication, and medical treatment, we can improve patient care. Nutritional support complements medical treatment to promote speedy and complete recovery.

BIBLIOGRAPHY

Abbott Laboratories: Clinical product sheets, North Chicago, Ill, November 1997.

Bella JA: Principles of nutritional therapy for dogs and cats, *Vet Tech* 10(3):152, 1989.

Case LP, Carey DP, Hirakawa DA: Geriatrics. In Duncan LL, ed: *Canine and feline nutrition,* St Louis, 1995, Mosby.

Case LP, Carey DP, Hirakawa DA: Growth. In Duncan LL, ed: *Canine and feline nutrition,* St Louis, 1995, Mosby.

Crowe DT: Enteral nutrition for critically ill or injured patients, part II, *Comp Cont Ed* 8(10):179, 1986.

Culp AM: Nasogastric tube feeding: indications and applications, *Vet Tech* 18(1):47, 1997.

Greene S: Anorexia and hospitalized cats. *Vet Tech* 13(8):580, 1992.

Guilford WG, Strombeck DR: Diseases of swallowing. In Guilford WG, Center SA, Strombeck DR, et al, eds: *Strombeck's small animal gastroenterology,* ed 3, Philadelphia, 1996, WB Saunders.

Lawrence AB: Keeping it down: canine megaesophagus, *Vet Tech* 18(9):616, 1997.

Levine PB, Smallwood LJ, Buback JL: Esophagostomy tubes as a method of nutritional management in cats: a retrospective study, *J Am Anim Hosp Assoc* 33:405, 1997.

Lewis LD, Morris ML Jr, Hand MS: Gastrointestinal, pancreatic, and hepatic diseases. In Lewis LD, Morris ML, Hand MS, eds: *Small animal clinical nutrition,* ed 3, Topeka, Ks, 1987, Mark Morris Assoc.

Mathews KA: Nutritional support: enteral feeding and parenteral. In Mathews KA, ed: *Veterinary emergency and critical care manual,* Guelph, Ontario, Canada, 1996, Lifelearn Inc.

Parkman A: Evaluating body condition in cats and dogs. *Vet Tech* 19(2):129, 1998.

Remillard RL, Armstrong PJ, Davenport DJ: Assisted feeding in hospitalized patients: enteral and parenteral nutrition. In Hand MS, Thatcher CD, Remillard RL, et al, eds: *Small animal clinical nutrition IV,* Topeka, Ks, 2000, Mark Morris Institute.

Box 7-1 Technical Tip: *Nasal Catheterization*

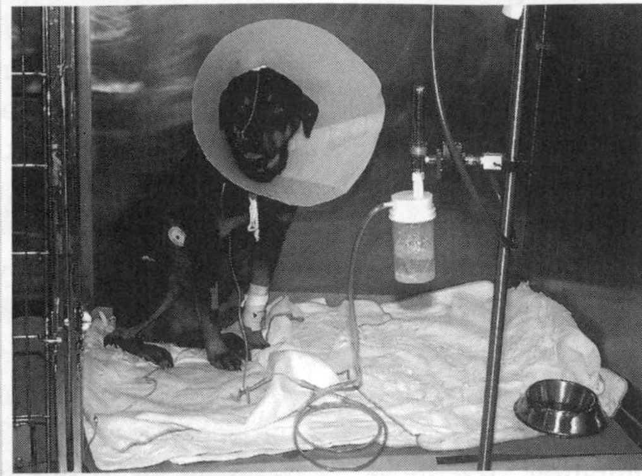

1. Catheter length is determined by measuring the distance from the tip of the nares to the second upper premolar or the medial canthus. Mark this distance on the catheter.
2. A suture should be placed close to the external nares, with long ends for tying the catheter in place.
3. Desensitize the nasal passages with a local anesthetic. Proparacaine solution or 2% lidocaine can be used. Instill 1 or 2 drops. Wait 30-60 seconds. Repeat if necessary.
4. Tip the head slightly upward and gently press the tip of the nose upward with your thumb.
5. Advance the lubricated catheter (surgical lube or lidocaine gel) into the ventral meatus in a ventromedial direction (not necessary in the cat) up to the mark indicated. Be gentle and do not force.
6. Suture the catheter in place using two additional points. The bridge of the nose and between the eyes are the most common sites. Suturing to the side of the face is another option. Secure to the oxygen tubing.
7. Place tape around neck and anchor tube.
8. Attach a disposable humidifier to the flowmeter.

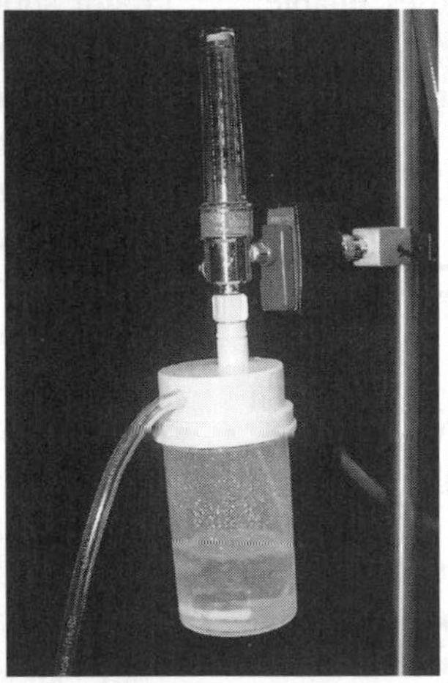

Flow Rates

These rates provide tracheal oxygen of approximately 40% to 50% (50-100 mL/kg/min). Oxygen should be administered immediately but gradually. A sudden burst of oxygen can be very uncomfortable for the animal.

Cats and small dogs <10 kg: 0.5-1.0 L/min
Dogs 10-20 kg: 1.0-2.0 L/min
Dogs 20-50 kg: 2-4 L/min
Dogs >50 kg: 5 L/min

dogs and cats tolerate 3- to 8-French catheters best. Larger and smaller catheters are available from various sources for use in other species (Technical Tip Box 7-1).

Nasal prongs also can be used to administer oxygen in some species. The determining factor in this instance would be the distance between the right and left nostril. This device is one of the most common oxygen administration devices in human oxygen therapy. The nasal prongs are placed at the nares so that each prong is aligned with the opening of one nostril. These devices can slip out of place easily because only the tips of the prongs are in the nares. Be sure to secure both prongs with suture or surgical staples, taking care not to obstruct the lumen. Oxygen flow rates of 3 to 6 L/min are common, with percentages of oxygen delivered similar to those delivered by nasal catheters. Although the prongs are not placed as far into the nasal cavity as the nasal catheter, it is advisable to use topical anesthetic, at least initially, to reduce mucosal irritation, particularly if flows higher than 3 L/min are used. Nasal prongs are available in newborn, pediatric, and adult sizes; the space between the prongs depends on the size selected. Check these devices frequently to ensure that proper position is maintained (Figure 7-1).

Nasal tracheal catheters are presented in many veterinary emergency training programs as a means of administering oxygen at percentages greater than 50%, especially for laryngeal paresis or paralysis or collapsing trachea. These devices are placed the same way as the nasal catheter except that the nasal tracheal catheter is advanced to the epiglottis and then slid into the trachea. These catheters are not tolerated well because they can cause the animal to cough frequently, which can dislodge the cannula from the trachea. A topical anesthetic is applied to the laryngotracheal area before insertion to minimize coughing, and a mild tranquilizer can be used to keep the animal sedated. These factors can be risky in patients with severe trauma or disease because they can cause hypoventilation. Also, because the catheter is left in the trachea, the epiglottis is propped open and the patient can aspirate vomitus or saliva.

A better approach might be transtracheal oxygen. The same catheter used for tracheal and nasal oxygen delivery can be used for transtracheal oxygen. In human medicine, cannulas designed for this purpose are available from various manufacturers. Silicone catheters are best for this purpose because silicone is softer, less irritating, and less damaging to the tracheal mucosa. These devices are placed surgically using a scalpel or a large-bore needle. The area between the 4th and 5th cartilaginous ring is prepped and anesthetized locally and a puncture slightly larger than the catheter is made in this space. The catheter is advanced into the trachea so that the tip of the catheter is directly above the carina. The catheter position can be verified by oral observation: a laryngoscope is used to lift the epiglottis and observe the catheter position. Connect the proximal end of the catheter to the oxygen source tube and turn on the flow to approximately 3 L/min. The flow rate is determined by the patient's minute ventilation. If the patient's breathing is deep and rapid, higher flow rates may be necessary. When oxygen is administered one should evaluate the effect of the intervention. The best means is arterial blood gas measurement, but if this is not available pulse oximetry should be used. This analysis should be made 15 to 20 minutes after the initial intervention or change in parameters to allow physiologic compensation to take place.

An oxygen collar is less restrictive than an oxygen mask and less invasive than a cannula. This

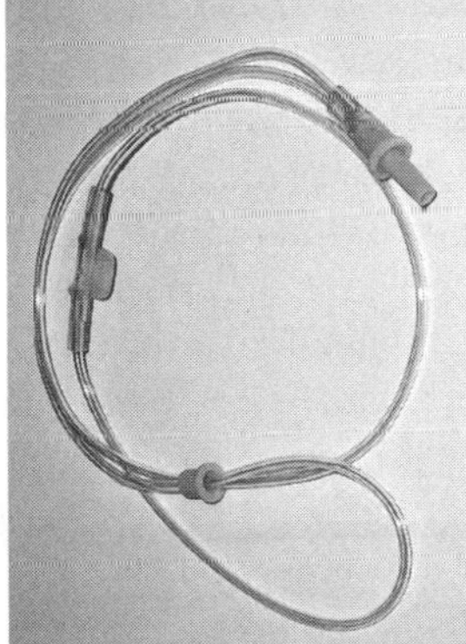

Figure 7-1

Nasal prongs for oxygen administration.

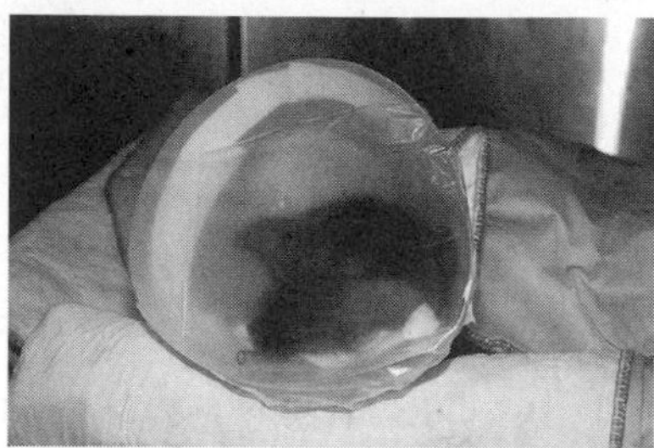

Figure 7-2
Oxygen collar.

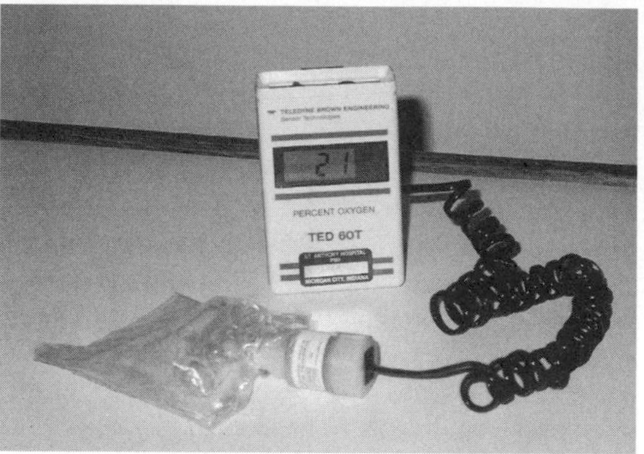

Figure 7-3
Oxygen analyzer.

is a very effective oxygen delivery method, and high levels can be reached very quickly using low flows. One can make an oxygen collar from an Elizabethan collar (Figure 7-2). An oxygen tube is taped at the base of the collar, with the tip approximately 2 inches from the end of the collar. Clear cellophane wrap is placed across the front of the collar, covering two thirds of the front and taped securely to the sides. The opening acts as a vent, which reduces the confining effect and releases the excess oxygen and exhaled carbon dioxide. This vent size can be increased or decreased depending on the desired oxygen percentage which should be monitored with an oxygen analyzer. Oxygen is heavier than air and will remain in the lower two thirds of the collar, which acts as an oxygen reservoir. Flow must meet the patient's ventilatory demand. Monitoring the oxygen saturation in the blood by using a pulse oximeter is a good way to determine the effectiveness of this method. It is also important to monitor the buildup of heat and humidity inside the collar. Oxygen is very drying to the mucous membranes. Lubricating the eyes periodically with ophthalmic ointment is recommended with this method of oxygen administration.

OXYGEN CAGES AND CRIBS

Oxygen cages and cribs are environmental control devices. They consist of a box, connecting tubes to an oxygen source, filters, and a circulating fan to move the air. Some may have climate controls for temperature and humidification. Because of their size, these devices are not the best choice when oxygen control and accurate delivery are critical. It takes time for the oxygen concentration to stabilize in this system. Flows as high as 15 L/min are needed to maintain 40% oxygen. These units also develop dead spaces, areas that are not saturated with the proper percentage of oxygen. The cage must be opened frequently to evaluate the patient, and the gas concentration decreases every time the door is opened. This creates an unstable environment for the animal and can be fatal when oxygen concentration control is critical. Oxygen concentration should be monitored with an oxygen analyzer to ensure that proper levels are maintained in the cage (Figure 7-3). Pulse oximetry should be used to ensure that adequate levels of gas are being delivered to meet the patient's physiologic demand.

Hypoxia can lead rapidly to anoxia, especially in a patient who has been sedated or anesthetized. Humidification systems also must be checked frequently for bacterial growth. Some older oxygen cages were equipped with passover humidifiers in which air flowed over a pan of water and humidity was derived from surface evaporation. It was difficult to clean these systems, and water often was not replaced frequently enough, leading to the growth of bacteria, particularly *Pseudomonas aeruginosa*.

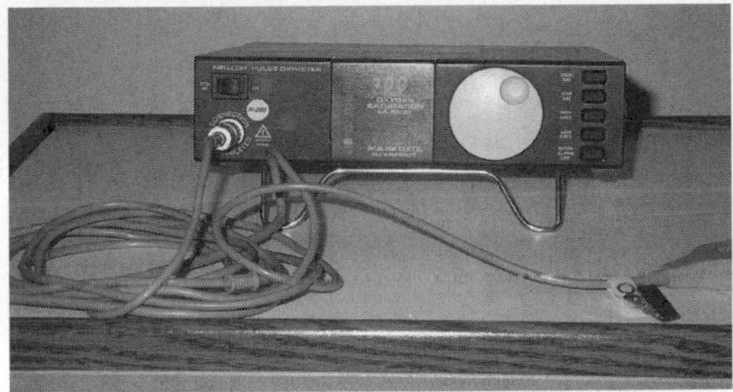

Figure 7-4

Pulse oximeter and oxygen analysis device.

There are many ways to administer oxygen to patients with respiratory compromise, and some work better than others. Whether a particular method meets the patient's physiologic demand can be assessed only by monitoring the oxygen support system used and the patient's physiologic response. Devices such as pulse oximeters, oxygen analyzers, and blood gas measuring devices are invaluable in treating the patient with respiratory compromise (Figure 7-4).

CONCLUSION

There are many ways to administer oxygen to a patient, and some are more effective than others. Understanding the available methods enables veterinary practitioners to choose the appropriate therapy. Some animals tolerate one type of delivery system better than another. Oxygen therapy should calm the patient and improve its condition. If it causes the animal to struggle and become anxious, another delivery system should be used.

Monitoring equipment is used to evaluate the animal's response to the treatment. Careful observation also is important in determining how well the patient is tolerating the therapy.

BIBLIOGRAPHY

Bistner SI, Ford DB: *Handbook of veterinary procedures and emergency treatment,* ed 6, Philadelphia, 1995, WB Saunders.

Crowe DT: Seminar notes, case-based discussion, 5th Annual Emergency Medical Conference, Kansas State University, March 1, 1997, Kansas State University Student Chapter of the Veterinary Emergency and Critical Care Society.

McPherson SP, Spearman CB: *Respiratory therapy equipment,* ed 3, St Louis, 1995, Mosby.

Shawver DM: *Clinical notes on airway management, Cambridge University, England,* Bloomington, Ind, 1995, Cook Veterinary Products Inc.

Spearman D, Sheldon RL, Egan DF: *Egan's fundamentals of respiratory therapy,* ed 4, St Louis, 1982, Mosby.

White GC: *Equipment theory for respiratory care,* ed 3, Albany, NY, 1998, Delmar.

Chapter 8

Mechanical Ventilation

Normal ventilation is the inspiration and expiration of air to and from the lungs. Downward movement of the diaphragm creates negative pressure, allowing air to enter the lungs. Mechanical ventilation is the act of assisting or controlling the patient's breathing by the use of a machine-driven or hand-operated device. Positive pressure in the lungs drives mechanical ventilation. Reversing the normal respiratory pattern stresses all body systems. The technician responsible for administering mechanical ventilation must understand the system being used and monitor the patient frequently at specific intervals.

WHEN TO MECHANICALLY VENTILATE

Trauma and various disease processes can impair an animal's ability to breathe properly. The animal in respiratory distress must be assessed quickly and treated immediately. Oxygen therapy is started immediately and the patient's response is assessed. Visual assessment includes observing the animal's ventilatory pattern, respiratory rate, and posture. Lung auscultation also is important (Table 8-1). If the patient does not have the muscular ability and control to breathe effectively and efficiently, administering oxygen alone will not be effective. The animal must be able to move the oxygen from the lungs to the tissues to maintain stable oxygen saturation. Cyanosis is not a good indication of when to begin mechanical ventilation; it is a late sign of hypoxemia.

Once the physical assessments are complete, response to oxygen therapy can be evaluated. Work of breathing and anxiety should decrease if treatment is effective. Pulse oximetry can be used to determine oxygen saturation but should not be used exclusively. Normal readings are approximately 95% to 98% depending on respiratory rate and O_2 flow rate, even low flows will result in ABGs above 100 mm Hg and O_2 saturations of 100% if the pulmonary system is working correctly. Arterial blood gas is the best indicator of oxygen therapy effectiveness.

It is beyond the scope of this text to cover all aspects of blood gas analysis, but it is important to know the normal values and understand what fluctuations in these parameters indicate.

Normal Values	
pH	7.35-7.45
$Paco_2$	35-45 mm Hg
Pao_2	94-100 mm Hg
HCO_3	22-26 mEq/L
Base excess	−2 to +2

The key ventilation parameter is $Paco_2$. Elevated $Paco_2$ indicates hypercapnia and a ventilation deficit. Decreased $Paco_2$ indicates hypocapnia, which could indicate hyperventilation or metabolic alkalosis. pH is a mathematical representation of the hydrogen ion concentration. It is inversely proportional to CO_2: an increase in pH means a decrease in CO_2 and a decrease in pH means an increase in CO_2. Elevated pH indicates alkalosis and a decreased pH indicates acidosis.

TABLE 8-1 Interpreting Chest Sounds

Sound	Possible Cause
Wheezes	Obstruction
Crackles	Fluid in airspace
Gurgles or bubbles	Heavy secretions in upper airway
Rhonchi, harsh or coarse sounds	Irritated bronchial mucosa
Quiet or diminished lung sounds	Collapsed air sacs, pneumothorax
Drum sound (tympanic resonance) to tapping	Possible pneumothorax or air trapping

Two systems maintain the acid-base balance: the renal system and the respiratory system. As respiratory acidosis occurs, the renal system retains HCO_3 to buffer the excess acid. As alkalosis occurs, the respiratory system compensates by slowing respiration to retain CO_2 and increase the body's acid level. Respiratory response occurs in minutes, but a renal response may take hours.

Metabolic status is indicated by the HCO_3 level and the base excess. Metabolic and respiratory alkalosis are indicated by an increase in HCO_3. Metabolic and respiratory acidosis are indicated by a decrease in HCO_3. PaO_2 is an indicator of oxygen status. PaO_2 is normal if ventilation is adequate.

Many texts on acid-base chemistry are available, and technicians should consider reviewing this material before attempting to administer mechanical ventilation.

If improvements are noted and the blood gas results are normal, mechanical ventilation may not be needed immediately. The animal remains on oxygen therapy and causes of its respiratory distress are analyzed.

If no improvements are noted or the patient's condition begins to decline, ventilation must be considered. An increase in $PaCO_2$ (more than 45 mm Hg) and a pH less than 7.4 indicate that the patient cannot maintain adequate ventilation. When hypoxia increases, the work of breathing increases. Total body and system fatigue can occur, which leads to death rapidly.

The first step is to choose the type of sedation, if needed, and establish an airway. The endotracheal tube is used most often, but for patients with upper airway trauma or those under mild sedation a tracheostomy tube may be necessary. The tube should be made of a material, such as silicone that will not cause additional irritation. Once the tube is placed, the minimal leak technique is used to prevent damage from an overinflated cuff. Once the tube is secured, it is connected to the functioning ventilator. The cuff is inflated slowly until air stops leaking. The cuff is then deflated until a slight hissing sound is heard. Cuff pressure can be measured with a Posey® cuff manometer.

TYPES OF VENTILATION

Complete understanding of the various ventilator types enables the technician to care for patients receiving mechanical ventilation.

Controlled ventilation is the total control of all ventilatory activity, used for apnea.

Assisted ventilation is the intermittent control of ventilation, used for periodic episodes of suppressed respiratory effort.

Positive end expiratory pressure (PEEP) is the elevated pressure maintained in the lung, during mechanical ventilation which increases the functional residual capacity (FRC). Spring valves or other devices are used to add expiratory resistance to continuous air flow.

Continuous positive airway pressure (CPAP) is the maintaining of an end expiratory pressure above ambient pressure during spontaneous breathing. This also increases FRC and diffusion.

Continuous positive-pressure ventilation (CPPV) involves applying positive pressure with every breath. This is necessary for animals that cannot breathe spontaneously.

Intermittent positive-pressure ventilation (IPPV) involves applying positive-pressure breaths intermittently during spontaneous breathing. This is necessary for animals that have a depressed respiratory drive or periods of apnea and is used often for administering gas anesthesia.

MOST COMMON TYPES OF VENTILATORS

MANUAL VENTILATOR

These are manual compression bags that can be connected quickly and easily to an endotracheal tube. Reservoir tubes or bags can be connected to the compressible bag to assist in short-term ventilation or cardiopulmonary resuscitation (CPR). Portability and availability are the main advantages of these units.

This device has some limitations. There is time limit for use due to the necessity of manual operation. Volume delivery and inspired oxygen cannot be controlled. These devices are best suited for short-term use. The Ambu-Bag is one type of manual resuscitation device (Figure 8-1).

PRESSURE-CYCLED VENTILATOR

These machines terminate inspiration based on a preset pressure. To control the percentage of oxygen to be delivered, a blender must be connected to the ventilator. Without a blender, the inspired oxygen levels can reach 90% continually. For long-term ventilation, the technician must be able to control the oxygen concentration.

Pressure-cycled ventilators are pressure limited. A control regulates the amount of pressure delivered to the patient's lungs and ventilator system. Tidal volume is the result of the flow of gas from the ventilator to the patient's lungs over a period of

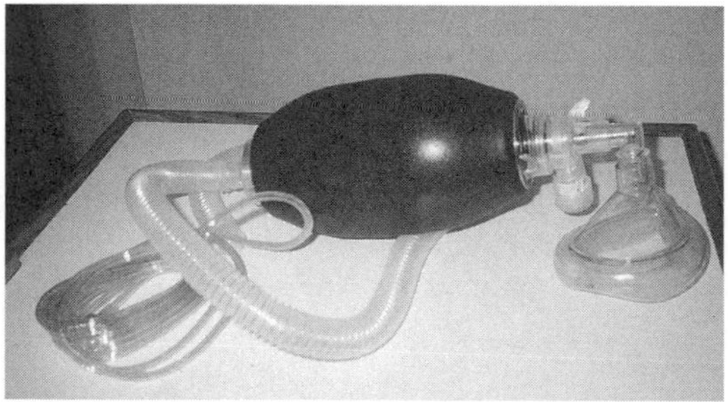

Figure 8-1

Manual resuscitator.

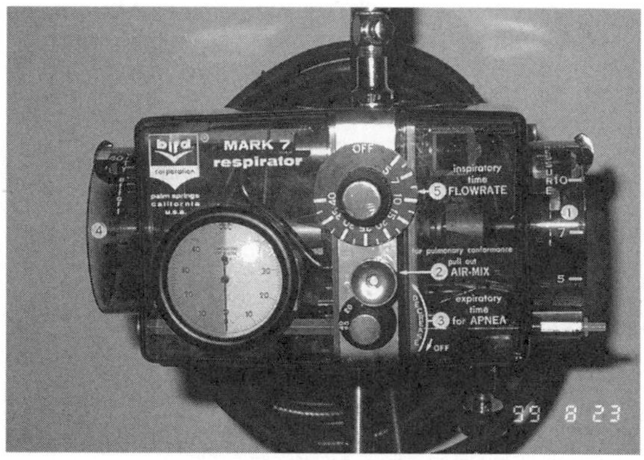

Figure 8-2

Bird Mark 7 IPPB.

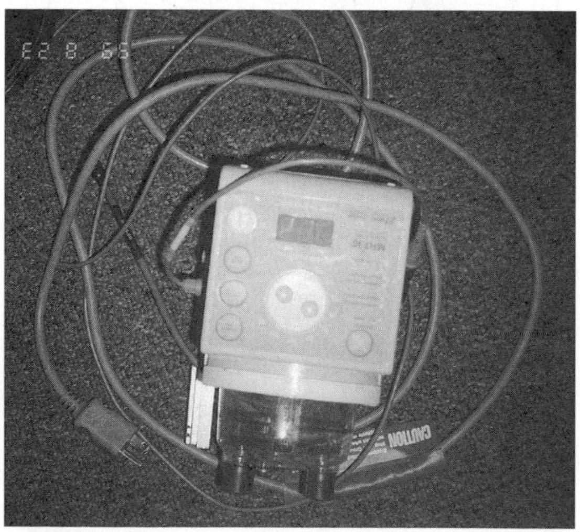

Figure 8-3

Oxygen blender.

time. The resistance and compliance of the ventilatory circuitry and the patient's physiology create pressure readings on the ventilator's manometer. When a patient needs a specific tidal volume to maintain a stable pH, this pressure limit can create a problem. Lungs can become less compliant and demand an increase in pressure to reach the desired tidal volume. The pressure-cycled ventilator may not be able to meet this demand due to premature inspiratory termination.

The advantage of these machines is that they are less expensive than others and more readily available. The disadvantage is that there is no way to ensure adequate tidal volume. Tidal volumes can be monitored with a spirometer.

The Bird Mark 7, Puritan Bennett PR II, and Puritan Bennett PR I are types of pressure-cycled ventilators (Figures 8-2 and 8-3).

Volume-Cycled Ventilators

The volume-cycled ventilator terminates inspiration when a predetermined volume is reached. The desired volume is delivered even if resistance in the system occurs.

Disadvantages include the high cost and low availability of these machines. The ability to control the inspired oxygen percentage (FiO_2) and tidal volume and the availability of PEEP, CPAP, and alarm systems are the benefits of the volume-cycled ventilator.

The Puritan Bennett MA1, MA11, Servo 300/400 (blender separate) and STAR ventilator are types of volume-cycled ventilators (Figure 8-4).

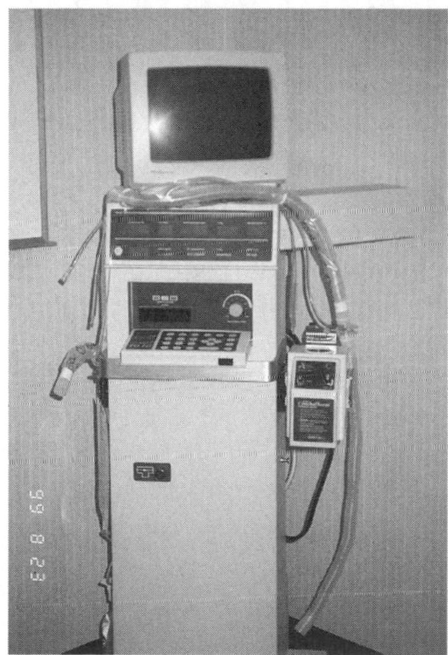

Figure 8-4
STAR model 300A.

Time-Cycled Ventilators

The time-cycled ventilator terminates the inspiratory phase after a set period of time. These are commonly used as anesthetic delivery devices. The Bird Mark 11 and the Hallowell Ventilator are examples of time-cycled ventilators.

High-Frequency Jet Ventilators

High-frequency jet ventilators (HFJVs) are highly specialized machines. They deliver the gases at a rapid rate so small volumes are stacked, forcing the gases to permeate the alveolar-capillary membranes. They are used primarily in cases of shock lung syndrome or fibrosis (Figure 8-5). The Sechrist IV-100B, Life Pulse Jet Ventilator, and Healthdyne Impulse Jet Ventilator are examples of HFJVs.

Parameters critical to the support of the patient must be monitored and maintained at all times. The type of ventilator chosen must be able to deliver adequate volumes in a given period of time at an oxygen saturation that meets the patient's physiologic demands.

The care and monitoring of the patient on the ventilator are important factors in successful treatment (Technical Tip Box 8-1).

TROUBLESHOOTING

Understanding the mechanics of the specific ventilator used enables the technician to support

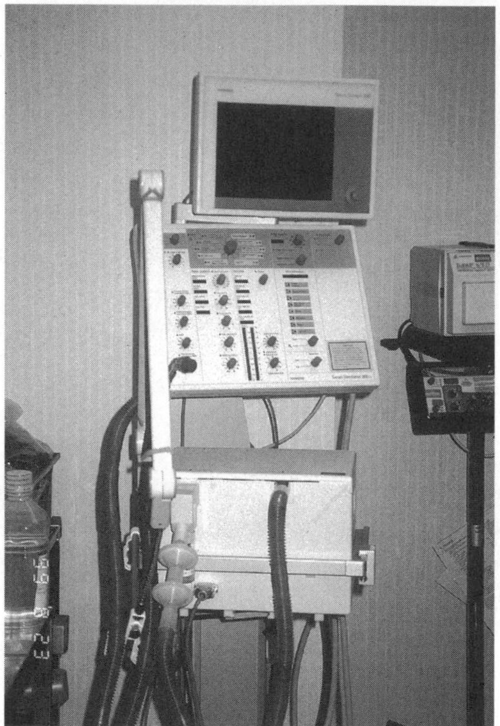

Figure 8-5
STAR jet ventilator model 3010.

the patient and solve problems as they arise. If the machine cycling begins to fail, gas and electrical sources should be checked first. Tanks should be filled and all electrical connections confirmed.

Most of these devices are pressure or volume limited, so leaks are the most common cause of malfunction. The leaks may be around hose connections or the cuff of the endotracheal tube. Feel around all connections and listen for air escaping.

Excess humidification in the system can cause problems. Water pooling in any of the hoses can increase pressure within the system.

The airway must be evaluated continually. Excess secretions, mucous plugs, or an improperly sized endotracheal tube can cause malfunctions.

True mechanical failure can occur, so a backup system must be available.

WEANING OFF THE VENTILATOR

When the patient is ready to be weaned and the acid-base status has been stabilized, the Fio_2 is decreased in 10% decrements. The patient's responses are observed and blood gases checked every 20 minutes. This is continued until the percentage of atmospheric air (21%) is reached.

The mandatory ventilation rate is decreased every 2 to 4 minutes by a couple of breaths. Observing for spontaneous breaths, inspiratory effort, and frequency is important.

Once the patient can breathe spontaneously with adequate effort, extubation can occur. Blood gas is checked after extubation and oxygen therapy may be necessary for minimal support if the patient is mildly hypoxic (Technical Tip Box 8-2).

COMPLICATIONS OF MECHANICAL VENTILATION

The decision to ventilate mechanically is not made lightly. It is a serious commitment by the care facility and the owners. It is time-consuming and expensive, and carries a risk of complications. Upper airway trauma can result if the type of tube used is wrong for the patient or if the cuff is inflated improperly. Pulmonary barotrauma and pneumothorax can result from high ventilatory pressures. Inadequate ventilation are caused by misplaced endotracheal tubes or improper use of the machine's functions. Insufficient monitoring can cause overhydration and renal insufficiency, and nasocomial infections can result from improper aseptic techniques.

Knowledge of respiratory physiology, mechanical ventilation, patient monitoring, and overall patient care enables the technician to minimize complications and administer mechanical ventilation successfully.

Box 8-1 Technical Tip: *Care of the Patient Receiving Mechanical Ventilation*

Mechanical ventilation is stressful for the patient, but the technician can alleviate some of the stress by using continuous monitoring equipment to optimize treatment. Many available monitors incorporate many features in one system, and some units can be upgraded.

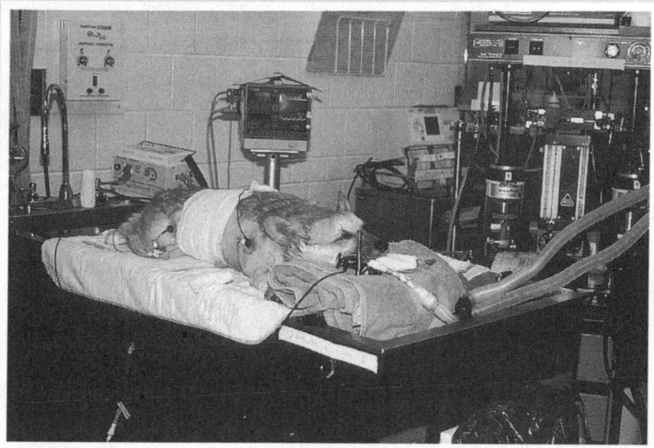

Continuous Monitoring Equipment

Electrocardiogram
Pulse oximeter
CO_2 analyzer
Thermometer (temperature probes)
IV fluid pumps
Blood gas analyzer
Suction
Stethoscope
Doppler

Supplies

Suction catheters
Endotracheal tubes (multiple sizes)
Manual resuscitator
Warming units
Syringe for cuff inflation
Items for padding
- Towels
- Blankets
- Support wedges
- Absorbent pads

Possible Indwelling Tubes to Maintain

Endotracheal tubes or tracheostomy tube
Intravenous catheters
- Jugular catheter
- Peripheral catheter
- Arterial catheter

Urinary catheter with closed system
Nasogastric feeding tube or stomach tube

Treatment List

1. Perform airway tube maintenance as needed.
2. Lubricate eyes every 4 hours with sterile ophthalmic ointment.
3. Wipe and moisturize nose as needed.
4. Apply olive oil to tongue as needed for moistening.
5. Rinse mouth clean of excess secretions as needed. Suction to collect solution.
6. Use a mouth gag to prevent clamping down on endotracheal tube and tongue. This is not necessary if a tracheostomy tube is in place.
7. Change the patient's position every 2 hours. Animals should not be placed in a complete lateral position.
8. Perform physical therapy every 2 hours. Massage legs. (This step must be performed very carefully. Depending on the type of sedation or depth of anesthesia, massage may be too stimulating.)
9. Perform catheter care every 24 hours or as necessary.
10. Check settings on ventilator and vital parameters every hour; adjust as needed.

Box 8-2 Technical Tip: *Airway Care*

Suctioning

The airway must be suctioned to remove secretions.

Tools needed: suction kit, sterile gloves and catheter, suction unit

1. Hyperventilate for 10 breaths or increase oxygen to 100%.
2. Disconnect. If the airway appears dry, inject 9% NaCl. If moist, do not infuse additional fluid. Insert lubricated suction catheter into endotracheal tube (sterile water can be used for lubricant). Do not apply suction during insertion. Insert 1 cm past distal end of endotracheal tube.
3. Apply suction and rotate catheter gently between thumb and finger. Slowly withdraw catheter, maintaining suction (maximum suction time 10-15 seconds).
4. Reconnect breathing system on original settings.
5. Observe secretions and note amount, consistency, and color.

Caution: Reduction of oxygen levels, trauma to the tracheal mucosa, and introduction of infection can occur during suction. All staff should understand the importance of suctioning and sterile technique.

Humidification

The patient's normal humidification system is bypassed during mechanical ventilation. It is important to humidify the air to maintain a healthy airway. Cold aerosol mists and warm water vapors usually are ancillary ventilator components. Nebulizers and artificial noses are connected to the breathing circuit to provide continual humidification.

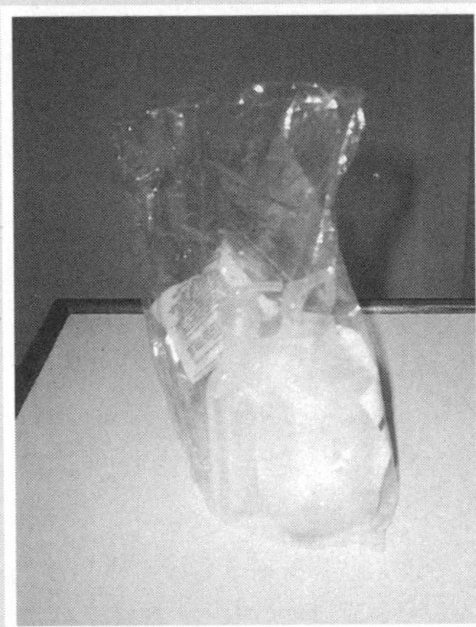

Changing the Airway Tube

The airway tube is changed only when necessary.

1. Suction internal lumen and upper airway. Suction the patient's mouth, including the area around the cuff, to remove debris.
2. Hyperventilate or increase oxygen to 100% for 10 breaths.
3. Suction upper airway above the cuff.
4. Deflate cuff and immediately but gently remove tube. Replace if hypoxia or apnea is apparent.
5. Reconnect ventilator if mechanical ventilation is to be continued.

Recordkeeping

One person should be assigned to each patient receiving ventilation to keep forms and observations consistent throughout the shift. Records must be accurate and detailed, especially with regard to ventilator settings and assessments made during treatment. Shift changes must overlap at least 30 minutes so the next technician has enough time to review updates and patient status.

The critical care team must be trained to operate each machine being used; each type has different features.

The veterinary technician also must understand blood gas analysis and respiratory therapy to maximize the patient's chances of survival and recovery.

CONCLUSION

Clients must understand the time demands, cost, and risks of mechanical ventilation before treatment can begin.

BIBLIOGRAPHY

Martz KV, Joiner JW, Sheperd RM: *Management of the patient-ventilator system,* ed 2, St Louis, 1984, Mosby.

McPherson SP, Spearman CB: *Respiratory therapy equipment,* ed 3, St Louis, 1985, Mosby.

West JB: *Respiratory physiology,* ed 3, Baltimore, 1985, Williams & Wilkins.

White GC: *Equipment theory for respiratory care,* Albany, NY, 1995, Delmar.

Chapter 9

Pain Assessment and Treatment

Philosophers and scientists have long debated the issues of animal pain. Until recently, practical pain treatment in veterinary patients has not been addressed. This oversight may have resulted from the following beliefs:

- Animals do not experience pain.
- Animals experience pain but not in a way that is detrimental to their well-being or that warrants treatment.
- The signs of pain in animals are too subjective to be assessed.
- Pain is good because it limits activity.
- Analgesia is bad because of adverse side effects or because it interferes with the ability to accurately monitor patients.

The veterinary community finally has recognized that animals experience pain. The emerging specialty of veterinary critical care has brought greater attention to pain management. Critically ill and injured patients are subjected to numerous painful treatments and diagnostic procedures. The commitment to treat critically ill animals must include alleviating or minimizing their pain throughout treatment.

Critically ill patients are the most likely to experience pain and in the greatest need of treatment, but they may be less able to express it. It has been suggested that these animals inspire less affection and greater detachment by caregivers than do healthier animals with "personality." This is thought to diminish attention paid to their pain needs. One might argue that to some caregivers, critically ill patients inspire greater compassion in response to an increased perception of helplessness.

The ambiguity in pain management rests largely in the subjective nature of pain assessment. Veterinary pain assessment is based solely on the ability to recognize often subtle, varying signs and symptoms of nonverbal patients. The study of pain in nonverbal patients (human neonates, infants, and animals) is fairly recent. The first human work examining pain manifestations in preverbal children was conducted in 1986. This research showed that healthy full-term newborns display painful distress in response to tissue damage. Crying, body movements, avoidant behaviors, and facial expressions were described as manifestations of pain in neonatal patients. Despite these acknowledgments, neonates were not routinely treated for pain for nearly 10 more years. The inability to distinguish pain from other stress, the extreme subjectivity of assessment, and persistent ambiguity about the existence of neonatal pain confounded clinicians' efforts. Even now, human neonatal pain assessment and management remains an area of research, growth, and ethical debate.

In veterinary medicine, the issue is further confounded by several factors. First, there is a natural variation in the experience and display of pain between species, breeds, and individual animals. We are expected to recognize pain in cats, dogs, and other small companion animals. There may appear to be very little similarity between a cat who sleeps curled in the back of its cage, avoiding movement or contact and a crying, restless dog. However, they both may be exhibiting signs of pain. Even within species, breed variations are strong. It has become customary to discriminate between perceived stoic and weak animals. Animals that do not display overt signs of pain are praised for their fortitude. Patients that show excessive signs of pain are assumed to be weak. Collies and borzois, for example, are stereotyped as fragile and without strong will to survive grave illness. Conversely, Labradors seem to be oblivious to pain and able to survive where other dogs might not. Although some may argue the specifics, most veterinary professionals probably have preconceived ideas about breed predisposition and ability to handle pain, stress, and illness. There probably are some actual differences in breed pain threshold and response, but it is dangerous to make general assumptions about pain rather than to consider each patient individually.

Second, veterinarians often make assumptions about which procedures are most painful. For example, most would agree that a thoracotomy is a painful procedure, whereas an ovariohysterectomy is not considered painful. It is useful to examine how these conclusions were reached. There is no valid reason to make generalizations about procedures other than to assume that invasive surgical or nonsurgical procedures are likely to cause some degree of pain. Each patient must be evaluated. Ultimately, pain treatment often is determined arbitrarily, based on a combination of limited information, subjective assessment, and personal beliefs. A scientific and humane course of pain assessment and treatment is best approached by studying the physiology of pain, how it is manifested in nonverbal patients, and when and how pain should be treated.

PHYSIOLOGY OF PAIN

There is a physiologic explanation for pain. Pain receptors, called nociceptors, in the nervous system are stimulated by noxious events. The stimulus may be chemical, mechanical, or thermal. For example, chemical injury often is caused by substances such as prostaglandins and histamines produced in response to inflammation. Once a painful stimulus reaches a nociceptor cell, the information is transmitted to the brain via the spinal cord and the pain response begins. This includes the release of endogenous opioid endorphins, which function as natural analgesia. Often, in both chronic and acute situations, the level of pain exceeds the body's ability to provide relief. Chronic pain is prolonged and persistent; the body becomes habituated to nervous system responses and no longer provides adequate endogenous pain control. Acute pain is of severe, sudden onset that overwhelms endogenous analgesic mechanisms. Because pain assessments generally are made at the acute onset of stress, less is known about the manifestations of chronic pain in animals. Acute pain is the predominant concern among critically ill patients.

ASSESSMENT AND RECOGNITION

What Does Pain Look Like?

In an effort to form a consensus on what animal pain looks like, several hundred veterinary personnel from four leading veterinary institutions were surveyed. The survey was a simple form asking the participant to list all criteria he or she used to determine whether a patient was experiencing pain. The results were tabulated and categorized by frequency of response and subcategorized by professional group (i.e., technician or clinician). The top responses, in order of frequency, were vocalization, increased heart rate, increased respiratory rate, restlessness, increased body temperature, increased blood pressure, abnormal posturing, inappetence, aggression, unwillingness to move, frequent changes in position, facial expression, trembling, depression, and insomnia. Also mentioned but less statistically significant were anxiety; nausea; pupillary enlargement; licking, chewing, or staring at site, poor mucous membrane color, salivation, decreased CO_2, and head pressing.

More than 50% of all participants cited "known painful condition or procedure" as a reason to treat for pain. Listed criteria other than physical manifestations were presence of one or more of the preceding signs without other attributable cause, intuition, and responsiveness to pain medication.

These findings are similar to those found in human neonates and infants, although there has been more attention to their facial expressions and measured hormonal responses. Increased heart rate and respiratory rate, vocalization, and increased body movements are listed among the top pain manifestations in both human and veterinary patients. Several things become clear from this study. Various types of veterinary personnel have similar criteria for evaluating pain in their patients. This means that there is agreement about what pain looks like, although it is not necessarily scientifically conclusive. It is also clear that the list of manifestations is extensive and at times contradictory (e.g., unwillingness to move and frequent position changes). The following signs and symptoms, in the absence of any other reasonable explanation, are reasons to suspect pain and consider treatment. These are the most common signs but by no means the only indicators of pain in veterinary patients.

- Increased heart rate
- Increased respiratory rate
- Increased blood pressure
- Increased temperature
- Vocalization
- Inability to rest or sleep
- Trembling
- Inappetence

When and How Should Pain Be Treated?

Scientific data support beneficial aspects of pain: it limits further aggravating activity, causes homeostatic regulating hormone release, and motivates the patient to seek medical attention. It has also been demonstrated that severe acute pain can have the following deleterious physiologic effects:

- Neuroendocrine responses such as excessive release of pituitary, adrenal, and pancreatic hormones, possibly resulting in nutritional, growth, development, and healing disturbances and immunosuppression.
- Cardiovascular compromise (increased arterial blood pressure, heart rate, and intracranial pressure and decreased perfusion).
- Respiratory rate increases accompanied by decreased po_2 or dyspnea.
- Coagulopathies such as thrombotic events, increased platelet reactivity, and disseminated intravascular coagulation.
- Complications associated with long-term recumbency caused by pain or depression.
- Poor nutritional intake and hypoproteinemia, resulting in slow healing.

Much less is known about the psychological effects of pain on animals, but it appears that these manifestations are numerous and detrimental and may include inappetence, insomnia, and depression.

Pain should be treated to inhibit its deleterious effects. Analgesia is not benign. Risks and potential complications are associated with most pain medications. The most common arguments for withholding analgesia are as follows:

- Pain medication may cause cardiovascular compromise in fragile patients.
- Sedation may inhibit movement and lead to respiratory complications.
- Anesthetics and analgesics may mask signs of progress or regression, complicating evaluation of patient status. Cardiovascular monitoring may be obscured by sedation.
- Pain is self-protective; that is, animals limit their own activity to minimize pain, and eliminating pain allows the patient to do further damage.
- Pain control measures may result in longer hospital stays and higher costs.

Because our interest is to alleviate animal pain, we must find ways to address these concerns without withholding analgesia. The expected changes in heart rate, respiration, blood pressure, and mentation that accompany analgesic use must be understood. Baseline assessments should be made before treatment. After treatment, follow-up assessments should be made at regular intervals.

More frequent cardiovascular monitoring may be needed in patients treated for severe pain. Pain treatment may result in diminished activity and a slower return to normal body functions (e.g., eating, drinking, walking), but these effects may be less detrimental than the recovery delays associated with persistent pain.

PAIN RELIEF

NONPHARMACOLOGIC INTERVENTIONS

Before pain medication is administered, every effort should be made to provide nonpharmacologic comfort to the patient. Differentiating between physical pain and other types of stress is the first step in assessment. Stressors such as boredom, thirst, anxiety, and the need to urinate or defecate can mimic the signs of pain. All these stressors must be addressed before one can determine whether the patient needs medication. In some cases, these efforts may obviate further treatment. Even when pain medication is administered, these comfort needs must be addressed continually.

Providing comfort includes attention to physical surroundings and perceived psychological needs. It should not be assumed that the patient will automatically assume a comfortable position. The patient may need to be placed in a position that reduces pressure on painful areas, facilitates adequate ventilation, and promotes sleep. Bedding, padding, and pillows can be used to provide additional support. Reducing light and sound can also encourage rest or sleep.

Assessing the patient's emotional needs may be more difficult because of the great variation in individual response to pain and stress. The critical care technician must become adept at recognizing the unique needs of each patient. Gentle stroking and calming speech can be potent means of easing stress. When distraction is more effective, the animal can be placed in an active area with many visual and auditory stimuli. In some cases, owner visits are very comforting to the patient. In others, the patient becomes too agitated by the visit or the apparent benefits are negated by the response to owner's leaving.

Patient comfort can also be improved by reducing painful events. Because many nursing interventions entail painful procedures (e.g., injections, venipuncture, catheter placement, suturing), increasing technical proficiency can prevent pain. Organizing treatments efficiently to reduce the total number of disturbances is another nonmedical pain reduction intervention.

Once the patient's physical and emotional needs have been addressed, the patient's comfort is reassessed. The following questions should be asked. Is the patient at an acceptable comfort level? Is it possible that the clinical signs are manifestations of pain? Are there any contraindications to giving pain medications? Can the patient be supported through any adverse effects of drug administration? What is the appropriate (safe and effective) medication for the patient? It is common practice in human and veterinary medicine for technicians to assess pain status and administer appropriately ordered analgesia by continually asking themselves these questions.

ANALGESIC DRUGS

The options for analgesia are increasing. Choosing the correct analgesic therapy involves understanding the pharmacokinetics of a wide range of drugs and the levels or type of pain associated with various conditions (Table 9-1). Also, great individual variation in human responsiveness to drugs has been recognized recently. In other words, the same drug can produce vastly different results in different patients. These differences are partly a result of individual genetic differences. They are also a result of the nonphysiologic factors that influence any pain state: anxiety, fear, sense of control, ethnocultural background, and meaning of the pain state to the patient. This phenomenon appears to hold true for animals as well. Individual personality, breed traits, and the psychological states of fear and anxiety all seem to play a role in the animal's perception of pain and response to treatment. This is one reason protocols for treating pain in veterinary patients have been difficult to develop. Ultimately, pain relief is the only true measure of successful treatment. The following

TABLE 9-1 Analgesic Drugs

	Indications	Dosage	Special Considerations
NSAIDs			
Aspirin	Mild analgesia and anti-inflammatory effects	Dogs: 10-25 mg/kg PO q 12 hr	GI side effects occur at higher dosages or with chronic use.
Carprofen (Rimadyl)	Long-term mild to moderate analgesia and good antiinflammatory effects	Dogs: 2.2 mg/kg PO q 12 hr	Safer than other NSAIDs; no adverse GI effects reported.
Flunixin meglumine (Banamine)	For orthopedic pain, musculoskeletal pain	Dogs: 0.5-1.0 mg/kg IV, IM, SQ, PO q 24 hr	Use limited to 3 consecutive days; causes GI ulceration.
Ketorolac tromethamine (Toradol)	Effective for acute pain	Dogs: 0.3-0.5 mg/kg IV, IM q 8-12 hr for 1-2 doses; 5-10 mg/dog PO Cats: 0.25 mg/kg IM q 8-12 hr for 1-2 doses	Do not exceed 10 mg total dosage. Do not use for >3 days in dogs or 1 day in cats.
Phenylbutazone	Chronic pain	Dogs: 15-20 mg/kg PO q 8-12 hr	Can cause bone marrow suppression, GI ulceration, kidney damage.
Opioids			
Buprenorphine	Moderate to severe pain	Dogs: 0.01-0.2 mg/kg SQ or IM q 8-12 hr Cats: 0.005-0.01 mg/kg IM q 12 hr	Partial μ-agonist. Difficult to reverse with naloxone.
Butorphenol (Torbutrol)	Moderate to severe pain	Dogs and cats: 0.2-1.0 mg/kg IM, IV, SQ, PO q 4-6 hr	κ-Agonist, μ-antagonist.
Fentanyl	Moderate to severe short-term pain	Dogs: 0.005-0.04 mg/kg IV, epidural q 0.5-1 hr	Short acting; can be given as CRI.
Fentanyl transdermal patch (Duragesic)	Persistent moderate to severe postsurgical pain	Dogs and cats (<10 kg): 25 μg/hr Dogs (10-20 kg): 50 μg/hr Dogs (20-30 kg): 75 μg/hr Dogs (>30 kg): 100 μg/hr	Long acting (up to 3 days); 12-24 hr until effective.
Meperidine (Demerol)	Moderate to severe pain, recommended for patients with pancreatitis	Dogs and cats: 2-10 mg/kg IM, SQ q 2-4 hr	Severe hypotension with IV use. Painful injection.
Morphine	Severe postoperative abdominal or orthopedic surgery–related pain	Dogs: 0.1-0.5 mg/kg IV, 0.5-1.0 mg/kg IM, SQ q 4 hr Cats: 0.1 mg/kg IM, SQ q 4 hr	Respiratory depression and vomiting. Use with caution in cats.

TABLE 9-1 Analgesic Drugs—cont'd

	Indications	Dosage	Special Considerations
Opioids—cont'd			
Naloxone	Reversal of opioid agonists	Dogs and cats: 0.04 mg/kg IM, IV, repeated as necessary	Pure opiate antagonist.
Oxymorphone	Severe, acute abdominal, thoracic, or orthopedic pain	Dogs: 0.005-0.2 mg/kg IM, IV, SQ, q 6 hr Cats: 0.1 mg/kg IM, IV, SQ q 6 hr	Excitatory in cats. Causes respiratory depression, auditory hypersensitivity, and altered thermoregulation.
Local anesthetics			
Bupivacaine	Long term (4-6 hr), good thoracic blocking action	Cumulative daily dosage not to exceed 8 mg/kg day 1 and 4 mg/kg thereafter, interpleural intercostal, epidural	Available as 0.25% to 0.5% with epinephrine.
Lidocaine	Short term (0.5-1.5 hr), can be given IV	Use as local block or as CRI at 25-35 μg/kg/min	Painful on injection. Can be mixed with $NaHCO_3$ 9:1 to reduce sting. Available in varying concentrations.

NSAIDs, Nonsteroidal antiinflammatory drugs; *GI,* gastrointestinal; *CRI,* constant-rate infusion.

information is meant as a guide to forming an initial treatment plan.

DRUG OPTIONS

Nonsteroidal Antiinflammatory Drugs. Nonsteroidal antiinflammatory drugs (NSAIDs) are among the most widely used analgesics in the treatment of chronic pain. However, they are not effective in treating acute pain. Patients with acute pain can be weaned to NSAIDs as their pain diminishes. NSAIDs are convenient to administer, are inexpensive, and provide long-lasting pain relief.

NSAIDs are also referred to as antiprostaglandins. Actually, NSAIDs do not directly inhibit prostaglandins but rather inhibit cyclooxygenase (COX), which synthesizes prostaglandin. There are two types of COX, type 1 (COX-1) and type 2 (COX-2). NSAIDs have effect on both types of COX. COX-2 gives rise to the group of prostaglandins that mediate the inflammatory response associated with pain. Therefore, COX-2 inhibition reduces inflammation, the desired effect of treatment with NSAIDs. However, COX-1 gives rise to the group of prostaglandins that maintain platelet function and gastrointestinal mucosal integrity. Therefore, the main disadvantage of extended NSAID administration is COX-1 inhibition resulting in mucosal sloughing, GI ulceration, and bleeding. Ideally, NSAID therapy should be directed at inhibiting only COX-2, thereby reducing inflammation while eliminating the negative effects. Many new NSAIDs have emerged recently, such as carprofen (Rimadyl) and etodolac (Etogesic), which have been targeted toward COX-2 inhibition only. Research and development moves us closer to COX-2–specific NSAIDs that will allow long-term, safe use. Other non–COX-specific NSAIDs commonly used are aspirin, phenylbutazone, and flunixin meglumide.

Narcotics and Opioids. Opioids are the most commonly used analgesics in hospitalized critically ill or injured patients because of their efficacy, rapid onset of action, and safety. The efficacy of various opioids is determined by the specific receptors in the brain and spinal cord they affect. The receptors are classified as μ, κ, and Σ; μ- and κ-receptors are responsible for sedation, analgesia, and respiratory depression. κ-Receptors are responsible for analgesia and sedation. Σ-Receptors are less clinically relevant and are thought to be responsible for the adverse effects of opioid administration such as dysphoria, excitement, restlessness, and anxiety. Opioid drugs are classified as agonists (meaning that they stimulate the opioid receptors) or antagonists (meaning that they block particular opioid receptors). There are also mixed agonist and antagonist opioids that stimulate some receptors while blocking others and partial agonists with lesser effects. In general, pure agonists are the most potent opioids but also have the most severe adverse side effects. Side effects include vomiting, constipation, excitement, bradycardia, and panting, but the most severe side effect is respiratory depression. Pure antagonists reverse the narcotic properties of agonists. The availability of opioid antagonists makes opioid use safe because the drug effects can be removed rapidly. Mixed agonist and antagonist and partial agonist opioids can provide reasonably good analgesia without many of the deleterious side effects of pure agonists. Opioids are metabolized by the liver and excreted via the kidneys and should be used with caution in patients with renal or hepatic disease.

PURE AGONISTS

Pure agonists are the most potent opioid drugs. They provide excellent analgesia but can have adverse effects including respiratory and CNS depression, gastric stimulation, bradycardia, and hypotension. A disadvantage of pure opioids is habituation, which necessitates ever-increasing dosages to achieve therapeutic effects. Regimented treatment, or dosing at regular intervals, is helpful in maintaining an analgesic plane. Otherwise, a rollercoaster effect occurs, leaving the patient in varying degrees of pain between treatment. Keeping a patient out of pain always is more efficacious than repeatedly taking the patient out of pain. The type of opioid is chosen based on the degree of analgesia needed and the specific needs or limitations of the individual patient.

OXYMORPHONE

Oxymorphone probably is the most often used narcotic in veterinary critical care. It has a potency approximately 10 times greater than that of morphine and long duration (4 to 6 hours). Oxymorphone may cause less respiratory depression and gastrointestinal stimulation than morphine. Some patients experience dysphoria, which may include vocalization, panting, and sensory hypersensitivity. The cost of oxymorphone also may be prohibitive. The typical dosage is 0.05 to 0.1 mg/kg intravenously or intramuscularly.

MORPHINE SULFATE

Morphine often is used to provide maximal analgesia and sedation. Its low cost and similar efficacy make it preferable to oxymorphone in some cases. However, it has additional side effects, particularly systemic hypotension and vomiting, that make it less desirable in many instances. Cats seem to be particularly sensitive to morphine. The typical dosage for dogs is 1.0 to 1.5 mg/kg intravenously.

MEPERIDINE HYDROCHLORIDE

Meperidine is one half to one third weaker than morphine and has a shorter action. It may have fewer adverse GI effects. Intravenous meperidine causes a profound histamine release, resulting in severe systemic hypotension.

FENTANYL CITRATE

Fentanyl is an extremely potent synthetic opioid with rapid onset but short duration of action when administered intravenously or intramuscularly. It is efficiently used as a transdermal patch for long-term (3 days) analgesia. Fentanyl is contained in an adhesive patch of varying concentration to deliver

25, 75, or 100 μg/hr. Once applied to shaved, cleaned skin, the drug is absorbed continuously. Onset of action is from 12 to 24 hours, so supplemental analgesia is recommended during the initial treatment period. Use of mixed agonist and antagonist opioids reverses the effects of the fentanyl patch and should be avoided.

ANTAGONISTS

Opioid agonist analgesia, sedation, and side effects can be reversed rapidly with antagonists such as naloxone hydrochloride. Antagonists work by blocking opioid action at the μ-receptors. Onset of reversal occurs within 1 to 2 minutes of intravenous administration and can last for 1 to 4 hours. Treatment can be repeated when reversing narcotics with a longer duration. The typical dosage is 2 μg/kg intravenously.

MIXED AGONIST AND ANTAGONIST OPIOIDS

Mixed agonist and antagonist opioids provide analgesia at some opioid receptors while inhibiting or decreasing stimulation at the μ -receptors. Their action results in diminished analgesia and decreased side effects. These drugs partially reverse pure agonists by blocking action at the μ-receptors.

BUTORPHANOL TARTRATE

Butorphanol is a κ-agonist and a μ-antagonist. The overall effectiveness of butorphanol is questionable. It is expensive compared to morphine but has a markedly lowered incidence of respiratory depression and dysphoria. Butorphanol is used in patients experiencing mild to moderate pain. It is available in oral and injectable forms. The typical dosage is 0.1 to 0.8 mg/kg intravenously.

BUPRENORPHINE

Buprenorphine is a partial μ-agonist that is 30 times more potent than morphine and of longer duration because of its slow dissociation from receptors. Although buprenorphine may have greater sedative properties than other opioids, its use is limited to patients with mild to moderate pain because at high dosages buprenorphine probably has antagonistic effects on the μ-receptors and, in effect, reverses itself. The typical dosage is 0.006-0.02 mg/kg intravenously.

Local and Regional Anesthetics. There has been a great deal of recent work in local or regional analgesia. Applying analgesia directly to the affected nerve endings can provide excellent pain control while reducing or eliminating the need for systemic drugs. Local anesthetics work by disrupting neural information transmission by axons at the treatment site. Blocking neuronal activity also results in an expected loss of sensation and function at the area. This loss of motor control is not seen with systemic analgesia. Local anesthesia should be used with caution in patients who are at risk for self-injury such as those who have undergone orthopedic surgery.

EPIDURAL ANESTHESIA AND ANALGESIA IN DOGS AND CATS

Lumbosacral epidural administration of local anesthetics and analgesics is a valuable way to produce segmental anesthesia or analgesia in dogs and cats. It is an easy, safe, and effective way to alleviate pain, especially after procedures involving body parts caudal to the ribs, and should be considered an adjunct or alternative to other drug administration methods.

ANATOMIC ASPECTS

Three different layers of protective and supportive sheets (meninges; singular meninx) surround the spinal cord. Firmly adhered to the cord, the pia mater is the deepest, most vascular layer. It is highly cellular and has attachments to the most external meninx, the dura mater, along the lateral margin of the spinal cord (denticulate ligaments). These ligaments suspend the spinal cord within the cavity formed by the dura mater.

The intermediate meninx is the arachnoid membrane, another mainly cellular layer that is connected to the pia mater by numerous membranous bridges, the arachnoid trabeculae. The space between the arachnoid and the pia mater contains cerebrospinal fluid (CSF). CSF pressure holds the arachnoid against the dura mater. The two are separated only by a very thin layer of fluid. This fluid film allows sliding of the arachnoid with respect to the dura mater. The depth of the subarachnoid space varies because the arachnoid contacts the dura mater, whereas the pia mater follows every irregularity of the spinal cord's surface.

The most superficial of the three layers, the dura mater, is a tough, fibrous sheath that encloses the spinal cord and the nerves that originate in the spinal cord. Around these nerve roots the dura mater forms protective cuffs, the dural sheaths that accompany the nerves traversing the vertebral canal.

The epidural space is located between the dura mater and the bony walls of the vertebral canal. This space contains loose connective tissue, blood vessels, and adipose tissue. In larger dogs, the spinal cord terminates approximately at the caudal margin of the sixth or the cranial margin of the seventh lumbar vertebra (L6-L7; Figure 9-1). In smaller dogs and in cats the spinal cord extends further caudad, about the length of one vertebral body (L7-S1, the lumbosacral junction); therefore, in these animals it seems to be safer to administer epidural injections at the sacrococcygeal junction or first intercoccygeal space. The cavity formed by the dura mater (dural sac) generally extends about two vertebral bodies more caudal than the spinal cord.

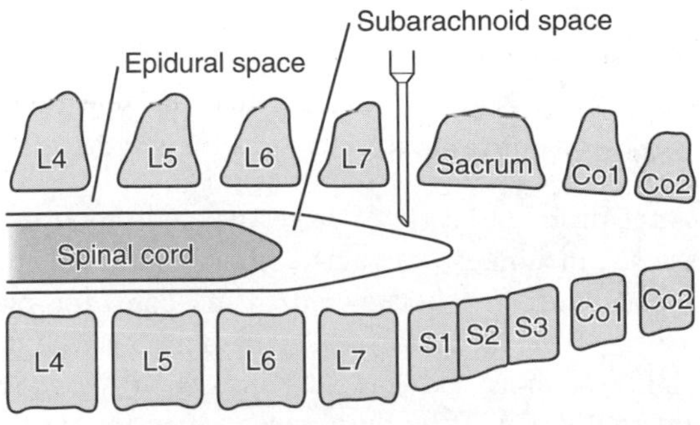

Figure 9-1

Spinal column of the dog at the lumbosacral junction.

Consequently, in larger dogs (more than 15 kg body weight) the dural sac, but not the spinal cord, is accessible at the level of the lumbosacral junction. In smaller dogs and in cats, the spinal cord probably is present at the lumbosacral junction.

Definitions and Clinical Implications

The epidural space occupies the large volume between the walls of the vertebral canal and the dura mater. The amount of fat in the epidural space is not necessarily correlated to the amount of body fat. In patients that have lost a lot of weight within a short period of time, there may still be a considerable amount of fat in the epidural space. The more fat in the epidural space, the more cranial the effects of epidurally administered drugs extend.

Old age also can influence the volume of injection necessary to produce a clinical effect. Calcified and fibrous tissue can occlude the intervertebral foramina (where the spinal nerves exit the vertebral canal) and decrease the amount of injectate that leaks from the epidural space, thereby increasing the cephalad distance over which a given volume will travel in the epidural space.

On the bottom of the vertebral canal are large venous plexi. In a patient with reduced venous return, these plexi are engorged, which increases the probability of injecting into the vascular bed. This can lead to increased and potentially toxic plasma levels of thc injected substances.

Spinal or intrathecal injection aims for the space filled with CSF that lies between the arachnoid and the pia mater. When drugs are injected into the spinal column, they can be administered inadvertently into this space. This is more likely in cats because of the more caudal spread of the subarachnoid space in this species. Most drugs that we administer epidurally can be injected safely into this subarachnoid space, but injection volumes have to be much lower (50% to 60%) to obtain the same spatial distribution because the subarachnoid space is much smaller, so injected substances are likely to be carried further cephalad with CSF flow.

In the literature about epidural techniques, the terms *epidural anesthesia* and *epidural analgesia* often are used interchangeably. For didactic reasons, the term *epidural anesthesia* should be for injection of local anesthetics into the epidural space and *epidural analgesia* used for administration of drugs that produce analgesia (e.g., opioids, α-2 agonists, ketamine).

Injection Volumes

Because of variations in age, nutritional status, and desired segment of anesthesia or analgesia, there is still no golden rule for determining epidural injection volume. However, most authors consider volumes of 1 ml/4.5 to 5 kg body weight (0.22 to 0.24 ml/kg) for anesthesia or analgesia of segments caudal to the umbilicus and 1 ml/3.5 to 3.8 kg (0.26 to 0.28 ml/kg) for the segments as cranial as the tenth to thirteenth thoracic vertebra (T10-T13) to be effective.

Calculating injection volumes based on body weight presents several problems. If the patient is obese, the calculated volume could be too large for the size of the vertebral canal because the large amount of adipose tissue in the epidural space could cause a given volume to spread further forward than expected.

For administering local anesthetics only, the injection volume can also be calculated by the following formula: $y = 0.13x - 3.8$, with y the injection volume in milliliters and x being the distance in centimeters between the occiput and the base of the tail.

The volume of the epidural space also varies between individuals. Some authors consider injection volumes to be safe up to approximately 6 ml for animals up to 35 kg. As in cats, the spinal cord is likely to extend to the lumbosacral junction or even further, so epidural administration could be performed more safely at the sacrococcygeal junction or the first intercoccygeal space with injection volumes of 0.3 to 0.9 ml total, although it has been done at the lumbosacral junction with volumes of 0.2 ml/kg.

For animals with an increase in intraabdominal pressure (ascites, pregnancy), the calculated volume should be reduced by approximately 25%. If the calculated dosage of a drug gives a smaller volume, then it should be made up to the calculated volume with 0.9% sterile saline solution.

Local Anesthetics

Local anesthetics are the substances most commonly injected into the epidural space and produce reliable, dose-dependent epidural anesthesia. They stabilize the axonal membrane of a nerve by blocking the influx of sodium and in this way interrupting the passage of nerve impulses. It is unclear where exactly this local anesthetic block has its effect after epidural administration. Three possibilities are considered: a paravertebral block after foraminal leakage, a block of the intradural spinal nerve roots (this seems to be the most prominent mechanism), and a spinal cord block. However, local anesthetics do not act on specific receptors, and their effects on different types of nerves are dose dependent. The smaller the diameter of a nerve fiber, the lower the local anesthetic dosage needed to produce a block of conduction. Therefore sympathetic nerves are the first, sensory nerves intermediate, and motor nerve fibers the last to be blocked with increasing concentrations of local anesthetics.

Local anesthetics administered epidurally may enter the CSF, the epidural venous blood, and lymph. A variety of local anesthetics have been used for epidural anesthesia, and the selection is based on the patient's size and the extent, onset, and duration of the desired anesthesia.

A 2% solution of lidocaine, procaine, or carbocaine produces anesthesia after 10 to 15 minutes for 60 to 90 minutes. The addition of 1:200,000 epinephrine or adrenaline to the local anesthetic may prolong the duration of action. Bupivacaine as a 0.75% solution has a slower onset (20 to 30 minutes) but a longer duration of action (about 4 hours). Etidocaine in a 1% solution has been shown to produce surgical anesthesia for 4 to 6 hours. Ropivacaine (0.75%) has a time of onset similar to that of bupivacaine, and the duration of motor blockade has been found to be about 1 hour and 40 minutes.

Epidural application of local anesthetics produces some loss of motor function. The extent and duration are dosage (concentration and volume) dependent, but at the suggested dosages, there is a nearly constant motor blockade for the hind limbs.

Epidural anesthesia as far cranial as the first thoracic segments (T4-T5) has been reported not to affect cardiovascular or respiratory function in healthy, awake dogs. However, in anesthetized, aged, or sick dogs, hypotension can occur, so under these circumstances intravenous fluids should be administered and vasopressors held on hand.

In general, the side effects that can be associated with epidural or subarachnoid administration of local anesthetics include hypoventilation (caused by respiratory muscle paralysis), sympathetic blockade–related hypotension, hypoglycemia, and Horner syndrome, and toxic plasma levels can cause muscle twitches, coma, convulsion, and circulatory depression (i.e., after inadvertent intravenous injection). The initial sign of hypoventilation usually is the change from thoracic to abdominal breathing as the intercostal muscles become paralyzed.

Opioids

Since the discovery of opioid receptors in the spinal cord (μ, κ, Δ, Σ), several opioids have been used for epidural or intrathecal administration, but still it is unclear whether they act directly on the opioid receptors of the spinal cord or after systemic absorption and redistribution.

Because they alleviate somatic and visceral pain (antinociceptive action) but do not block impulses of sensory, motor, or sympathetic function, their effect is called selective spinal analgesia. This and the prolonged duration of analgesic effects compared to other drugs and compared to other methods of administration are the major advantages of epidurally administered opioids. Furthermore, epidural administration of opioids produces a lower level of sedation than does intramuscular administration.

The analgesic efficacy of opioids increases if they are given preemptively. Therefore preoperative epidural administration is recommended. In addition, epidurally administered opioids reduce the need for inhalant anesthetics.

For a better understanding of the different times of onset and duration of action of the single opioids, it is important to understand that their lipid solubility affects the spread of the administered solution in the epidural and subarachnoid space. The less lipid soluble an opioid, the longer it is present in an unbound form in the spinal canal and consequently the more time is available for cephalad distribution. This explains why low-efficacy (low–lipid solubility) opioids, such as morphine, must be injected very slowly into the spinal canal (over 1 to 2 minutes). Moreover, low–lipid solubility opioids have been found to produce a greater magnitude of tolerance. On the other hand, low–lipid solubility opioids have a longer duration of action.

The most important side effect of epidural opioids is respiratory depression, which can be biphasic or delayed (for up to 12 hours). This may be even more marked for the less lipid-soluble opioids such as morphine. Animals that have been given epidural or intrathecal morphine should be held in a controlled environment (intensive care unit, dyspnea watch) and observed for at least 24 hours. Centrally mediated increases in vagal tone are responsible for the bradycardia sometimes associated with systemic absorption of epidural opioids. Urinary retention has been found to be present in 15% to 100% of people who received epidural morphine, and although the incidence in animals has not been studied so far, the bladder should be emptied before recovery from general anesthesia. Delayed gastrointestinal motility and nausea seem to be related to epidural morphine in people as well, but it is not clear whether these side effects also occur in animals. Pruritus has been reported as a side effect in dogs as well as in humans (Table 9-2).

The opioids shown are ordered with increasing lipid solubility. The lower end of the dosage ranges

TABLE 9-2 Epidural Opioids: Dosages and Time Factors in Dogs

Opioid	Dosage (mg/kg)	Onset (min)	Duration (hr)
Morphine sulfate PF	0.05-0.15	30-60	10-24
Meperidine hydrochloride	0.5-1.5	10-30	5-20
Oxymorphone hydrochloride	0.05-0.15	20-40	7-10
Fentanyl citrate	0.001-0.01	15-20	4-6

PF, Preservative free.

is more applicable to larger breed dogs, and the higher dosages are for smaller dogs. Because cats occasionally have adverse reactions to higher opioid dosages, the lower dosages should be applied to cats. In cats morphine has been given successfully to produce epidural analgesia at 0.1 mg/kg.

OTHER DRUGS

α_2-Adrenergic agonists act primarily by stimulating α_2 adrenoceptors, inhibiting neurotransmitter release. In the human spinal cord there is a high density of α_2 adrenoceptors. This primary site of activity may be augmented by a secondary local anesthetic–like effect blocking axonal conduction.

Xylazine given epidurally or intrathecally is an effective analgesic in cattle, horses, and sheep.

At a dosage of 0.2 to 0.25 mg/kg given epidurally to dogs, xylazine has analgesic effects but only minimal cardiovascular side effects.

Medetomidine has been given to dogs epidurally at a dosage of 0.005 to 0.015 mg/kg. It can provide analgesia similar to that of epidural oxymorphone, but bradycardia and second-degree atrioventricular block are common side effects. Enhanced analgesia has been found when medetomidine is given with an opioid.

CONTRAINDICATIONS

Absolute contraindications for epidural or subarachnoid injection are infection at or near the injection site, hypovolemia, bleeding disorders and anticoagulation thereof, central or peripheral nervous diseases, anatomic abnormalities of the spinal column, and spinal trauma. Bacteremia, sepsis, and neurologic disorders are relative contraindications (Technical Tip Box 9-1).

TOPICAL ANALGESIA

Applying topical analgesia to the surface skin or mucosa can reduce pain associated with minor procedures such as wound suturing, venipuncture, arterial puncture, or nasal cannulization. Solutions of lidocaine, bupivacaine, tetracaine, and epinephrine can be used alone or in various combinations to desensitize the application site. Gauze pads soaked with solutions can be applied directly to the site. Alternatively, several commercially prepared topical anesthetic creams and jellies can be applied as a thick paste. Regardless of application method, 20 to 30 minutes of direct contact time is needed to ensure effective analgesia.

LOCAL INFILTRATION

Injecting lidocaine or bupivacaine into local tissue can reduce pain associated with various painful procedures. This technique is useful for arterial catheter placement, thoracocentesis, abdominocentesis, and bone marrow sampling. The entry area is infiltrated with small amounts of anesthetic. Pain reduction is expected at 5 to 10 minutes after injection.

INTRABODY CAVITY

Infusing local anesthetics directly into body cavities provides nonsystemic analgesia at the site of injury. Lidocaine or bupivacaine generally is used.

Box 9-1 Technical Tip: *Epidural Anesthesia and Analgesia*

Increasing the percentage of inspired oxygen with a face mask or endotracheal tube helps prevent the sedated or anesthetized patient from becoming hypoxic. Intravenous fluids should be administered (crystalloids, 10 ml/kg/hr) to help prevent hypotension that may result from autonomic blockade. The animal should be placed on a padded surface and temperature should be measured and if necessary corrected. The monitoring should include respiratory frequency and adequacy, heart rate, pulse quality, and blood pressure.

The animal is placed on the surface in sternal recumbency (or lateral if a more ipsilateral effect is desired) with the legs bent forward (to expose the lumbosacral junction). For ipsilateral anesthesia or analgesia the patient must be left for the duration of onset in an unchanged position.

Items Needed

- Clippers
- Sedatives, if animal is not anesthetized
- Antiseptic solutions for surgical preparation
- Sterile gloves
- Sterile drapes
- Sterile saline solution (0.9%)
- Local anesthetic (2% lidocaine) for infiltration at the puncture site if the patient is not anesthetized
- New vial of the preservative-free drug(s) to be administered
- 3 Sterile syringes (1 for infiltration of anesthesia, 1 for sterile saline, 1 for drugs to administer epidurally) and suitable sterile needles
- Spinal needle (18- to 22-gauge Tuohy, Crawford, or Quincke)
- Epidural catheter tray

Procedure

1. Clip area generously, surgically prepare, and drape.
2. Place thumb and middle of finger of one hand on the iliac crests. With the index finger palpate the dorsal processes of the lumbar and sacral vertebrae in a cranial and caudal direction. The dorsal process of the seventh lumbar vertebrae is identified and the three fingers should form a triangle with its base between thumb and middle finger. Just caudal to this is the lumbosacral junction, which generally is perceivable as the deepest depression between the midline bone structures. In obese dogs, it can be helpful to mark (with an indelible marker) iliac crests, seventh lumbar, and first sacral dorsal spinal processes before the surgical preparation is done.

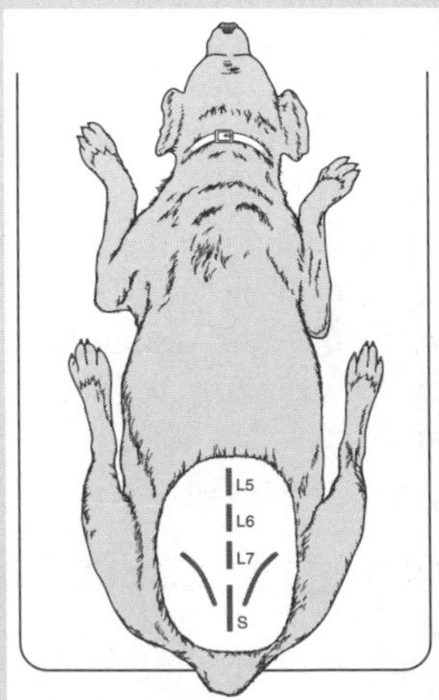

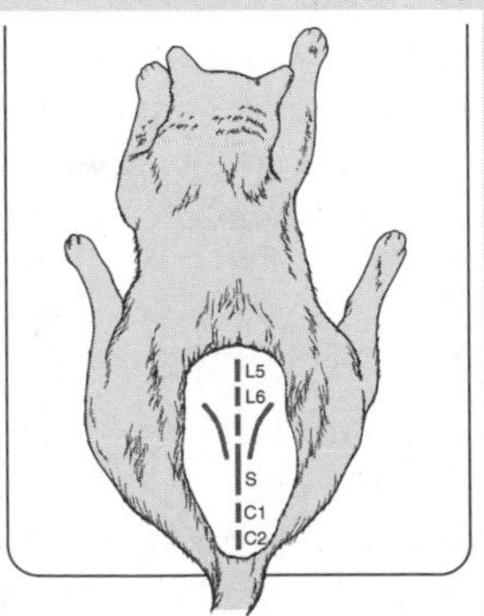

Box 9-1 Technical Tip: *Epidural Anesthesia and Analgesia—cont'd*

Procedure—cont'd

3. Surgically prepare the area.
4. Infiltrate puncture site with 1 to 2 ml of 2% lidocaine solution.
5. Insert needle caudal to the spinal process of the seventh lumbar vertebra (where the index finger is) and strictly on midline advance until a distinct popping sensation is felt. This resistance results from penetration of the interarcuate ligament (ligamentum flavum), which the needle should penetrate perpendicularly (this causes less damage). There are two ways to identify the positioning in the epidural space:
   Loss of resistance test: a test injection of 2 to 3 ml with air or 0.9% sterile saline should be feasible with no resistance.
   Hanging drop test: a few drops of sterile saline are placed in the hub of the needle. If the positioning is correct, the saline should be drawn into the epidural space. This method is not always a reliable indicator and is not applicable with an animal in lateral recumbency.
6. Allow 30 to 60 seconds to observe the needle for outflow of CSF or blood. The presence of CSF indicates a puncture of the subarachnoid space. Under these circumstances, the injections could still be made, but with a 50% dosage reduction. Presence of blood flow from the needle indicates the puncture of a vessel or hematoma. Epidural injection should not be made.
7. If the needle has been positioned correctly, the injection can be made slowly (over 60 to 90 seconds). This should avoid stinging (bupivacaine) or patchy anesthesia or analgesia.

If a sacrococcygeal or intercoccygeal injection is planned (i.e., in cats), the procedure is analogous. The sacrococcygeal junction can be identified easily by slightly moving the tail up and down. (Draping of the tail is necessary.)

If epidural analgesia is necessary for continued pain control, the catheter is inserted through the needle, directed cranially. This can be secured to the animal and left in place for intermittent injections or a slow continual drip of the chosen drug.

Joint Space

Effective analgesia before and during orthopedic surgery has been achieved by injecting local anesthetics directly into the joint space. Intraarticular morphine has also been shown to reduce joint pain. It has been suggested that applying a tourniquet above the joint for 10 minutes after injection greatly enhances drug efficacy.

Peritoneal Space

Patients with abdominal pain, generally from abdominal surgery or acute pancreatitis, may benefit by local anesthetic infusion. The anesthetic must be delivered in fairly large volumes of saline to provide maximum interperitoneal surface contact. Risks of the increase in abdominal pressure must be weighed against the benefit of analgesia.

Pleural Space

Interpleural bupivacaine infusion after thoracotomy surgery may have some analgesic benefit. Bupivacaine (1.5 to 2 mg/kg) is injected via an indwelling chest tube into the pleural space. Analgesia is thought to occur by direct blocking of the intercostal nerves. For maximum coverage, the affected side must be down 10 minutes after injection to allow the analgesic to follow gravity and be around the pain site. Drug absorption through the pleural tissue should be considered.

Sedatives and Tranquilizers

Although tranquilizing agents are not considered analgesics, their concurrent use in pain management should not be overlooked. Combining sedatives such as acepromazine or a benzodiazepine with opioid analgesia can reduce stress and anxiety. The analgesic effects often are enhanced, reducing the opioid analgesic dosage needed.

Monitoring Drug Effects

Perhaps the most confounding aspect of pain management is assessing pain and pain relief after treatment. The abatement or cessation of clinical signs associated with pain is the best indicator of successful treatment. Careful monitoring of cardiovascular status and mentation are vital to achieving good pain management without detrimental side effects. Effective treatment may result in cardiovascular or respiratory depression, diminished movement, inability to eat or drink, urinary and fecal incontinence, and hypothermia. Supportive care is integral to pain management. The complications and side effects of treatment are monitored and corrected aggressively. Temperature, heart rate, pulses, respiratory rate and effort, mucous membrane color, and capillary refill time should be measured frequently. Treatment may include fluid volume and hydration support, nutritional supplementation, urinary catheterization, external warming, and even oxygen augmentation. Veterinary critical care professionals must eliminate pain and stress wherever possible and treat the adverse consequences as needed.

PAIN MANAGEMENT CHECKLIST

Veterinary technicians play a vital role in pain management. The technician is most likely to first detect signs of pain and request pain treatment. Critical care technicians can improve pain management practice in the following ways.

- Establish pain alleviation as a standard of care.
- Recognize the signs of pain.
- Respect clients' observations and assessment of pain in their pets.
- Understand and overcome the barriers to assessment and treatment.
- Be aware of known painful procedures and surgeries and encourage preemptive and immediate postprocedure treatment.
- Reduce incidence of painful procedures by combining treatments efficiently.
- Use techniques to minimize pain (e.g., use ECG snaps instead of alligator clips and use indwelling catheters to obtain blood samples).
- Minimize pain associated with critical care techniques by improving technical skill and helping to develop new technologies that minimize pain.
- Differentiate pain from other distress such as confinement, boredom, separation from owners, insomnia, fear, and need to urinate or defecate.
- Understand the treatment options and encourage appropriate types of therapy.
- Monitor the effects of various drugs in a coherent manner to evaluate treatment efficacy.
- Educate other animal caregivers about pain management issues.

BIBLIOGRAPHY

Anand KJS, McGrath PJ: Pain in neonates, *Pain Res Clin Manage* 5, 1993.

Bradley R, Withrow S, Heath R, et al: Epidural analgesia in the dog, *Vet Surg* 9:153, 1980.

Branson KR, Ko JC, Tranquilli WJ, et al: Duration of analgesia induced by epidurally administered morphine and medetomidine in dogs, *J Vet Pharmacol Ther* 16:369, 1993.

Bromage P, Camporesi E, Durant P, et al: Rostral spread of epidural morphine, *Anesthesiology* 56:431, 1982.

Broome ME, Tanzillo H: Differentiating between pain and agitation in premature neonates, *J Perinat Neonat Nurs* 4(1):53, 1990.

Craig KKD et al: Pain in the preterm neonate: behavioral and physiological indices, *Pain* 52:287, 1993.

Day T, Pepper W, Tobias T, et al: Comparison of intra-articular and epidural morphine for analgesia following stifle arthrotomy in dogs, *Vet Surg* 24:522, 1995.

Dodman N, Clark G, Court M: Epidural opioid administration for postoperative pain relief in the dog. In Short C, Pozrak A, eds: *Animal pain,* New York, 1992, Churchill Livingstone.

Durant P, Yaksh T: Epidural injections of bupivacaine, morphine, fentanyl, lofentanyl, and DADL in chronically implanted rats: a pharmacologic and pathologic study, *Anesthesiology* 64:43, 1986.

Fletcher T: Spinal cord and meninges. In Evans H, Christensen G, eds: *Miller's anatomy of the dog,* Philadelphia, 1979, WB Saunders.

Golder F, Pascoe P, Bailey C, et al: The effect of epidural morphine on the minimum alveolar concentration of isoflurane in cats, *J Vet Anaesth* 25, 1998.

Greene S, Keegan R, Weil A: Cardiovascular effects after epidural injection of xylazine in isoflurane-anesthetized dogs, *Vet Surg* 24:283, 1995.

Heath RB: Lumbosacral epidural management, *Vet Clin North Am Small Anim Pract* 22:417, 1992.

Hellyer PW: Management of acute and surgical pain. In Murtaugh RJ, ed: *Seminars in veterinary medicine and surgery (small animal),* vol 12, no 2, 1997.

Hendrix P, Raffe M, Robinson E, et al: Epidural administration of bupivacaine, morphine, or their combination for postoperative analgesia in dogs, *J Am Vet Med Assoc* 209:598, 1996.

Keegan RD, Greene SA, Weil AB: Cardiovascular effects of epidurally administered morphine and a xylazine-morphine combination in isoflurane-anesthetized dogs, *Am J Vet Res* 56:496, 1995.

Klide AM: Anatomy of the spinal cord and how the spinal cord is affected by local anesthetics and other drugs, *Vet Clin North Am Small Anim Pract* 22:413, 1992.

Maierl J, Reindl S, Knospe C: Observations on epidural anesthesia in cats from the anatomical viewpoint, *Tierarztl Prax* 25:267, 1997.

Mathews KA: *Veterinary emergency and critical care manual,* Eden Mills, Ontario, 1996, Lifelearn.

McMurphy RM: Postoperative epidural analgesia, *Vet Clin North Am Small Anim Pract* 23:703, 1993.

National Academy Press: *Recognition and alleviation of pain and distress in laboratory animals,* 1992, National Academy of Sciences.

Nolte J, Watney C, Hall L: Cardiovascular effects of epidural blocks in dogs, *J Small Anim Pract* 24:17, 1983.

Otto K, Piepenbrock S, Rischke B, et al: Effects of epidural xylazine on EEG responses to surgical stimulation during isoflurane anaesthesia in dogs, *J Vet Anaesth* 24:33, 1997.

Papich MG: Principles of analgesic drug therapy. In Murtaugh RJ, ed: *Seminars in veterinary medicine and surgery (small animal),* vol 12, no 2, 1997.

Pascoe PJ: Local and regional anesthesia and analgesia. In Murtaugh RJ, ed: *Seminars in veterinary medicine and surgery (small animal),* vol 12, no 2, 1997.

Pascoe PJ: Advantages and guidelines for using epidural drugs for analgesia, *Vet Clin North Am Small Anim Pract* 22:421, 1992.

Popilskis S, Kohn D, Laurent L: Efficacy of epidural morphine versus intravenous morphine for post-thoracotomy pain in dogs, *J Vet Anaesth* 20:21, 1993.

Pybus D, Torda T: Dose-effect relationships of extradural morphine, *Br J Anaesth* 54:1259, 1982.

Rollin BE: *The unheeded cry,* New York, Oxford University Press, 1989.

Sackman JE: Pain management. In McCurnin DM, ed: *Clinical textbook for veterinary technicians,* Philadelphia, 1994, WB Saunders.

Short CE, Van Poznak A: *Animal pain,* New York, 1992, Churchill Livingstone.

Skarda R: Local and regional anesthetic and analgesic techniques: dogs. In Thurmon J, Tranquilli W, Benson G, eds: *Lumb & Jones' veterinary anesthesia,* ed 3, Baltimore, 1996, Williams & Wilkins.

Stevens BJ et al: Issues of assessment of pain and discomfort in neonates, *J Obstet Gynecol Neonatal Nurs* 849, 1995.

Tyler DC, Krane EJ: Pediatric pain, *Adv Pain Res Ther* 432, 1990.

Valverde A, Dyson D, McDonell W, et al: Use of epidural morphine in the dog for pain relief, *Vet Compar Othopaed Trauma* 2:55, 1989.

Vesal N, Cribb PH, Frketic M: Postoperative analgesic and cardiopulmonary effects in dogs of oxymorphone administered epidurally and intramuscularly, and medetomidine administered epidurally: a comparative clinical study, *Vet Surg* 25:361, 1996.

Yaksh T, Sosnowski M: Spinal opioid analgesia: characterization of acute tolerance in an animal model. In Estefanous F, ed: *Opioids in anesthesia II.* Stoneham, Mass, 1991, Butterworth-Heinemann.

Chapter 10

Anesthesia

Anesthesia is defined as the loss of sensation. The goal of general anesthesia is to provide a state of reversible unconsciousness with adequate analgesia and muscle relaxation in such a way that it does not jeopardize the patient's health. Delivering safe anesthesia to a critically ill small animal is one of the most important and often one of the most challenging and stressful tasks of a veterinary technician. In many emergencies, under direct supervision of the attending veterinarian the technician must provide both anesthesia and technical assistance in the operating room. This practice often is necessary but is not recommended. Critically ill or unstable patients demand the undivided attention of one anesthetist.

The old adage that there is no safe anesthesia, just safe anesthetists holds true especially for anesthesia of critically ill or injured patients. Referring to the American Society of Anesthesiologists' classification of the risk of death as a complication of anesthesia (from class I, the lowest risk, to class V, the highest; Box 10-1), critically ill or injured patients often are in class IV or V and are unstable. It would be ideal to be able to stabilize all patients before anesthetizing them; however, this may not be possible. Some patients cannot be stabilized or treated successfully without surgery. The patient who cannot breathe because of a diaphragmatic hernia, the patient who was hit by a car and has a severe hemoabdomen that continues to bleed, and the patient with septic peritonitis are all examples of animals that need surgery even though they are at high risk. The technician must be familiar not only with anesthetic agents and their use but also with invasive and noninvasive monitoring of critically ill and injured patients. These patients may have little in the way of reserves, and the anesthetist must understand respiratory and cardiovascular physiology and the pathophysiology of the disease process. Only in this manner can they provide anesthesia safely and support the patient effectively.

Some of these patients may need anesthesia as they arrive in the emergency room. Some of them may need surgery within the first few minutes or hours. This chapter attempts to provide an overview of anesthesia for these critically ill or injured patients. The focus is on balanced anesthesia, which involves administering multiple drugs to the patient, each for a specific purpose. It is assumed that the reader has a basic understanding of anesthetic equipment, anesthetic drugs, and basic monitoring, and the reader is referred to general anesthesia texts for these specifics.

GOALS FOR SUCCESS

Maintaining the ABCs of airway, breathing, and circulation is as important in the anesthetized patient as in the awake patient. Each of these goals is discussed throughout this chapter. The goals are to establish and maintain a patent airway, ensure that breathing is as normal as possible, and ensure adequate circulation while the patient is anesthetized. This helps maximize the delivery of oxygen and nutrients to the tissues at all times. Young, healthy patients undergoing elective surgery usu-

Box 10-1 Classes of Anesthesia Risk

Class 1: No systemic disease, elective procedure considered not life-threatening.
Class 2: Very mild systemic disease or age >5 yr, elective procedure, procedure not life-threatening.
Class 3: Mild systemic disease or illness, procedure >2 hr long, or possibly life-threatening procedure.
Class 4: Moderate systemic disease or illness, procedure >5 hr long, or life-threatening procedure.
Class 5: Severe systemic disease or illness.
Class 5: Unstable, includes patients that are unstable; also:
E: Emergency; any procedure done on a non-elective emergency basis.
C: Catastrophic; any procedure considered catastrophic or immediately necessary.
The higher the classification, the more morbidity and mortality is expected:
Class 1: 0.01% morbidity or complication rate, 0.001% death rate
Class 2: 0.1%-1% complication rate, 0.01%-0.1% death rate
Class 3: 5%-10% complication rate, 0.1%-1% death rate
Class 4: 10%-30% complication rate, 1%-5% death rate
Class 5: 30%-50% complication rate, 10%-25% death rate
Class 5 Unstable E: 50%-80% complication rate, 25%-50% death rate
Class 5 Unstable C: 80%-95% complication rate, 50%-75% death rate

ally can cope with the adverse effects of general anesthesia. This may not be so for the critically ill or injured patient. There are five physiologic goals of general anesthesia with regard to the cardiopulmonary system: ensure adequate hemoglobin levels, ensure adequate preload (venous volume returning to heart), ensure adequate cardiac contractility, ensure adequate oxygen delivery at the capillary level, and ensure adequate cellular oxygenation uptake and elimination of cellular waste products.

The critically ill or injured patient must be intubated and maintained on 100% oxygen when general anesthesia is provided. Assisted ventilation always is indicated—either using mechanical ventilation or hand-bagging the patient—and may make the difference between adequate and inadequate oxygen delivery to the alveoli and carbon dioxide removal. Excess carbon dioxide levels secondary to hypoventilation cause acidosis, which leads to vasodilation, poor cardiac function, and dysfunction of metabolic enzyme systems. There must be sufficient hemoglobin to carry the oxygen. The hemoglobin should be kept between 7 and 10 g/dl (hematocrit of 20% to 30%). Cardiac output, or the blood that carries the oxygen to the peripheral tissues, depends on adequate preload and an effective pump (heart muscle). Very high heart rates do not allow the heart to fill properly before pumping (diastolic time) and therefore decrease cardiac output and coronary circulation. Irregular rhythms may indicate poor coordination of the heart muscle as it contracts. Decreased preload can result from inadequate circulating volume, vasodilation or venodilation, or a combination of the two. Thus, if surgery is to be successful, the goals before, during, and after anesthesia must be to keep each of these physiologic parameters as normal as possible.

Critically ill or injured patients respond to analgesics, sedatives, and anesthetics differently than do healthy animals, for a variety of reasons, including decreased distribution volume, decreased plasma protein levels and acidosis leading to higher concentrations of the active form of the drug, and decreased metabolism secondary to decreased hepatic function, acidosis, and hypothermia. For these reasons, dosages of most anxiolytics, analgesics, and anesthetics should be reduced to 25% to 50% of normal and titrated to effect. In general, all drugs should be given intravenously or via the epidural route in the critically ill or injured patient because absorption from the oral and subcutaneous routes is unpredictable. If needed, intramuscular injections should be given in the epaxial muscles (the muscles dorsal and lateral to the vertebra in the region of the thoracolumbar spine) because of more sustained blood flow to these muscles. Intraosseous drug administration can be effective in very small patients, birds, and exotic animals (Box 10-2).

PREANESTHETIC EXAMINATION, EVALUATION, AND READINESS

Physical Examination and Preanesthetic Diagnostics

All patients must undergo physical examination. The anesthetist and veterinarian need a baseline of physical parameters from which to work. Only in this manner can early changes in the patient's status be noted. The focus on the physical examination obviously varies somewhat depending on the reason for presentation. There should be close communication between the veterinarian and the technician in regard to the underlying disease or injury and anesthesia concerns.

The patient's respiratory rate and effort should be noted, and both tracheal and bilateral thoracic auscultation should be performed. This will help localize the source of any disease or problem that may be encountered during intubation or anesthesia. It is especially important if trauma to the airway is suspected. The presence of respiratory distress, stridor or very loud airway sounds (indicating at least a 75% loss of airway diameter), wheezing, crackles, areas of dullness, and subcutaneous emphysema indicate ventilatory compromise, which may be worsened under anesthesia. Guttural or sonorous noises indicate pharyngeal disease. High-pitched or stridorous sounds indicate laryngeal or tracheal disease. Lung sounds should be compared on both sides of the thorax. Heart tones should be auscultated and pulses palpated for both strength and the presence of any deficits. Jugular veins should be clipped and evaluated for distention. A flat jugular vein that does not distend with digital pressure at the thoracic inlet is consistent with hypovolemia. The jugular vein that is distended with the patient standing or sitting may indicate a pneumothorax, pericardial effusion, or other causes of right-sided heart failure. The presence of abdominal distention should be noted. Distended superficial epigastric veins suggest high intraabdominal pressure. When this patient is placed in dorsal recumbency, additional pressure can be placed on the vena cava, thus compromising venous return to the heart. If severe enough, it can cause significant hypotension and potentially cardiac arrest. Mucous membranes should be evaluated for color, capillary refill time, and presence of petechiae.

An accurate weight (in kilograms for drug dosages) should be recorded whenever possible to ensure that accurate drug dosages are administered. However, in some patients an approximation of the weight may be all that is possible because moving

Box 10-2 Principles of General Anesthesia

- There is no such thing as a safe general anesthetic agent; there are only safe anesthetists.
- Be prepared with equipment, drugs, O_2, emergency drugs, knowledge, skills, and support.
- Each patient handles drugs differently (uptake, distribution, effect, metabolism).
- Choose drugs, dosages, and techniques based on each patient's age, condition, and surgery needed.
- Monitoring is essential to preventing complications (observe, record, report, act).
- Practice, practice, practice (this also includes drills) to be effective and efficient with rapid setup, monitoring, and contingency plans.
- Preemptive sedation and analgesia should be used when possible.
- Preoxygenate and perform induction rapidly for patients with airway or respiratory compromise.
- All patients under general anesthesia will hypoventilate and need ventilatory support.
- Maintaining equipment and understanding how it works are as vital as monitoring.
- The anesthesia does not end when the surgery ends. Preoperative support must continue through the postoperative period.
- All patients need physiologic support to prevent secondary decompensation of various body systems (including the pulmonary, cardiovascular, renal, and gastrointestinal systems).

the patient to the scale may compromise care. Vital signs including a blood pressure should be taken. If there are any concerns about cardiac injury or disease, a lead II electrocardiogram should be run. Thoracic radiographs are indicated in every patient with a history of trauma, in any patient with suspected or proven cardiorespiratory disease, in and any patient going to surgery for suspected neoplasia. Required laboratory analysis varies among patients; however, most critically ill or injured patients should have a minimum database evaluation including packed cell volume, total solids, electrolytes (sodium, chloride, potassium, phosphorus), blood gas (when available), glucose, blood urea nitrogen, creatinine, albumin, liver enzymes, activated clotting test, and platelet count. A buccal mucosal bleeding time should be evaluated in breeds with a high risk of von Willebrand's disease. A urinalysis, complete blood count with differential, and complete chemistry panel can be evaluated if time permits.

Vascular Access

One or two peripheral large-bore catheters (depending on the underlying disease) should be placed in all patients going to surgery. The diameter of T-port tubing may be less than that of the catheter and may interfere with rapid fluid infusion. A jugular catheter should be placed in any patient that is hemodynamically unstable to monitor central venous pressure, if possible. Jugular catheters also are indicated in patients with pulmonary disease, when pulmonary hypertension is a concern, or when fluid overload may be disastrous (e.g., pulmonary contusions, severe pneumonia, history of heartworm disease, or pulmonary neoplasia). Maintaining adequate preload while avoiding fluid overload is paramount to the survival of these patients. This is best accomplished using the appropriate combination of crystalloids and colloids. An indwelling arterial catheter for direct blood pressure monitoring and arterial blood gas determination is ideal in any patient when it is suspected that accurate intraoperative and postoperative monitoring of these parameters will be needed.

Preanesthetic Stabilization

Every attempt should be made to get the patient as stable as possible before inducing anesthesia. However, the patient may have to be anesthetized before abnormalities can be corrected. In fact, in many cases the abnormalities may not be correctable without surgery. The ABCs must be maintained. Oxygen should have been administered to patients that need it. Patients with severe pulmonary edema may need diuretics. Bilateral thoracenteses should be performed in patients with fluid in the pleural space. A chest tube is indicated in all patients with a pneumothorax when a thoracotomy is not being performed. Blood pressure should be normal if possible (unless hypotensive resuscitation is being performed). Venous volume should be adequate. Potentially life-threatening arrhythmias should be controlled. The exception to this may be mild ventricular premature contractions, which may resolve when the patient is intubated and ventilated on 100% O_2. Body temperature should be normal. (Rectal temperatures should be avoided in the respiratory-compromised or bradycardic patient because a vagally mediated hypotensive episode may be stimulated.) All laboratory abnormalities should have been corrected or should be in the process of being corrected. For instance, the patient with signs of a coagulopathy should be receiving a fresh frozen plasma transfusion. The transfusion can be continued intraoperatively if the patient is not stable enough to wait for surgery until the transfusion is completed.

Setting Up for Anesthesia

The anesthetic machine should be ready to be used at a moment's notice because patients may need anesthesia as part of their resuscitation (Box 10-3). Oxygen tanks should contain enough oxygen for a 6-hour procedure. The carbon dioxide absorption canister and hoses should be in good working order. The vaporizer should be full of inhalant anesthetic. A variety of sizes of clear endotracheal tubes and a laryngoscope must be available. Endotracheal tubes should be clear rather than opaque or red. This allows visualization of any

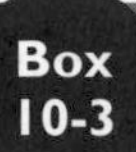

Box 10-3 Technical Tip: *Setting Up for Anesthesia*

The area for administering anesthesia should be ready at all times. The small animal emergency facility may not need surgical capability routinely, but sedation is needed for many of the procedures necessary for stabilization. Sedation in the critically ill or injured animal may necessitate intubation and further stabilization. Consider the following before anesthetizing or sedating the critically ill or injured animal.

Preparing the Anesthetic Machine

Hoses should be clean and checked for cracks routinely.
An oxygen source should be maintained for a possible 6-hour procedure.
The vaporizer must be kept full with inhalant anesthetic at all times.
Carbon dioxide absorption granules must be changed as indicated.

Items Needed for Induction

Anesthetic plan
- Patient positioning
- Emergency drug dosages and volume calculated and recorded on back of anesthetic flow sheet
- Type of intravenous fluid and rate
- Dosages and volume of induction drug

Clear, cuffed endotracheal tubes of a variety of sizes
Laryngoscope

Monitoring Equipment

Esophageal stethoscope
Blood pressure monitor
Electrocardiogram with printer
Pulse oximeter
Thermometer
Capnometer (especially for mechanically ventilated patients)

Miscellaneous Supplies

Warming blanket
Fluid or syringe pumps to regulate fluid and drug rates
Emergency crash cart

Airway

Laryngoscope and two to four blades
Stylets and lubricating jelly
Clear, low-pressure, high-volume cuffed endotracheal tubes in 3-10 mm, 12 mm
Intravenous line for securing tubes and syringe for inflating cuffs

Suction

Ear syringe
Hand-held and automated suction devices

Box 10-3 Technical Tip: *Setting Up for Anesthesia—cont'd*

Tracheal Suction

Yankauer tonsil or dental suction tip
Additional tubing and connectors for floor or wall suction
Ventilation
AMBU bag with reservoir and positive end-expiratory pressure (PEEP) valve (2 to 20 cm)
Infant AMBU bag with reservoir and PEEP valve
Oxygen tubing to connect to the oxygen supply
Oxygen E-tank with regulator and flowmeter
60-ml syringe attached to a stopcock and this attached to an extension set for chest taping

Vascular Access

Hypodermic needles (22, 20, and 18 gauge)
Syringes (3, 6, 12, and 35 ml)
Over-the-needle catheters (24, 22, 20, 18, 16, and 14 gauge)
Feeding tubes (3, 5, and 8 French) with additional three-way stopcocks
Small thumb forceps, iris scissors, mosquito hemostats, and catheter introducer
Intraosseous cannulas

Drugs

Syringes (1 ml and 6 ml) with needles attached for each of the following drugs:
- Epinephrine
- Norepinephrine
- Dobutamine
- Dopamine
- Isoproterenol
- Calcium chloride or gluconate
- Lidocaine
- Atropine
- Sodium bicarbonate
- Glucose
- Diphenhydramine
- Methylprednisolone sodium succinate
- Diltiazem

secretions (e.g., blood, mucus) that can obstruct the airway. Red tubes also are prone to cracking and are more difficult to clean and sterilize than clear endotracheal tubes. They are less flexible than clear tubes. If red tubes are placed incorrectly, they can cause deviation of the trachea. All patients should have cuffed endotracheal tubes placed because ventilation cannot be provided effectively without a good seal. To help prevent iatrogenic injury to the trachea, high-volume, low-pressure cuffs should be used. Red tubes have higher-pressure cuffs, which may increase the likelihood of injury to the tracheal mucosa.

Monitoring equipment should be handy and in good working order. Basic equipment should include an esophageal stethoscope, a blood pressure device (preferably a Doppler ultrasonic blood flow detector so that flow can be monitored), an electrocardiogram with continuous readout, a pulse oximeter, and a thermometer. A capnometer is extremely helpful in all patients, especially those who are being artificially (manually or mechanically) ventilated. If the patient has a chest tube, a large syringe should be available for aspiration.

Each patient must have an anesthetic plan. Planning helps the technician anticipate and prevent potential complications. Planning should include consideration of patient positioning. For instance, patients with head trauma should not be positioned with the head lower than the heart, and patients with a diaphragmatic hernia should be positioned with the thorax higher than the abdomen. Standard drugs to be given in case of emergency should be recorded on the back of an anesthesia flow sheet, with the drug dosage and the volume needed for the particular patient. In emergencies there is no time to perform these calculations. Consideration should be given to the types of fluids to be administered intraoperatively. Because many of these patients need fluid volumes delivered at precise rates, fluid pumps should be available. If it is suspected the patient may need a certain drug, such as a dopamine infusion, it is much better to set up the infusion in advance. Syringes, needles, and all medications should be present. A flow sheet should be used to record all drugs administered and the patient's vital signs.

Setting Up for Surgery

The operating room should be kept in a constant state of readiness. Surgical packs, gowns, and gloves should be laid out. A warm water circulating blanket or other safe, active warming device should be on the surgical table. The ground plate for the electrocautery should be in place and the electrocautery unit plugged in. Suction should be plugged in and ready to receive tubing from the surgeon.

For all patients, but especially the critically ill or injured patient, time under anesthesia must be minimized. Clipping and surgical prepping should be as complete as possible before anesthesia induction. Some patients with a severe hemoabdomen may be close to exsanguination from their injury or disease. In these patients, preparation may be limited to clipping the area of the incision and wiping with the surgical scrub before draping to save time. Surgeons should be gowned and gloved and instrument packs opened before induction, which should be performed in the operating room. This will allow the surgeon to enter the abdomen immediately and gain control of the hemorrhage.

RESERVES IN CRITICAL CARE: WHY BALANCED ANESTHESIA IS NECESSARY

Balanced anesthesia involves delivering specific drugs for analgesia or amelioration of pain, sedation, hypnosis or a loss of recognition and concern about the procedure in the patient's mind, and muscle relaxation. Recommendations and suggested protocols for each of these measures are outlined in this section.

Because critically ill or injured patients often need to be taken to surgery in the face of an unstable respiratory or cardiovascular system, the use of balanced anesthesia becomes vital. To provide balanced anesthesia, the anesthetist must be familiar with many different drugs and their effects in the patient with altered metabolism or organ function. The critically ill patient may have no reserves left, so the patient should receive only enough drugs to achieve the analgesia and anesthesia necessary to complete the surgery. The patient may develop tachycardia in an attempt to maintain blood pressure. When a drug such as isoflurane, which causes significant vasodilation and secondary hypotension, is administered, the patient may have no further cardiac reserves to draw on and blood pressure may plummet further, potentially leading to cardiac arrest.

ANALGESICS, LOCAL ANESTHETICS, AND PREANESTHETIC AGENTS

Analgesia

The primary goal of anesthesia is to eliminate pain. Pain has been shown to have detrimental effects on cardiopulmonary function, metabolism, endocrine status, and immune function (Box 10-4). This not

Box 10-4 Principles of Safe Anesthesia in Critical Care

- Use local anesthesia when appropriate.
- Use preemptive analgesia to prevent windup and to decrease the dosage of induction drugs.
- Always titrate medication to effect.

only can lead to serious physiologic effects such as ventricular premature contractions, hypoxia, muscle weakness, and delayed tissue healing but also can affect the patient's well-being. Clinical studies in children have demonstrated a 25% increase in mortality when pain is not controlled effectively.

Analgesia is vital in the surgical patient because every surgical procedure causes pain. There is almost no situation in which analgesics cannot be administered. It is important to avoid the windup phenomenon by providing preemptive analgesia. Windup, or a resetting of the pain threshold that makes the patient more sensitive to pain, occurs when pain is induced before adequate analgesia is provided. Dosages should be adjusted and titrated slowly to effect because in critically ill patients the effective dosage may be only 25% to 50% of normal.

Opioids are the most common analgesics used because of their effectiveness and safety. These include buprenorphine, butorphanol, fentanyl, meperidine, morphine, and oxymorphone. All opioids cause varying degrees of sedation, respiratory depression, and bradycardia. These effects are dose-related and can be avoided to a large extent by using lower dosages than would be used in the healthy, active patient. Bradycardia may decrease cardiac output and lead to secondary hypotension. If significant bradycardia develops (i.e., if it is affecting the blood pressure), an anticholinergic such as atropine or glycopyrrolate will counteract this effect and should be given. Because bradycardia is uncommon, it is not recommended to give the anticholinergic as a premedication because the tachycardia that may ensue can be very detrimental to the patient.

Opioids cause respiratory depression; however, at low dosages this rarely is a clinically significant issue. Whenever opioids are administered to critically ill or injured patients, the respiratory rate and depth should be monitored. Critically ill or injured patients under general anesthesia ideally should be positive-pressure ventilated, in which case the respiratory depression will not be a problem. The respiratory depression seen with oxymorphone and fentanyl can be reversed with butorphanol without decreasing the analgesic qualities of the opioids. Opioids and inhalant anesthetics routinely are used together; however, their effects are synergistic and the combination may lead to significant decreases in heart rate, blood pressure, and cardiac output. In the critically ill or injured patient the dosages of both must be decreased to avoid these complications. Opioids act to decrease intracranial pressure, but the concurrent respiratory depression may lead to hypercarbia and cerebral vasodilation and secondary hypertension. Therefore, if opioids are to be used when a change in intracranial pressure is a concern, positive-pressure ventilation should be provided. Opioids are metabolized by the liver, and a decrease in liver function may prolong the effects of the opioids.

The choice of opioid used depends on availability and familiarity with the drug. Buprenorphine probably is the only one not often indicated in the critically ill or injured patient because with its longer duration of effect it is harder to titrate. Morphine is a short-acting opioid that has excellent analgesic qualities. Its drawbacks include emesis and possible vasodilation secondary to histamine release when given intravenously. These side effects are not common with the low dosages used in critically ill or injured patients and often can be avoided by giving the morphine slowly. Morphine can be delivered effectively as a constant rate infusion (Table 10-1). Butorphanol is a short-acting analgesic that is useful because it has very minimal sedative and respiratory depressant effects. Oxymorphone is an intermediate-acting opioid that can be used effectively in the critically ill or injured patient. Fentanyl is a very short-acting opioid that is most

Table 10-1 Anesthetic Drugs

Drug	Dosages (Intravenous Unless Otherwise Indicated)
Preoperative and postoperative analgesia	
Atropine	0.02-0.04 mg/kg
Glycopyrrolate	0.01-0.02 mg/kg
Acepromazine	0.005-0.2 mg/kg (maximum 3 mg)
Ketamine	3.0-8.0 mg/kg
Oxymorphone	0.04-0.3 mg/kg
Fentanyl	5.0-10.0 mg/kg
Fentanyl patch	One half covered 25 μg/hr patch if <5 kg
	25 μg/hr 5-10 kg
	50 μg/hr 10-20 kg
	75 μg/hr 20-30 kg
	100 μg/hr >30 kg
Morphine*	0.5-2.2 mg/kg; 0.05-1.0 mg/kg/hr constant-rate infusion
Butorphanol	0.2-0.4 mg/kg
Buprenorphine	5.0-20.0 μg/kg
Induction	
Thiopental	6.0-10.0 mg/kg 2% solution
Ketamine	5.0-10.0 mg/kg
Etomidate	0.5-2.0 mg/kg
Propofol	3.0-6.0 mg/kg
With diazepam use	0.2-0.5 mg/kg
Propofol with diazepam	1.0-3.0 mg/kg
Oxymorphone with diazepam*	0.2 mg/kg
Fentanyl with diazepam*	20 μg/kg
Etomidate with diazepam	0.25-0.4 mg/kg
Maintenance	
Oxymorphone	0.05-0.1 mg/kg q 20 min
Fentanyl	0.5-1.0 μg/kg/min
Propofol	0.1-0.6 mg/kg/min
Diazepam	0.2-0.5 mg/kg/hr
Midazolam	0.5-1.5 μg/kg/min
Pentobarbital	0.05-2.6 mg/kg
Ketamine with diazepam	1.25-2.5 mg/kg
Diazepam	0.05-0.2 mg/kg
Neuromuscular blockers	
Atracurium	0.25 mg/kg load; 0.1 mg/kg redose; 2.0-8.0 μg/kg/min
Pancuronium	0.04-0.11 mg/kg; 0.04 mg/kg/hr
Succinylcholine	0.22-0.44 mg/kg; 0.2 mg/kg/hr
Reversal	
Naloxone	0.01-0.02 mg/kg 50% IV, 50% IM; 0.02-0.04 mg/kg IM
Nalbuphine	0.03-0.1 mg/kg IV
Buprenorphine	10-20 μg/kg IV 20 min before reversal
Atropine with edrophonium	0.01-0.02 mg/kg followed by 0.5 mg/kg IV
Atropine with neostigmine	0.04 mg/kg followed by 0.06 mg/kg IV

*Use 50% of dose for cats.

TABLE 10-1 Anesthetic Drugs—cont'd

Drug	Dosages (Intravenous Unless Otherwise Indicated)
Local anesthesia	
Epidural	If spinal or cerebrospinal fluid, decrease dosage by 50%-75%; 0.3 ml/kg volume; 1 ml/15 kg will block to T5; maximum volume 6 ml
Oxymorphone	0.1 mg/kg
Morphine	0.1 mg/kg
Buprenorphine	0.03 mg/kg
Bupivacaine	2 mg/kg 0.5% solution (1 ml/4.5 kg)
Lidocaine	2-4 mg/kg 2% solution (1 ml/4.5 kg)
Intercostal	
Bupivacaine*	2 mg/kg 0.5% solution; 0.5 ml/nerve
Intrapleural	
Bupivacaine*	1.5-2 mg/kg diluted to 1 ml/kg q 6 hr
Local	
Lidocaine*	0.5-2.0% maximum, 6 mg/kg with bicarbonate 1 ml per 10 ml lidocaine

Opioids	μ	κ	Σ
Analgesia	+	+	–
Respiration	Depression	Depression	Stimulation
Behavior	Euphoria	Sedation	Dysphoria
Dependency	+	–	–

	Duration	Receptors	Potency
Morphine	4-6 hr	μ, κ, Σ agonist	
Fentanyl	30-45 min	μ, κ, Σ agonist	100 × morphine
Oxymorphone	1-6 hr	μ, κ, Σ agonist	10 × morphine
Buprenorphine	10-12 hr	slow μ dissociation	30 × morphine
Butorphanol	3-4 hr	weak μ, strong κ	3-5 × morphine

*Use 50% of dose for cats.

useful as a constant-rate infusion during anesthesia. Fentanyl also can be administered in small boluses intravenously to effect. Significant bradycardia can be seen with fentanyl but is rare if appropriate dosages are used.

In general, nonsteroidal antiinflammatory agents are contraindicated in patients with hypotension or decreased tissue perfusion, gastrointestinal or renal disease or dysfunction, and/or thrombocytopenia or platelet dysfunction. For these reasons, they should not be administered to critically ill or injured patients.

LOCAL OR REGIONAL ANESTHESIA

Infiltration of nerve endings using local anesthesia is a very effective way to provide analgesia and is recommended highly. Because the systemic effects of anesthetic agents used to produce local or regional anesthesia are minimal, often this is a safer technique to use in the compromised patient. Recovery is quicker, resulting in a shorter hospital stay. Intrapleural analgesia has been shown to restore normal pulmonary function more quickly than parenteral opioids. Local or regional anesthesia can be used in combination with sedation, systemic analgesia, and anxiolysis. In the severely debilitated patient, local anesthetics in combination with systemic analgesics and sedation may be sufficient for performing the necessary surgery.

Lidocaine and bupivacaine typically are used for local, regional, and epidural anesthesia. Lidocaine can be placed directly onto the wound surface as well as into the skin edges to help decrease the pain associated with debridement, flushing, and suturing. Infiltration of surgical incisions with bupivacaine or lidocaine as a line block preoperatively or postoperatively helps decrease the pain associated with the incision. These are very acidic drugs and can cause irritation when injected locally. This effect can be lessened by adding sodium bicarbonate into the syringe with the local anesthetic. Up to one fifth the volume (usually one-tenth the volume) can be given as sodium bicarbonate. Also, if lidocaine is warmed to body temperature the sting is reduced. In wounds where a large volume of local anesthetic may be needed, 1% lidocaine can be used instead of 2%. The lidocaine can be diluted in any fluid with an acidic or neutral pH.

Regional Anesthesia

Examples of regional analgesia in the critically ill or injured patient include bolus injection of local anesthetic at the brachial plexus as an axillary block, anesthetic infiltration at the base of the scrotum as a block for castration, intrapleural analgesia by infusion into the pleural space, and intraarticular anesthesia using lidocaine or an opioid such as oxymorphone or morphine.

Epidural Analgesia and Anesthesia

Epidural analgesic and anesthetic agents are effective in controlling pain. When they are given preoperatively, the amount of analgesic agents needed postoperatively decreases significantly. Epidural anesthesia significantly decreases or even eliminates the need for inhalant anesthesia in unstable patients.

Local anesthetics such as lidocaine and bupivacaine in combination with morphine typically are used to deliver epidural anesthesia. Oxymorphone is thought to bind to receptors near the site of injection better than morphine because it is lipophilic. Therefore oxymorphone is more likely to have direct effects at the site of injection than morphine. Bupivacaine and morphine in combination are more effective than morphine alone, and bupivacaine alone has been shown to be more effective than morphine alone. Onset of action is approximately 30 to 60 minutes and duration is from 6 to 24 hours.

Potential complications of epidural anesthesia include hypotension from sympathetic blockade, respiratory depression, motor paralysis, hypothermia, urinary retention, and infections. The higher the epidural, the greater the likelihood of respiratory depression and hypotension.

Premedication

Premedication typically involves administering tranquilizers, sedatives, hypnotics, analgesics, and anticholinergics. Use of premedication decreases the dosages needed for induction and maintenance anesthesia and ensures a smoother recovery from anesthesia. Many of these drugs may not be indicated in or tolerated by the critically ill or injured patient; however, opioids can be used safely in fragile patients. Premedication always should involve an analgesic even if other agents are not administered.

Anticholinergics include atropine and glycopyrrolate. They are effective at reversing bradycardia secondary to increased vagal tone and decreasing airway secretions, and their direct effects dilate the airway. However, the increase in heart rate increases the myocardial oxygen demands, which can be detrimental in critically ill or injured patients. Tachycardia leads to decreased diastolic time for filling and decreased perfusion of the coronary vessels (which occurs during diastole). In the critically ill or injured patient the increased demands may cause myocardial hypoxia and malignant arrhythmias, and anticholinergics should not be given to these patients routinely. Exceptions include animals with high resting vagal tone (when it is anticipated that surgical manipulation will lead to increased vagal tone), significant bradycardia, significant liquid airway secretions, or increased salivation. Cats are more predisposed to salivation than dogs, and anticholinergics should be available. Anticholinergics given to a patient with restricted blood flow or pneumonia can be very detrimental and should be given only if bradycardia becomes pronounced. If in doubt, it is always better to administer the anticholinergic once the effects of the other administered drugs are known.

Phenothiazines, administered as a sole agent, generally are not indicated in critically ill or injured patients because of their vasodilatory and hypotensive side effects. These side effects can be a significant problem when normal or high dosages are administered. However, low dosages may have several beneficial effects. The vasodilatory effects improve microcirculatory flow or perfusion. When they are used in combination with opioids, the effects of both drugs are synergistic. Some of the clinical signs exhibited by the ill or injured patient may be interpreted as pain; however, they may be signs of anxiety. Acepromazine is an excellent anxiolytic and may help reduce stress (and its detrimental effects on patient metabolism). A dosage of 0.01 to 0.025 mg/kg body weight can be used safely in many patients to help decrease anxiety, increase the effectiveness of the opioid, and help decrease the dosage of induction and maintenance agents. This dosage also has been shown to reduce chance of arrhythmias while minimally affecting blood pressure. Phenothiazines have no effect on cerebral blood flow in the face of normal systemic blood pressure, but the vasodilatory effects can be detrimental to cerebral blood flow if the patient becomes hypotensive.

Some of the side effects of acepromazine are reported in the literature but rarely are a clinical problem, especially at low dosages. However, because many critically ill or injured patients may be unstable and may be unable to deal with side effects of drugs, the anesthetist should be aware of potential complications. Acepromazine causes a decrease in the hematocrit secondary to erythrocyte sequestration in the spleen. This may be especially important in the anemic patient. If it is anticipated that the patient will need a splenectomy, acepromazine should be avoided to minimize loss of red cell mass once the splenectomy has been performed. There is a decrease in the total plasma protein level secondary to vasodilation and hemodilution after acepromazine administration. Acepromazine can interfere with platelet function. Although controversial, phenothiazines may lower the seizure threshold and should not be used in patients with a history of seizures. Phenothiazines are metabolized in the liver.

ANESTHETIC AGENTS

General Concerns

General anesthesia can be provided with injectable drugs that are given systemically. It can be achieved also through the use of a combination of injectable drugs with or without inhalational agents, or it can be produced via the administration of inhalational agents alone.

Critically ill and injured patients have limited reserves and should be anesthetized using drugs that allow rapid airway control. All anesthetic agents affect respiratory and cardiovascular reserves, and it is very important to gain rapid control of the airway via endotracheal tube insertion and to be able to institute positive-pressure ventilatory support. Mask or tank inductions should not be performed. The only exception may be the extremely fractious cat that has been injured but cannot be approached to give even an intramuscular injection. Preanesthetic oxygenation should be performed for 5 minutes in all critically ill or injured patients after they have been premedicated.

Neuroleptanalgesia

Neuroleptanalgesia implies a tranquil, dissociative analgesic state produced by the synergism between an opioid and a tranquilizer. The combination of the two drugs allows lower dosages of each drug to be administered. Neuroleptanalgesia can provide anesthesia in the severely debilitated patient. In less debilitated patients, inhalant dosages can be reduced significantly. Awake intubation often can be performed with these combinations. Awake intubation involves placing an orotracheal tube in the patient that is not unconscious but rather is in a dissociative state. Examples of neuroleptanalgesic combinations include butorphanol and diazepam, butorphanol and acepromazine, oxymorphone and diazepam, and oxymorphone and acepromazine.

ETOMIDATE

Etomidate is an imidazole derivative that is classified as a nonbarbiturate, nonnarcotic sedative-hypnotic agent. It has poor analgesic qualities, and opioids or other means of providing analgesia should be administered if etomidate is being used. It causes mild respiratory depression but minimal change in cardiopulmonary function even in hypovolemic dogs. It does have mild negative inotropic effects, but these are not significant. This makes it a very useful drug in patients with severe cardiovascular instability. Vomiting, excitement, tremors, and apnea can be seen on induction. The neurologic signs are thought to be caused by disinhibition of subcortical neural activity and are not seizures. Etomidate decreases cerebral blood flow and metabolic oxygen needs, as barbiturates do, and can be used in patients with intracranial disease. Etomidate causes cortisol suppression for up to 6 hours in dogs and cats after a single injection. This effect is of unknown significance but may be a concern in the critically ill or injured patient. Even though etomidate is metabolized in the liver, liver disease does not seem to affect its metabolism.

KETAMINE-BENZODIAZEPINE COMBINATIONS

Ketamine in combination with a benzodiazepine such as diazepam or midazolam is excellent for inducing anesthesia in critically ill or injured patients. Midazolam is a water-soluble benzodiazepine with effects similar to those of diazepam but a shorter half-life. Midazolam and diazepam can be used in titrated dosages under anesthesia to decrease the amount of inhalant needed. Or, by using intravenous dosages titrated to effect, they can be used to help maintain anesthesia. Midazolam is significantly more expensive than diazepam.

Ketamine is a dissociative anesthetic that has good musculoskeletal analgesic properties, weak visceral analgesic qualities, and poor muscle relaxant properties. It exerts a positive inotropic effect on the myocardium and increases heart rate, cardiac output, blood pressure, pulmonary artery pressure, and central venous pressure. For these reasons it may be contraindicated in patients with elevated left atrial pressures or pulmonary hypertension. It should be avoided in cats with hypertrophic cardiomyopathy.

Because it increases myocardial oxygen demands, it should be used with caution in patients with significant myocardial dysfunction. The cardiovascular effects can be prevented or diminished by concurrently administering a sedative such as a benzodiazepine or acepromazine. Ketamine can cause seizures, an increase in cerebral metabolic rate, an increase in intracranial pressure, and a decrease in cerebral perfusion pressure. For these reasons ketamine should be used with caution in patients with intracranial disease or head trauma. Nystagmus is common, so it is a poor choice for patients needing ocular surgery. Ketamine increases airway secretions, and anticholinergics may be indicated, especially in the cat. Again, anticholinergics should not be used until indicated because of the potential detrimental side effects.

Benzodiazepines are metabolized in the liver and should be used with caution in severe liver disease. Ketamine is metabolized in the liver in the dog; however, in the cat it is excreted largely unchanged in the urine.

MEDETOMIDINE

α_2 Agonists such as xylazine and medetomidine usually are contraindicated in critically ill or injured patients. They cause a decrease in heart rate of up to 50% of baseline. They can also cause atrioventricular block and ventricular premature contractions. Medetomidine has a diuretic effect lasting up to 4 hours, which may be detrimental in the dehydrated or hypovolemic patient. For this reason it should be avoided if there is any concern about urinary tract obstruction.

Propofol

Propofol is an alkyl phenol classified as nonbarbiturate, nonnarcotic sedative-hypnotic that has poor analgesic qualities. Its advantages lie in rapid induction and recovery with no cumulative effects even after multiple doses. Disadvantages include a high rate of apnea on induction and systemic hypotension. The hypotension is secondary to a decrease in myocardial contractility as well as vasodilation and venodilation. This effect, which is similar to that seen with thiopental, is of greater significance in hypovolemic patients. Ventricular premature contractions may be seen. It also causes hypothermia. Tremors and opisthotonus may be seen and are thought to be caused by disinhibition of neural activity and are not seizures. These effects can be prevented by premedicating the patient with anxiolytics. It is a good choice in patients with intracranial disease as long as they are not hypotensive because it decreases cerebral metabolic oxygen requirements. It is metabolized extensively in the liver, but its effects do not appear to be prolonged in patients with significant liver dysfunction.

Barbiturates

Both thiobarbiturates (thiopental) and oxybarbiturates (pentobarbital) can be used to provide general anesthesia. However, because they have significant respiratory depressant qualities as well as negative inotropic properties, which can cause hypotension, they must be used with caution. The negative effects are intensified in the presence of shock, acidosis, hypothermia, and hypoproteinemia. Pentobarbital can be used very effectively at low dosages throughout anesthesia as part of a balanced anesthesia regimen, but because of their severe depressant effects barbiturates should not be used for induction without premedication. Barbiturates have no analgesic qualities and must be used in combination with opioids. Advantages include rapid induction, which allows rapid intubation and control of ventilation. They also decrease cerebral metabolic oxygen consumption and can be used safely in patients with intracranial disease. Lack of body fat and liver dysfunction significantly prolong recovery from thiobarbiturates, and they should be used with caution in thin patients or patients with liver disease.

Inhalants

Inhalant anesthetics most commonly used include halothane and isoflurane. Both cause significant dose-dependent decreases in blood pressure and cardiac output, which can be life threatening in the critically ill or injured patient. This is related to a combination of negative inotropic effects and vasodilatory properties. These result from the calcium channel blocking effects. Injectable anesthesia has been recommended when hypotension develops with inhalational agents. Halothane has less respiratory depressant effect than isoflurane and causes less of a decrease in blood pressure than isoflurane, although cardiac output is better maintained with isoflurane. Halothane is more likely to sensitize the myocardium to the arrhythmogenic effects of catecholamines. Arrhythmias include ventricular premature contractions, ventricular tachycardia, and ventricular fibrillation. Halothane has some analgesic qualities, whereas isoflurane has none; however, isoflurane is a better muscle relaxant. Both are effective at reversing bronchoconstriction; however, isoflurane is an airway irritant and can cause airway spasm. Both can be used with intracranial disease; however, isoflurane causes a greater decrease in cerebral metabolic rate than halothane and is a better choice. Halothane is metabolized by the liver and should not be used in patients with significant liver dysfunction.

Halothane rarely causes malignant hypothermia. Malignant hyperthermia occurs when the body temperature is greater than 39.5° C (102.5° F), often greater than 41° C (106° F) secondary to excessive metabolic activity within the muscle. It occurs in genetically susceptible patients and is characterized by a significant acidosis (respiratory and metabolic). Hypoxic cellular damage to all organs ensues, with subsequent organ failure and death.

Sevoflurane is a new inhalant that may have indications in the critical patient. Although it has cardiovascular effects similar to those of isoflurane, it sensitizes the myocardium less to the arrhythmogenic effects of catecholamines, and recovery is more rapid. It causes marked respiratory depression, both centrally and through its direct effects on the diaphragm. Many of its cardiovascular effects are attributed to its calcium channel blocking properties.

NEUROMUSCULAR BLOCKING AGENTS

GENERAL

Neuromuscular blocking agents are very useful in the critically ill or injured patient. They help gain airway control without inducing gagging, coughing, or laryngospasm. They do not affect the cardiovascular system, so the patient remains more stable under anesthesia. There is good muscle relaxation, which increases chest compliance and allows more effective ventilation with lower peak inspiratory pressures. The muscle relaxation is useful during reduction of luxations and fractures. Neuromuscular blockers do not cause central nervous system depression.

Patients are paralyzed but aware, and they must receive both analgesics and sedatives or dissociative agents. However because movement is eliminated, amounts of other drugs are decreased. Because the patient is paralyzed, positive-pressure ventilatory support is needed.

DEPOLARIZING MUSCLE-BLOCKING AGENTS

There are two classes of neuromuscular blockers: depolarizing and nondepolarizing. Depolarizing agents act like acetylcholine at the neuromuscular junction, causing the muscle to contract. Their effect is longer than that of acetylcholine, which leads to persistent contraction (muscle paralysis). Depolarizing agents are broken down by plasma cholinesterase. There are no antagonists for these drugs.

Succinylcholine is the most common depolarizing neuromuscular blocking agent used in veterinary medicine. It has a rapid onset of action (within 30 to 60 seconds) and rapid recovery (within 5 to 20 minutes). Muscle fasciculations may be seen as the membranes depolarize. It can cause a transient increase in potassium levels of 0.5 to 1 mEq/L and should not be used if this level of potassium would be detrimental to the patient. Because of its rapid onset of action, it is an effective drug to use if rapid airway control is needed. It should be used with caution in patients with renal disease, severe liver dysfunction, myopathy, penetrating eye injury, or chronic debilitating disease. Succinylcholine is not recommended in patients in whom increased intraabdominal or increased intrathoracic pressures are undesirable (e.g., tension pneumothorax, gastric dilation volvulus). Hypokalemia, hypothermia, and exposure to organophosphates prolong the effects of succinylcholine. Succinylcholine may cause malignant hyperthermia.

NONDEPOLARIZING NEUROMUSCULAR BLOCKING AGENTS

Nondepolarizing neuromuscular blocking agents bind to acetylcholine receptor sites at the muscle end plate, thus preventing acetylcholine from binding with the receptor sites. This prevents muscle contraction and causes a flaccid paralysis. Nondepolarizing drugs are not metabolized by cholinesterase, but they can be antagonized by anticholinesterase drugs such as edrophonium or neostigmine.

Atracurium and pancuronium are the two most common nondepolarizing neuromuscular blockers used in veterinary medicine. Some anesthesiologists use vecuronium and have found it to be effective. These drugs have a slightly later onset of action. They may not be the best choice if rapid airway control is being attempted using solely the neuromuscular blocker because there will be a period of time when the patient cannot breathe properly but is not paralyzed sufficiently to be intubated. A patient should never be allowed to struggle with its airway. Hypokalemia, hypocalcemia, hypothermia, most anesthetic agents (benzodiazepines, opioids, barbiturates, ketamine), and antibiotics such as aminoglycosides and clindamycin can prolong the effects of nondepolarizing neuromuscular blockers. Atracurium is degraded by Hoffman elimination, which is spontaneous degradation that is not dependent on hepatic metabolism or renal excretion. However, atracurium's effects are prolonged by acidosis and hypothermia. Pancuronium is metabolized in part in the liver and is excreted renally. It is contraindicated in hepatic or renal disease.

Atracurium has an onset of action of 1 to 5 minutes and a duration of effect of 20 to 45 minutes. A loading dose can be followed by repeat intravenous doses (using 40% of the initial dosage) or a constant-rate infusion. At high levels atracurium can cause histamine release. Pancuronium has an onset of action of 2 to 3 minutes and a duration of effect of 40 to 45 minutes. Unlike atracurium, repeated doses are cumulative. Pancuronium causes an increase in heart rate.

Nondepolarizing neuromuscular blockers can be reversed with drugs that inhibit acetylcholinesterase such as neostigmine. Administering this drug can cause parasympathetic side effects such as bradycardia, salivation, miosis, and increased gastrointestinal motility. Reversal is effective only if at least some muscle function has returned.

Monitoring with Neuromuscular Blocking Agents

Peripheral nerve stimulators using a train of four should be used to monitor neuromuscular blockade, if available. The stimulator can be attached to the facial or ulnar nerve. If a peripheral nerve stimulator is not available, it is impossible to assess the depth of the block until muscle function starts to return. The patient must be ventilated artificially until good ventilatory function returns, and the patient should never be extubated until it is able to sit up. It is more difficult to monitor patients under anesthesia with neuromuscular blockade because the normal neuromuscular reflexes are abolished. Lacrimation, salivation, slight muscle movement of the limbs or face, curling of the tip of the tongue, increased resistance to ventilation, and increased blood pressure may indicate that the patient is aware of its surroundings or is in pain.

INTUBATION

General

All critically ill or injured patients should be preoxygenated before induction. This can be done by placing a mask over the patient's face or simply placing a tube from an oxygen source in front of the patient's face (flow-by). In gasping patients, the tube should be placed into the patient's mouth. High flow rates should be used.

An endotracheal tube can be used as a pharyngeal airway if necessary. The tube is placed in the animal's mouth. The mouth is closed over the tube. An attempt is made to extrude the tongue and close the teeth over the tongue to prevent airway blockage by the tongue and to prevent the patient from breathing around the tube. By pushing dorsally on the cricoid cartilage the technician can occlude the esophagus partially and the patient can be ventilated via this pharyngeal airway.

All patients should be intubated with the largest endotracheal tube that fits comfortably in the trachea. The anesthetist should feel comfortable intubating a patient in lateral, dorsal, and sternal recumbency. Intubating the patient in dorsal recumbency allows insertion of a tube one half size to one size larger than can be placed with the patient in sternal recumbency. It also allows the patient to be intubated unassisted. To avoid aspiration, do not intubate a patient in dorsal recumbency if its stomach is distended.

For very unstable patients, an awake intubation may be indicated. This is done by administering an opioid and a benzodiazepine to provide mild sedation and anxiolysis. A neuromuscular blocking agent also may be needed to allow the animal to tolerate the endotracheal tube. The patient is sedated only, so a general anesthetic agent, which may decompensate the patient, is avoided.

Resistance to respiration is determined primarily by the diameter of the endotracheal tube. The larger the tube, the less the resistance. Cuffed endotracheal tubes should be used in all patients because ventilation cannot be provided effectively without a good seal. The cuff should be inflated to provide a seal at 15 to 20 cm H_2O. If there are concerns about tracheal disease, the cuff should be inflated to provide a seal at 10 to 12 cm H_2O. Care always should be taken not to overinflate the cuff, especially in cats. Overinflation can lead to mucosal injury and ischemia, and in cats can lead to tracheal disruption via tearing of the dorsal tracheal membrane. Whenever the patient is turned, the endotracheal tube should be disconnected from the anesthetic machine to avoid torquing the endotracheal tube. This may tear the dorsal tracheal membrane if the cuff is overinflated.

A laryngoscope should be used in all patients, and topical lidocaine (0.2 ml 2% lidocaine per 5 kg body weight) should be used on the arytenoid cartilages if laryngospasm, gagging, or coughing on induction must be avoided. If topical lidocaine is used, the anesthetist should wait at least 10 seconds before intubating. Cetacaine must not be used. It contains benzocaine, which can cause significant methemoglobinemia. Nontraumatic intubation is most important. Stimulating the larynx can invoke a vagally mediated bradycardia and potentially an arrest in the hypoxemic patient. In the severely hypotensive patient, the head should not be raised during intubation. This may decrease cerebral blood flow to the point of causing cardiorespiratory arrest. This patient should be intubated in dorsal or lateral recumbency in this situation. If a stylet is used, the tip must not protrude past the end of the endotracheal tube because it can damage the trachea.

Lidocaine can be given intravenously as part of an induction protocol to help decrease arrhythmias and decrease the gag or cough response to intubation. This also allows a decrease in the dosages of other induction agents. It is particularly useful in patients with preexisting ventricular premature contractions or suspected elevated intracranial pressure.

Once the patient is intubated and the tube is secured, the lungs should be ausculted bilaterally. This allows the anesthetist to confirm that the tube is in the trachea, not the esophagus, and that the tip of the tube has not been inserted into a mainstem bronchus.

Intubating the Patient with a Suspected Airway Disruption

Intubating a patient with a suspected airway disruption is more complex than regular intubation. Cervical bite wounds can tear the cervical trachea, and the tip of the tube must project past the suspected area of injury. In cats, a suspected tracheal membrane tear secondary to an anesthetic complication may progress from the mid-cervical or distal cervical region to the bifurcation of the bronchus. In these patients the tube should be passed more distally than normal, generally to the level of the bronchial bifurcation. Artificial ventilation of this patient should be avoided until the tear is located and it is confirmed that the tube projects past the injury. If the patient must be ventilated, it should be monitored closely for signs of a developing tension pneumomediastinum. Clinical signs include loss of Doppler blood flow sounds, low blood pressure, increasing difficulty in ventilation, and advancing subcutaneous emphysema.

Intubating the Patient with Upper Airway Swelling or Obstruction

If there are any concerns that the airway is too edematous or disrupted to intubate orotracheally, an awake tracheostomy should be performed under local anesthesia (and sedation if needed) before induction. If there is considerable edema, as in the case of the bulldog with suspected laryngeal paralysis, a single intravenous dose of dexamethasone sodium phosphate (0.5 mg/kg intravenously) may alleviate some of the swelling.

MAINTAINING THE PATIENT UNDER GENERAL ANESTHESIA

Critically ill or injured patients should be maintained on 100% oxygen and controlled ventilation. Metabolic oxygen requirements are approximately 5 ml/kg body weight per minute, and oxygen flows should not be less than this. With semiclosed anesthesia, oxygen flow rates of 100 to 300 ml/kg body weight per minute are indicated. Low-flow anesthesia is ideal for the critically ill or injured patient because there is less moisture loss from the airways, and because oxygen flow rates are low, there is less heat loss. During low-flow anesthesia the oxygen flow rates are by definition slightly greater than metabolic oxygen requirements. Because critically ill or injured patients may have a higher oxygen demand, low-flow anesthesia should provide no less than 10 ml/kg body weight per minute. Many anesthetic machines have small leaks that lead to losses of 100 to 200 ml/minute, and flow rates should rarely decrease below this level. During low-flow anesthesia the canister that traps carbon dioxide should be checked more often because this method relies more on carbon dioxide removal by the canister than on flow. Monitoring end-tidal carbon dioxide levels via capnography is very important during low-flow anesthesia.

Critically ill or injured patients under anesthesia often need modifications in their anesthetic protocols and fluid rates because they are not stable. Most of these patients develop severe hypotension with normal concentrations of inhalant anesthesia. As a result, injectable drugs often are needed intraoperatively. When patients appear to be responding to surgical stimulation, they may be perceiving pain. For this reason analgesics should be used judiciously throughout the surgical procedure. This allows the anesthetist to lower significantly the amount of other anesthetic agents used. It may be necessary to redose opioids such as butorphanol or oxymorphone every 15 to 20 minutes. If benzodiazepines are being used to create neuroleptanalgesia, it may be necessary to redose these drugs every 15 to 20 minutes. In most cases, subsequent doses should be given at increasing intervals and lower amounts because hypothermia and acidosis prolong the effects of many anesthetic agents.

CONTROLLED VENTILATION

All anesthetic agents are ventilatory depressants, so ventilatory support is essential in the critically ill or injured patient. In general, tidal volumes should be set at 7 to 10 ml/kg at a rate of 10 to 15 breaths/min. Peak inspiratory pressures should be kept below 15 cm H_2O whenever possible. Tidal volumes as high as 20 ml/kg and peak inspiratory pressures as high as 25 cm H_2O may be needed. Tidal volumes are adjusted based on observation of chest movement during ventilation, lung auscultation, blood gases, capnometry, and blood pressure. To avoid complications, the lowest volumes and pressures that the patient will tolerate should be used.

Ventilator parameters must be adjusted according to the patient's condition. For instance, patients with less compliant lungs or masses pushing on the diaphragm may need higher tidal volumes and peak inspiratory pressures than patients with compliant chest walls. In addition, the tubing from the anesthetic machine to the patient absorbs some of the pressure from the ventilator. If a lot of tubing is used or the tubing is compliant, higher than expected tidal volumes and pressures may be needed in smaller patients. The tubing becomes less of a factor in larger patients. If higher-frequency ventilation is being used, then tidal volumes can be decreased. Overventilation can lead to a decrease in preload and a secondary decrease in cardiac output and blood pressure. Increased tidal volumes or inspiratory pressures may be needed in patients with a large amount of dead space (large amount of anesthetic tubing compared to the tidal volume), restrictive pulmonary disease, or impaired diaphragmatic movement (e.g., gastric dilation volvulus, obesity). It also can be needed in patients restrained in dorsal recumbency with limbs stretched because chest wall movement is restricted.

Manual ventilation is provided by hand bagging. Respiratory and ventilatory parameters should be monitored. Mechanical ventilation is recommended to provide consistent, continuous ventilatory support in all critically ill or injured patients. It also enables the technician to provide positive end-expiratory pressure (PEEP). Mechanical ventilation frees the technician to monitor the patient. Many economical ventilators are available that are simple to use.

PEEP increases the lung's functional residual capacity by sustaining alveolar volume during exhalation. The primary concern with the use of PEEP is decreased cardiac output, so blood pressure or pulse pressure should be monitored closely. PEEP ideally should be kept between 5 and 10 cm H_2O. At the very least, physiologic PEEP (2 to 3 cm H_2O) should be instituted. This will help prevent atelectasis.

An AMBU bag with a reservoir and 100% oxygen should be used to ventilate all patients during transport from the prep area to the operating room or to radiology.

MONITORING

TEAMWORK IN ANESTHESIA

The circulating nurse, anesthetist, surgeon, and assistant surgeon must work together to treat the critically ill or injured patient. There must be constant communication between team members. For example, if the anesthetist notices that the lingual pulses do not feel very strong, the surgeon should be asked to inspect internal blood pressure (i.e., aortic pulsation). If the surgeon notices that the tissues are starting to look pale, he or she should ask the anesthetist to check vital signs and perhaps laboratory work such as a packed cell volume.

Respiration, Doppler blood flow sounds, and cardiac rhythm as recorded by the electrocardiogram must be monitored continuously. Most parameters should be recorded every 5 minutes in the unstable patient to every 15 minutes in the stable patient. The exception may be temperature, which can be recorded every 15 minutes. All vital signs, ventilatory parameters, and drugs administered should be noted on an anesthesia flow sheet (Box 10-5).

ESSENTIALS OF HANDS-ON PHYSICAL PARAMETER MONITORING

The anesthetist should not rely solely on monitoring equipment but should check the patient physically at regular intervals using eyes, ears, and hands to confirm that the machine readouts are accurate. In addition, changes such as cyanosis and pallor cannot be picked up by a machine. The seriously ill or injured patient who is undergoing surgery is at risk for serious complications such as airway compromise, respiratory depression, hypercarbia, hypoxemia, arrhythmias, coagulopathy, metabolic acidosis, and even cardiac arrest. Absolute numbers are vitally important, but often the trend of change is an early indicator of whether the patient is beginning to decompensate. This section discusses monitoring of the patient under anesthesia.

The respiratory rate should be measured. The lungs should be auscultated using an esophageal stethoscope if appropriate (if drapes prevent direct auscultation). The earliest way to detect pulmonary edema is with an esophageal stethoscope. With

Box 10-5 Monitoring Checklist for Anesthesia in Critical Care

Continuous monitoring by devices (able to see numeric values and waveforms at a glance)
- Electrocardiogram, respiratory rate and effort (by impedance), $ETCO_2$, SpO_2, arterial and central venous blood pressure
- Doppler blood flow qualitative evaluation by listening to sounds generated

Monitoring as often as needed and recording every 5 minutes
- Heart rate, pulse rate, eye position, blood pressure by Doppler or indirect via oscillometric method, color, capillary refill time
- Muscle tone by estimating tone in muscles of mandible (jaw tone test)

Monitoring as often as needed and recording generally every 15 minutes
- Lung sounds and heart tones, urinary output, toe versus core temperature
- Core temperature, estimated amount of blood loss by observation of sponges, reservoir, table
- Stage of operation, manipulations done, and amount of fluids, plasma, and blood given

Monitoring as often as needed and recording generally every hour
- Packed cell volume, total solids, venous blood gas, arterial blood gas, glucose, sometimes electrolytes

interstitial pulmonary edema the breath sounds change, normally from a very quiet exhalation sound to that of breath sounds getting louder on exhalation. As alveolar edema becomes evident, crackles become audible, first just on exhalation, and later crackles are heard on both inhalation and exhalation. An esophageal stethoscope can be used to assess lung sounds as well as heart tones. Abnormalities such as crackles that are consistent with pulmonary edema and dullness consistent with obstruction or atelectasis can be heard.

Chest excursions should be assessed with both spontaneous respiration and mechanical ventilation (both by hand bagging and mechanical ventilation).

Electronic Monitoring of Ventilation and Oxygenation

More sophisticated methods of assessing ventilatory function include the following.

- Pulse oximetry (Spo_2) readings should indicate an oxygen saturation (Sao_2) above 98%. The most accurate location for oxygen sensor placement is on the tongue. A good pulse signal (indicated by either waveform or signal intensity light) is necessary to get valid Spo_2 readings. Tongue clips often apply sufficient pressure to the tongue to interfere with circulation and cause inaccurate readings. This can be corrected by moving the clip at regular intervals to a slightly different location on the tongue. Oxygen saturation reaches 100% at an arterial pressure (Pao_2) of about 95 mm Hg. The Pao_2 should be 4.5 to 5 times the fraction of inspired oxygen (Fio_2). Therefore with an Fio_2 of 1 (100% O_2, which is the concentration given during anesthesia) the Pao_2 should be 450 to 500. The Spo_2 will read 100% from a Pao_2 of 500 to below about 95 mm Hg. This makes Spo_2 a very inaccurate means of monitoring oxygenation in the patient that is receiving 100% O_2. Therefore if there are any concerns about pulmonary function, arterial blood gases should be assessed. Pulse oximetry is a very important tool when the patient is not on supplemental oxygen (i.e., is breathing room air) or is receiving low levels of oxygen supplementation (nasal, nasopharyngeal, or nasotracheal) during recovery.
- Capnography or capnometry should be assessed in all critically ill or injured patients. Ideally, waveform analysis with capnography is preferred to capnometry, which gives only a number that corresponds to peak end-tidal carbon dioxide ($ETco_2$). Waveform analysis allows the anesthetist to detect changes in ventilatory mechanics. For example, a steep slope means a clear airway, whereas a slow rise in the slope indicates an obstructive airway problem. Peak or $ETco_2$ corresponds to air exhaled from the lung's alveolar segments. It should be on the plateau of the air coming from the alveolar space, which is equilibrated with capillary blood. It is the only way to assess adequacy of ventilation. Assuming normal perfusion to the lungs and no airway obstruction, $ETco_2$ correlates with the arterial pressure of carbon dioxide ($Paco_2$). Therefore this is the only way to monitor ventilation effectiveness in the anesthetized patient. $ETco_2$ levels generally are about 5 mm Hg lower than $Paco_2$. The $ETco_2$ should remain between 25 and 35 mm Hg.
- A respirometer can be placed between the endotracheal tube and the breathing circuit to determine tidal and minute volume. By the "weather-vane" principle, as each breath is exhaled a measurement of the volume of that breath is determined. A more sophisticated electronic unit measures flow and volume and determines flow-volume loops. Tidal volume should be kept as close to 7 to 10 ml/kg as possible. The volume being delivered by the ventilator should be compared with the calculated value.
- The peak inspiratory pressure (PIP) must be monitored whenever the patient is being ventilated. Peak airway pressure should be

kept no higher than 20 cm H_2O whenever possible. Higher pressures may lead to barotrauma with subsequent air trapping in the alveoli, pneumothorax, or pneumomediastinum. Periodic sighing every 2 to 5 minutes with pressures from 20 to 30 cm H_2O also is recommended to prevent atelectasis in patients who are not being mechanically ventilated.

- Electronic sensors of breaths are small devices that sound when air passes through the endotracheal tube or Y-connector. They are activated by temperature changes of the exhaled air. They may whistle or beep and are useful for indicating breath rate and in some cases breath volume. Mechanical whistles also are available but appear to be less sensitive than electronic devices.
- More sophisticated monitoring can be accomplished using a device that determines compliance, graphs flow-volume loops, and calculates dead space fractions. Another device measures the volume of CO_2 gas exhaled with each breath and therefore provides more accurate information on respiratory mechanics, dead space, and the amount of carbon dioxide generated and exchanged at the pulmonary circuit.

Monitoring Cardiovascular Parameters

Heart rate should be measured by esophageal auscultation or a Doppler blood flow detector. Low heart rates can be associated with a low cardiac output and hypotension. High heart rates can lead to inadequate cardiac filling and low cardiac output, with subsequent hypotension. High heart rates also lead to increased myocardial oxygen demands and may lead to arrhythmias.

To assess cardiovascular status adequately there must be a way to measure blood pressure, either directly or indirectly. Systolic blood pressure should be maintained above 100 mm Hg and mean arterial pressure should be kept above 60 mm Hg to ensure adequate renal and splanchnic perfusion.

- A Doppler ultrasonic blood flow detector is recommended because it allows accurate determination of blood pressure. Also, the listener can assess flow based on the strength of the sound. Arrhythmias also are audible. Oscillometric blood pressure monitors are accurate but cannot be used to assess flow. If the patient is small, there are significant arrhythmias; if the signal is weak, readings may be inaccurate.
- An oscillometric blood pressure monitor detects pulse waves under a cuff that is placed around the limb. Systolic, diastolic, and mean arterial pressures are then displayed on the screen. It is simpler to use than the Doppler method, but its major disadvantage is that flow cannot be evaluated. It is also very sensitive to motion artifact.
- Central venous pressure correlates with right atrial pressure, which correlates with the volume reaching the right atrium during diastole. Ideally it should be 4 to 8 cm H_2O. Central venous pressure is falsely elevated in any condition that increases intrathoracic pressure (e.g., positive-pressure ventilation, pneumothorax). If a jugular catheter is not present, jugular distention, filling, and relaxation should be evaluated.
- If an indwelling urinary catheter is in place, the patient should be producing a minimum of 1 ml/kg body weight per hour. If a catheter is not present and abdominal surgery is being performed, the surgeon should monitor the urinary bladder for signs of urine production. This helps confirm adequate blood pressure and circulating blood volume.
- An electrocardiogram allows monitoring of electrical rhythm only. Therefore it is a vital tool for detecting arrhythmias but indicates nothing about cardiac function. Changes in the ST segment and T-wave configuration can be used to detect possible myocardial ischemia. The anesthetist must be able to identify sinus tachycardia, sinus bradycardia, atrioventricular block (first, second, and third degree), ventricular premature contractions, atrial fibrillation, and ventricular fibril-

lation. Arrhythmias noted on the electrocardiogram can be confirmed by esophageal auscultation. In addition, electrical equipment such as electrocautery equipment can interfere with the electrocardiogram. In cases of malfunction, the esophageal stethoscope can be used.

- Mucous membrane color and capillary refill time should be monitored. Lingual pulse strength and rhythm should be compared with blood pressure measurements and the electrocardiogram. Jaw tone should be assessed along with eye position; however, neither is a very accurate assessment of depth; they depend on the drugs administered to the patient. One of the best guides to general anesthetic depth when a neuromuscular blocker is not being used is jaw tone. It should always be present to some extent. Extreme laxity of the jaw and extreme ventral strabismus suggest a depth of anesthesia that may be excessive.

Temperature

This is best monitored by direct thermometry with thermistors that attach to physiologic recorders so that every few seconds the temperature is recorded and displayed. Many different physiologic recorders can accomplish this. The thermistors are placed in the esophagus, rectum, and ear canal or taped to the patient's toe web space. This allows core and peripheral temperature monitoring. Temperature monitoring also can be accomplished by the use of indoor-outdoor temperature probe devices. These are much less expensive, but they do not provide longevity, they are less accurate, and the data cannot be recorded. But they do allow simpler and more accurate temperature monitoring than simple rectal thermometry. The last option is to use a hypothermic thermometer, available from emergency medical supply companies. Hypothermic thermometers measure temperatures as low as 21° C. The regular rectal thermometer measures no less than 34.8° C. Therefore hypothermic thermometers are needed if only rectal or oral (buccal mucosa) thermometry is being performed.

SUPPORTIVE MEASURES NEEDED DURING ANESTHESIA

Temperature Conservation and Preventing Hypothermia

Hypothermia can cause prolonged coagulation times and peripheral vasoconstriction, leading to increased peripheral tissue acidosis secondary to anaerobic metabolism. Ventricular fibrillation and asystole can start to develop at 28° C. Hypothermia should be avoided in critically ill or injured patients unless the patient is undergoing surgery that would benefit from induced hypothermia such as certain types of cardiac surgery, neurosurgery, or surgery that can cause splanchnic organ ischemia. In these cases the decreased metabolic rate may help reduce cellular ischemia and apoptosis. Metabolic oxygen needs decrease 7% between 37° C and 30° C, so anesthetic needs decrease as the patient's temperature decreases.

A toe web temperature also can be measured. The difference between core and toe web temperature should be no greater than 3° C, and the core temperature should not drop below 37° C. Sometimes this is difficult to prevent.

The use of plastic wrap, bubble wrap, infrared heating lamps, warm irrigation fluids, warm intravenous fluids, hot water circulating blankets, and Bair huggers can be used to reduce hypothermia. The patient should not be placed on a cold surface; using warm water to perform the surgical scrub and avoiding overwetting the patient may help. Low-flow anesthesia helps slow hypothermia development. Using a heating circuit in the patient's anesthetic tubing is a very good way to decrease heat loss during anesthesia. Care should be taken with any item used to supply supplemental heat because it can cause burns. Wrap all warm water bottles and warm water circulating blankets in a towel before placing them next to the patient.

Fluid Support

Fluid therapy is much more important for the critically ill or injured patient under anesthesia than for the healthy patient, but the endpoints are the same. The goal of fluid therapy is to maintain an adequate circulating blood volume, adequate hemoglobin levels, and adequate clotting factors. Crystalloids are redistributed primarily to the interstitium, so if intravascular volume is needed, a combination of colloids (both synthetic and biologic) and crystalloids is indicated. Hemoglobin levels should be maintained above 7 g/dl using red cells or oxyhemoglobin. Albumin levels should be maintained above 2.0 g/dl using plasma. If albumin levels are low and the patient is not hemodynamically stable, synthetic colloids such as hetastarch or dextran 70 should be administered.

Based on normal fluid requirements and evaporative fluid losses under anesthesia (with major body cavities opened), a maintenance rate of 10 ml/kg body weight per hour of a balanced electrolyte solution should be administered. If major body cavities are not open, the rate generally can be decreased by 50%. This is based on studies in dogs. The authors are not aware of any studies in cats, but it seems logical that the rate requirements might be slightly less. If the patient has significant heart or liver disease, it may be important to use a half-strength sodium solution to avoid sodium and thus fluid overload.

If the patient is hypoglycemic, glucose should be supplemented in the fluids. Dextrose supplementation should be considered in any patient when it is anticipated that the patient might become hypoglycemic during the procedure. This includes patients with liver disease or endotoxemia and all pediatric patients. If the patient is significantly hypokalemic, potassium should be supplemented to help with muscle strength and cardiac function and to avoid prolonging the effects of drugs such as neuromuscular blockers. If potassium supplementation is being performed, the potassium level must not be allowed to rise above normal, and intraoperative serum potassium level monitoring may be indicated.

SPECIAL CONSIDERATIONS

Sight Hounds

Sight hounds tend to have prolonged recovery for several reasons. They have less body fat than many breeds, and drugs that are redistributed, such as thiobarbiturates, have a prolonged effect. They have decreased hepatic microsomal enzyme activity, which prolongs the effects of any drugs metabolized in the liver. Sight hounds also tend to have low plasma protein levels, which increases the concentration of the active form of some anesthetics. It is always safer to use drugs that require minimal hepatic metabolism, but in general similar drugs can be used in sight hounds as in other breeds. Neuroleptanalgesia combinations of opioids and diazepam can be used, as well as ketamine and diazepam and inhalants such as isoflurane and sevoflurane. The difference is that the dosage should be reduced. Propofol causes similar effects in sight hounds as in other breeds. The recovery period is longer than for other breeds, but propofol appears to be a safe anesthetic agent.

Cesarean Section

The important factors in choosing an anesthetic protocol relate as much to familiarity with the technique as the drugs that are used. Hypothermia, hypoxia, and hypotension should be avoided. Barbiturates should be avoided because they readily cross the placenta. Epidural anesthesia is considered the most beneficial, but postoperative paralysis may be undesirable. The combination of propofol and isoflurane has been shown to be as acceptable in terms of survival of the pups as an epidural. Neuromuscular blocking agents generally do not cross the placental barrier because of their large size. The combination of oxymorphone, a line block with lidocaine, and succinylcholine for muscle relaxation can be used effectively. To avoid overdosing, the dam should be dosed according to her lean body weight, minus the pups.

ANESTHETIC EMERGENCIES AND COMPLICATIONS

Any complications that can arise during general anesthesia of the healthy patient can occur in the critically ill or injured patient under anesthesia. Of course, the best treatment is prevention. The following section focuses on complications specific to critically ill or injured patients and problems that may pose more of a risk to these patients in the intraoperative or perioperative period. Hypoventilation and severe hypotension probably are the two most important complications. If left unresolved, they can lead to respiratory and cardiac arrest. If even moderate hypotension is allowed to persist for short periods of time, there may be significant postoperative morbidity.

Hypoventilation can be caused by anesthetic drugs, central nervous system disease, airway obstruction, space-occupying intrathoracic mass, pneumothorax (either from the injury or secondary to barotrauma), severe abdominal distention (gastric dilation volvulus, severe ascites), musculoskeletal disease, obesity, and body position. If a ventilator is being used, the cause may be inappropriate ventilator settings, air leak in the system (endotracheal tube cuff, anesthetic hoses), lack of oxygen in the tank, airway obstruction, or resistance to lung expansion.

The patient may develop a more rapid respiratory rate or ventilatory effort. This is not always because the patient is becoming more aware, and deepening the level of anesthesia may be disastrous for the patient. Hypercarbia secondary to hypotension with inadequate pulmonary circulation, airway obstruction, or depleted soda lime is the most common cause. This is commonly seen secondary to hypovolemia, pneumothorax, or pericardial tamponade. Other causes of increased ventilatory rate or effort include hypoxia, pain, opioid pant, hyperthermia, pressure buildup in the rebreathing bag, and space-occupying lesions.

Pneumothorax may occur secondary to barotrauma from artificial ventilation. Clinical signs include hypotension, bradycardia or tachycardia, greater resistance to ventilation, cyanosis, a thoracic cage that does not deflate on expiration, loss of lung sounds on auscultation, subcutaneous emphysema, and distended jugular veins. If a pneumothorax is suspected, thoracentesis should be performed immediately.

Hypotension generally is caused by hypovolemia or anesthetic drugs (leading to bradycardia or vasodilation). The hypovolemia can be an actual volume deficit, as occurs with severe blood loss. It can also be caused by the lack of venous return to the heart. This may occur when a patient with a large abdominal mass or a gravid uterus is placed in dorsal recumbency. The pressure on the vena cava can cause partial occlusion of the vessel. In a small percentage of patients, cardiac arrhythmias may be the cause. Primary signs of hypotension include an increasing heart rate (assuming the baroreceptor reflex has not been overridden), vasoconstriction, poor pulses, and signs of deepening anesthesia.

Cardiac arrhythmias that appear under anesthesia usually are caused by anesthetic drugs, hypoxemia, hypotension, hypothermia, acidosis, anemia, hyperthermia, toxemia, or cardiac trauma. They must be identified rapidly and treated accordingly (Table 10-2).

POSTOPERATIVE ANALGESIA, VENTILATORY, AND CARDIOPULMONARY SUPPORT

Critically ill or injured patients should be kept on oxygen until they are extubated. The patient should be monitored during trials on room air via pulse oximetry or arterial blood gases for signs of hypoxemia and hypercarbia. If hypoxia is present the patient may need supplemental oxygen, and a nasal, nasopharyngeal, or nasotracheal oxygen tube may be indicated. Nasopharyngeal oxygen provides higher concentrations than nasal oxygen. To place a nasopharyngeal catheter, the tube is premeasured from the naris to the lateral canthus of the eye. The tube is inserted in the same manner as a nasal oxygen cannula; however, the tip rests in the rostral nasopharynx. Nasotracheal intubation decreases the work of breathing in patients with upper airway compromise that would otherwise have increased respiratory effort. If the patient is significantly hypercarbic, especially in the face of hypoxemia, continued ventilatory support may be needed.

The patient should be kept intubated until it shows signs of a strong gag response. In addition, the cuff should remain inflated until extubation. Regurgitation and aspiration may occur during recovery, and the airway must be protected. If there is evidence of regurgitation, the oropharynx should

Text continued on p. 152

TABLE 10-2 Complications That Can Occur Under Anesthesia

Complication	Cause	Diagnostic Test	Treatment
Anaphylaxis*	Drugs	Check clinical signs (hypotension, facial edema).	Discontinue drug. Treat for allergic reaction.
Perivascular injection	Perivascular drug administration	Check clinical sign (perivascular swelling).	Dilute with saline 5-10 × volume (± sodium bicarbonate).
Regurgitation or vomiting	Decreased lower esophageal sphincter tone Drugs	Check clinical sign.	Suction ± Nasal irrigation. ± Esophageal lavage. ± Nasogastric tube placement. Extubate with cuff partially inflated.
Air embolism*	Vessel or vascular sinus open to air pneumocystogram	Check for severe bradycardia progressing to asystole.	Position patient so air floats to apex of heart and aspirate. Consider hyperbaric O_2.
Malignant hyperthermia*	Halothane, succinylcholine	Check rectal temperature. Check electrolytes, blood gas.	Provide 100% O_2. Discontinue anesthetic. Perform active cooling. Administer dantrolene 3 mg/kg IV.
Cyanosis	Lack of oxygen supply Airway obstruction	Check O_2 tanks and flowmeter. Check endotracheal tube. Auscultate lungs.†	Provide 100% O_2. Unkink, suction, or replace as indicated.
	Pulmonary failure	Auscultate lungs.†	Increase peak inspiratory pressures, respiratory rate, positive end-expiratory pressure.
	Inadequate pulmonary circulation secondary to hypotension, pneumothorax, or pericardial tamponade	Auscultate lungs.† Check blood pressure. Check for jugular distention.	Correct underlying cause.
Lack of thoracic expansion	Hypoventilation	See causes of hypoventilation.	Correct underlying cause.
	Barotrauma and pneumothorax	Auscultate lungs. Check for jugular distention. Perform thoracentesis.	Perform thoracentesis.

*Rare complication.
†Using esophageal stethoscope.

TABLE 10-2 Complications That Can Occur Under Anesthesia—cont'd

Complication	Cause	Diagnostic Test	Treatment
Hypoventilation	Anesthetic drugs	Check drugs dosages.	Decrease drug dosages. Discontinue inhalant temporarily. Administer positive-pressure ventilation.
	Airway obstruction	Check endotracheal tube and hoses.	Unkink, suction, or replace as indicated.
	Pneumothorax	Auscultate lungs. Check for jugular distention. Perform thoracentesis.	Perform thoracentesis.
	Body position		Loosen limb restraints. Change position if possible.
	Ventilator problems (inappropriate settings, air leak, lack of O_2)	Check ventilator settings. Check for air leak in cuff, hoses.	Correct underlying problem.
Need for increased PIP	Airway obstruction	Check endotracheal tube and hoses.	Unkink, suction, or replace as indicated.
	Underlying pulmonary disease (e.g., space-occupying mass, fibrosis)		Consider increasing PIP or RR or allowing permissive hypercapnia.
	Barotrauma and pneumothorax	Auscultate lungs. Check jugular distention. Perform thoracentesis.	Perform thoracentesis.
Decreased SpO_2	Insufficient O_2	Check O_2 supply.	Provide 100% O_2.
	Esophageal or bronchial intubation	Visualize, auscultate.	Reposition tube.
	Obstructed endotracheal tube	Check tube.	Replace tube.
	Poor perfusion	Check blood pressure.	Correct hypotension.
	Poor sensor contact	Check tongue clip.	Reapply clip.
	Bronchospasm	Check for tachypnea. Auscultate lungs. Check response to treatment.	Treat with bronchodilator.
	Aspiration pneumonia	Check oral cavity.	Suction airway.
	Severe anemia	Check mucous membranes and PCV.	Perform blood transfusion.
Decreased $ETCO_2$	Hyperventilation	Check ventilation. Auscultate lungs. Check thoracic expansion.	Correct underlying problem.
	Esophageal or bronchial intubation	Visualize, auscultate.	Reposition tube.
	Obstructed endotracheal tube	Check tube.	Replace tube.
	Poor pulmonary circulation	Check for lung overinflation. Check blood pressure.	Decrease ventilation. Correct hypotension.

PCV, Packed cell volume; *PIP*, peak inspiratory pressure; *RR*, respiratory rate.

Continued

TABLE 10-2 Complications That Can Occur Under Anesthesia—cont'd

Complication	Cause	Diagnostic Test	Treatment
Increased $ETCO_2$	Hypoventilation.	Check ventilation. Auscultate lungs. Check thoracic expansion.	Correct underlying problem.
	CO_2 absorber not working	Check CO_2 absorber.	Change absorber.
	Increased dead space	Check for tachypnea, increased inspired CO_2 level.	Increase or institute ventilation. Consider neuromuscular blocker.
		Check anesthesia circuit.	Correct underlying problem.
	Lung disease	Take history. Auscultate lungs.	Change ventilation parameters. Treat underlying disease.
	Moisture in sensor	Check sensor and tubing.	Replace sensor or tubing.
Hypertension	Underlying disease Drugs	Systolic >180 mm Hg. Diastolic >120 mm Hg.	Increase inhalant dosage. Consider nitroprusside.
Hypotension	Hypovolemia	Check blood pressure. Check lingual pulses.	Administer colloid and crystalloid.
	Too deep a plane of anesthesia	Check vaporizer settings.	
	Inadequate preload from pressure on vena cava	Consider underlying disease.	Increase fluids. Correct underlying disease.
	Bradycardia	Check heart rate.	See Bradycardia below.
	Poor cardiac contractility	Check heart rhythm.	Infuse dobutamine. Administer antiarrhythmics.
	Refractory vasodilation	Rule out other causes.	Administer dopamine at vasopressor dosages.
	Peripheral vasoconstriction, hypothermia	Check temperature.	Warm patient.
Severe hypotension (arrest pending)	Severe hypovolemia Cardiac failure Extreme depth of anesthesia	Check blood pressure. Check heart rate and ECG.	Discontinue anesthetic agents. Perform fluid resuscitation. Surgeon to place pressure on cranial abdominal aorta if abdomen open. Positive inotropic and vasopressor support.
Bradycardia	Too deep a plane of anesthesia	Check anesthesia depth.	Decrease or discontinue drugs. Administer atropine.‡
	Opioids		Administer atropine.‡

ECG, Electrocardiogram.
‡High atropine dosages (0.05-0.2 mg/kg IV) should be used because lower dosages can lead to a second-degree atrioventricular block and worsening of the problem. If the patient does not respond, consider dosages up to 0.5 mg/kg IV or epinephrine to effect (start at 0.001 mg/kg/min).

TABLE 10-2 Complications That Can Occur Under Anesthesia—cont'd

Complication	Cause	Diagnostic Test	Treatment
Bradycardia—cont'd	Severe hypotension	Check blood pressure.	Discontinue anesthetic agents.
		Check heart rate and ECG.	Perform fluid resuscitation.
			Surgeon to place pressure on cranial abdominal aorta if abdomen open.
			Positive inotropic and vasopressor support.
	Surgical manipulation of vagus nerve or organs innervated by vagus	Check with surgeon.	Decrease surgical stimulation.
Tachycardia	Pain	Check level of anesthesia.	Administer analgesics.
	Hypoxia	Check for airway obstruction.	Unkink, suction, or replace as indicated.
		Check for tension pneumothorax or mediastinum from barotrauma.	Perform thoracentesis.
Supraventricular tachycardia	Idiopathic heart disease	Check ECG.	Treat underlying disease. Administer diltiazem.
	Pulmonary disease		Administer adenosine.
	Pain		Avoid β-blockers.
Multifocal ventricular premature contractions, ventricular tachycardia	Myocardial hypoxia (traumatic myocarditis)	Check ECG. Check blood pressure. Check electrolytes.	Ensure O_2 is being provided. Administer lidocaine 2 mg/kg followed by CRI at 25-75 μg/kg/min. If unresponsive consider procainamide 6-8 mg/kg over 5 min or magnesium chloride 1 mEq/kg over 30 min.
	Splenic disease	Check ECG. Check blood pressure. Check electrolytes.	Administer lidocaine 2 mg/kg followed by CRI at 25-75 μg/kg/min.
	Acidosis	Check $ETCO_2$. Check blood gas. Check blood pressure. Check electrolytes.	Improve perfusion. Administer lidocaine 2 mg/kg followed by CRI at 25-75 μg/kg/min.
Sinus arrest, severe or second-degree AV block		Check ECG.	Administer atropine 0.05-0.2 mg/kg IV.‡

AV, Atrioventricular; *CRI*, constant-rate infusion.

Continued

TABLE 10-2 Complications That Can Occur Under Anesthesia—cont'd

Complication	Cause	Diagnostic Test	Treatment
High CVP	Hypervolemia	Check CVP.	Administer diuretics.
	Pneumothorax, pneumomediastinum	Auscultate lungs. Check jugular distention. Perform thoracentesis.	Perform thoracentesis.
	Pericardial tamponade	Auscultate heart. Check ECG.	Perform cardiocentesis.
Low CVP	Hypovolemia		Increase fluid administration.
Pallor	Anemia	Check PCV.	Administer blood transfusion.
	Hypotension	Check blood pressure.	See Hypotension above.
	Hypothermia and vasoconstriction	Check temperature.	Warm patient.

CVP, Central venous pressure.

be suctioned (along with the esophagus if there is a lot of liquid) and the tube should be removed with the cuff partially inflated.

Patients should be rewarmed aggressively if they are hypothermic; proceed cautiously to prevent burns. Vital signs, including blood pressure, should be checked every 5 to 10 minutes until the patient is sternal. The patient should not be left unattended until it is sternal. Fluid support should be continued as needed to maintain normal central venous pressure and urine production. Any positive inotropes, vasopressors, or antiarrhythmics should be continued as needed to maintain normal blood pressure and cardiac rhythm.

Analgesia is vitally important in the postoperative period, and the patient should be given medication according to need, not a set schedule. Often in the critically ill or injured patient constant-rate infusions are needed and dosage reduction may be needed. A syringe pump is recommended. Regional and epidural analgesia can be repeated postoperatively as needed.

These patients often have received a number of drugs and large amounts of fluids during anesthesia. There may be significant metabolic abnormalities in combination with the underlying disease. Laboratory work should be checked immediately after surgery. Tests should include packed cell volume, total solids, and glucose. Ideally, they should also include blood urea nitrogen, albumin, electrolytes, and venous or arterial blood gas. Abnormalities should be corrected as indicated.

CONCLUSION

The veterinary technician must understand respiratory and cardiovascular physiology and the pathophysiology of the disease process to administer anesthesia successfully.

Items necessary for inducing anesthesia must be available in the emergency room at all times. A source of oxygen that can last for 6 hours must be available, with a fully functioning anesthetic machine. A variety of clear endotracheal tubes, at least two laryngoscopes, and basic monitoring equipment also are necessary.

Ventilatory and cardiovascular support must be maintained during anesthesia. Monitoring the anesthetized patient throughout the procedure allows the technician to determine whether the patient is being supported properly. The monitoring is continued after the patient is extubated, including laboratory work to determine the effects of the procedure on the patient.

Teamwork is essential for a positive outcome. Establishing protocols and checklists for the anesthetized patient promotes good communication and recordkeeping.

BIBLIOGRAPHY

Branson KR, Gross ME: Propofol in veterinary medicine, *J Am Vet Med Assoc* 204:1888, 1994.

Brock N: Premedication of fragile dogs and cats, *Can Vet J* 36:474, 1995.

Brock N: Feline anesthesia, *Can Vet J* 37:751, 1996.

Burton S, Lemke KA, Ihle SL, et al: Effects of medetomidine on serum osmolality; urine volume, osmolality and pH; free water clearance; and fractional clearance of sodium, chloride, potassium, and glucose in dogs, *Am J Vet Res* 59:756, 1998.

Carpenter RL, Caplan RA, Brown DL, et al: Incidence and risk factors for side effects of spinal anesthesia, *Anesthesiology* 76:906, 1992.

Cornick JL: Anesthetic management of patients with neurologic abnormalities, *Compend Contin Educ Pract Vet* 14:163, 1992.

Dyson DH: Influence of oxygen flows during anesthetic management, *Can Vet J* 32:752, 1991.

Dyson DH: Combating hypothermia, including recommendations for the use of oat bags, *Can Vet J* 38:517, 1997.

Dyson DH, Pettifer GR: Evaluation of the arrhythmogenicity of a low dose of acepromazine: comparison with xylazine, *Can J Vet Res* 61:241, 1997.

Funkquist PME, Nyman GC, Lofgren A, et al: Use of propofol-isoflurane as an anesthetic regimen for cesarean section in dogs, *J Am Vet Med Assoc* 211:313, 1997.

Green W: The ventilatory effects of sevoflurane, *Anesth Analg* 81:S23, 1995.

Harkin C, Pagel P, Kersten J, et al: Direct negative inotropic and lusitropic effects of sevoflurane, *Anesthesiology* 81:156, 1994.

Hatakeyama N, Momose Y, Ito Y: Effects of sevoflurane on contractile responses and electrophysiologic properties in canine cardiac myocytes, *Anesthesiology* 82:559, 1995.

Hendrix K, Raffe MR, Robinson EP, et al: Epidural administration of bupivicaine, morphine or their combination for postoperative analgesia in dogs, *J Am Vet Med Assoc* 209:598, 1996.

Herperger LJ: Postoperative urinary retention in a dog following morphine with bupivicaine epidural analgesia, *Can Vet J* 39:650, 1998.

Ilkiw JE, Pascoe PJ, Haskins SC, et al: Cardiovascular and respiratory effects of propofol administration in hypovolemic dogs, *Am J Vet Res* 53:2323, 1992.

Ingwersen W, Allen DG, Dyson DH, et al: Cardiopulmonary effects of halothane/oxygen combination in cats, *Can J Vet Res* 52:386, 1988.

Jacobson JD, McGrath CJ, Smith E: Cardiorespiratory effects of induction and maintenance of anesthesia with ketamine-midazolam combination with and without prior administration of butorphanol or oxymorphone, *Am J Vet Res* 55:543, 1994.

Ko JCH, Thurmon JC, Benson GJ, et al: Hemodynamic and anesthetic effects of etomidate infusion in medetomidine-premedicated dogs, *Am J Vet Res* 55:842, 1994.

Lukasik V: Neuromuscular blocking drugs and the critical care patient, *Journal of Vet Emergency and Critical Care* 5:99, 1996.

Martinez EA, Hartsfield SM, Melendez LD, et al: Cardiovascular effects of buprenorphine in anesthetized dogs, *Am J Vet Res* 58:1280, 1997.

Mathews KA: Nonsteroidal anti-inflammatory analgesics in pain management in dogs and cats, *Can Vet J* 37:539, 1996.

McCrackin MA, Harvey RC, Sackman JE, et al: Butorphanol tartrate for partial reversal of oxymorphone-induced postoperative respiratory depression in the dog, *Vet Surg* 23:67, 1994.

Moon PF: Cortisol suppression in cats after induction of anesthesia with etomidate, compared with ketamine-diazepam combination, *Am J Vet Res* 58:868, 1997.

Muir WW, Gadawski JE: Respiratory depression and apnea induced by propofol in dogs, *Am J Vet Res* 59:157, 1998.

Muir WW, Gadawski J: Cardiorespiratory effects of low-flow and closed circuit inhalation anesthesia using sevoflurane delivered with an in-circuit vaporizer and concentrations of compound A, *Am J Vet Res* 59:603, 1999.

Pascoe PJ, Ilkiw JE, Haskins SC, et al: Cardiopulmonary effects of etomidate in hypovolemic dogs, *Am J Vet Res* 53:278, 1992.

Pettifer GR, Dyson DH, McDonnell: An evaluation of the influence of medetomidine hydrochloride and atipamezole hydrochloride on the arrhythmogenic dose of epinephrine in dogs during halothane anesthesia, *Can J Vet Res* 60:1, 1996.

Remedios AM, Wagner R, Caulkett NA, et al: Epidural abscess and discospondylitis in a dog after administration of lumbosacral epidural analgesic, *Can Vet J* 37:106, 1996.

Roberts FL, Dixon J, Lewis GTR, et al: Induction and maintenance of propofol anesthesia, *Anesthesiology* 43:14, 1988.

Sawyer DC, Rech RH, Durham RA: Does ketamine provide adequate visceral analgesia when used alone or in combination with acepromazine, diazepam, or butorphanol in cats? *J Am Anim Hosp Assoc* 29:253, 1993.

Servin F, Cockshott ID, Farinotti R, et al: Pharmacokinetics of propofol infusion in patients with cirrhosis, *Br J Anaesth* 65:177, 1990.

Smith JA, Gaynor JS, Bednarski RM, et al: Adverse effects of administration of propofol with various preanesthetic regimens in dogs, *J Am Vet Med Assoc* 202:1111, 1992.

Southwick FS, Dalglish PH: Recovery after prolonged asystolic arrest in profound hypothermia, *JAMA* 243:1250, 1980.

Stobie D, Caywood DD, Rozanski EA, et al: Evaluation of pulmonary function and analgesia in dogs after intercostal thoracotomy and use of morphine administered intramuscularly or intrapleurally and bupivicaine administered intrapleurally, *Am J Vet Res* 8:1098, 1995.

Torske KE, Dyson DH, Pettifer G: End tidal halothane concentration and postoperative analgesia requirements in dogs: a comparison between intravenous oxymorphone and epidural bupivicaine alone and in combination with oxymorphone, *Can Vet J* 39:361, 1998.

Venugopalan CS, Holmes EP, Fucci V, et al: Cardiopulmonary effects of medetomidine in heartworm-infected and noninfected dogs, *Am J Vet Res* 55:1148, 1994.

Yao FF: Ischemic heart disease and coronary artery bypass grafting. In *Anesthesiology/problem-oriented patient management,* ed 2, Philadelphia, 1988, JB Lippincott.

Section

Emergency Care for Small Animals

This section discusses the importance of an organized work space in the emergency room and the types of emergencies seen in the small animal emergency facility. The technician plays a vital role in stabilizing these animals.

Chapter

Managing Shock

The veterinary technician plays an integral role in the management of the emergent or critically ill patient. Many of these patients suffer a disease process associated with inadequate tissue perfusion resulting in poor oxygen delivery. The condition often is assessed as shock. Shock typically is classified in several categories (e.g., cardiogenic, septic, hypovolemic), and the causes of shock are numerous. Regardless of the form of shock, the goal is to optimize oxygen delivery. This chapter discusses the determinants of oxygen delivery, the pathophysiology of hypovolemic shock, and shock management.

Equipment List

Oxygen delivery system
Variety of short, large-gauge over-the-needle catheters
Fluid administration sets
Intravenous fluids (crystalloids and colloids)
Pressure bag to increase fluid delivery
Steroids
Antibiotics
Electrocardiogram
Doppler
Supplies for quick assessment tests (packed cell volume, total solids, blood urea nitrogen, blood glucose)

OXYGEN DELIVERY

Oxygen delivery is the amount of volume of oxygen transported to the tissues each minute. Oxygen delivery is the product of cardiac output and oxygen content. In most practice situations it is not possible to calculate oxygen delivery. However, the concept is important, and there are several components of oxygen delivery (Figure 11-1). Cardiac output is the product of stroke volume and heart rate. To improve or increase cardiac output, the heart rate and/or stroke volume must increase. Stroke volume is the amount of blood pumped out of the heart with each beat, and there are three primary determinants of stroke volume: (1) Stroke volume is increased in proportion to the stretch of the walls of the ventricles during diastole (preload); (2) the strength of contraction (contractility); and (3) decreases in the forces that oppose blood flow from the heart (afterload, i.e., in the absence of valvular stenosis, arterial blood pressure).

Oxygen content is the amount of oxygen in arterial blood. Oxygen is either dissolved in plasma or bound to hemoglobin. Oxygen content is defined by the equation in Figure 11-2. Hemoglobin is the main carrier of oxygen in the blood. Each gram of hemoglobin has the capacity to carry 1.34 ml O_2 (20.1 ml O_2/dl blood when the hemoglobin is 15 g/dl). Only 0.3 ml O_2/dl blood is dissolved in the plasma when the PaO_2 is 100 mm Hg (Figure 11-3).

DEFINITIONS OF SHOCK

Many different categorization schemes have been used to define shock, and there is some overlap between categories. For the purposes of this discussion, shock is divided into four different categories based on the causative pathophysiologic

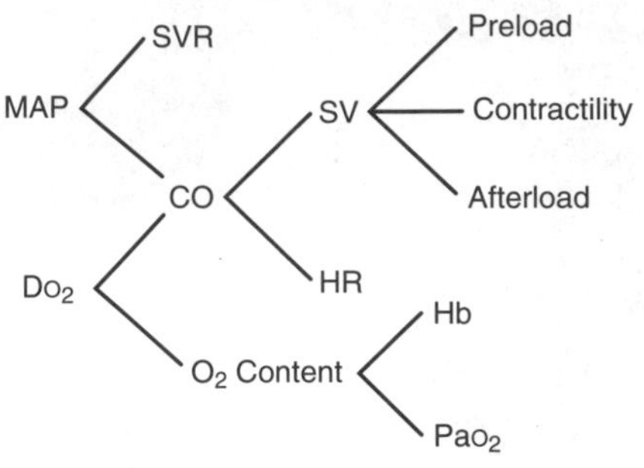

Figure 11-1

Determinants of O_2 delivery *(Do_2)*. *CO,* Cardiac output; *Hb,* hemoglobin; *HR,* heart rate; *MAP,* mean arterial pressure; *SV,* stroke volume; *SVR,* systemic vascular resistance.

$$Cao_2 = (1.34 \times Hb \times Sao_2) + (Pao_2 \times 0.003)$$

Figure 11-2

Oxygen content *(Cao_2)* equation.

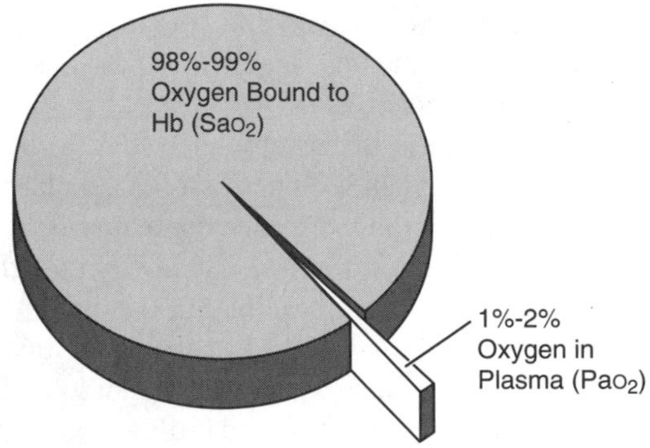

Figure 11-3

Percentage of oxygen bound to hemoglobin and dissolved in plasma.

mechanism. Ultimately the focus of therapy is to optimize oxygen delivery. Cardiogenic shock results from heart failure but excludes factors that are outside the heart (i.e., cardiac tamponade, caval syndrome). Pump failure may be caused by hypertrophic or dilative cardiomyopathy, valvular insufficiency or stenosis, arrhythmias, or fibrosis. Distributive shock often is used to describe shock states that are associated with flow maldistribution. Initiating causes for this form of shock include sepsis, anaphylaxis, trauma, and neurogenic causes. Obstructive shock results from a physical obstruction in the circulatory system. Heartworm disease, pericardial effusion, pulmonary embolism, and gastric torsion can impair blood flow. Hypovolemic shock is the result of decreased intravascular volume. The decreased volume may result from blood loss, third space loss, or fluid losses caused by excessive vomiting, diarrhea, and diuresis. Hypovolemic shock is the most common form of shock in small animals.

PATHOPHYSIOLOGY OF HYPOVOLEMIC SHOCK

Shock is a complex and dynamic process involving many compensatory mechanisms. An initiating cause results in a decreased intravascular volume. As a result of the decreased intravascular volume, venous return and ventricular filling (preload) decrease. With the decreased ventricular filling, stroke volume and cardiac output decrease. The result is inadequate tissue perfusion and oxygen delivery.

Decreased cardiac output and hypotension cause a baroreceptor-mediated sympathoadrenal reflex that activates the patient's compensatory mechanisms to help maintain perfusion. Norepinephrine, epinephrine, and cortisol are released from the adrenal gland. Epinephrine and norepinephrine cause an increase in heart rate and contractility and arteriolar constriction, which increases systemic vascular resistance and redirects blood flow to the heart and brain and away from skin, muscle, kidneys, and gastrointestinal tract. Cortisol enhances the effects of the catecholamines on arterioles. Sodium and water are conserved because of renin-angiotensin-aldosterone activation, increasing intravascular volume.

INITIAL ASSESSMENT AND RECOGNITION

The initial recognition of hypovolemic shock is based on historical and physical findings (Table 11-1). Historically, the owner may be able to provide information that supports a reason for hypovolemia such as trauma, excessive urination, diarrhea, or vomiting. Typically the physical findings indicate sympathoadrenal activation (tachycardia and vasoconstriction). In the early stage or compensatory phase of shock, tachycardia, decreased pulse quality, prolonged capillary refill time (CRT), pale mucous membrane color, and cool extremities are seen. This may be called stage 1, or compensated shock. In stage 2, decompensated shock, the patient has tachycardia, decreased pulse quality, variable CRT, muddy mucous membrane color, decreasing blood pressure, and obtunded mental status. When the patient is suffering from severe systemic hypoperfusion and therapies cease to be effective, the patient is said to be in stage 3, irreversible shock. The stages of shock are a continuum. Progression through the stages is based on patient-related factors and the timeliness and effectiveness of therapy.

TABLE 11-1 Nursing Assessment Parameters for Shock

Parameter	Assessment
Level of consciousness	Alertness, obtundation, stupor, or coma
Pulse	Rate, rhythm, strength, and quality
Respiratory	Rate, depth, effort, breath sounds
Cutaneous	Temperature (rectal or extremity), mucous membrane color and moistness, capillary refill time, skin turgor
Urine production	Output, specific gravity
Blood pressure	Changes in values

THERAPY

The goal of therapy is to improve oxygen delivery (Box 11-1). Our energies should be directed at correcting or improving the components of the oxygen delivery algorithm (see Figure 11-1).

OXYGEN THERAPY

Maintaining oxygen saturation is one of the primary goals in maintaining blood oxygenation. If there is any question about a patient's blood oxygenation, supplemental oxygen should be provided until assessment of arterial blood gases or hemoglobin saturation confirms that oxygen supplementation is not necessary. When this equipment is not available, assessment must be based on clinical dyspnea or auscultatable abnormalities and clinical signs of hypoxia (cyanosis of the mucous membranes or dark-colored blood, tachypnea,

Box 11-1 Summary of Therapy to Improve Oxygen Delivery

Correct primary problem: control fluid loss, treat infection.
Oxygenation: provide supplemental oxygen via mask, nasal or transtracheal catheter, or cage.
Fluid resuscitation
- Crystalloids
  - Dogs 80-90 ml/kg
  - Cats 50-55 ml/kg
- 7.5% hypertonic saline 4-6 ml/kg
- Synthetic colloids
  - Dogs 10-40 ml/kg
  - Cats 5-ml/kg increments over 15-20 minutes
- Plasma 10-40 ml/kg
- Whole blood 10-30 ml/kg
- Red blood cells 5-15 ml/kg, all fluids given to effect
- Oxyglobin® 10-30 ml/kg, not to exceed 10 ml/kg/hr

Consider sympathomimetics: dopamine 5-10 μg/kg/min.
Consider steroids: dexamethasone $NaPO_4$ 4-8 mg/kg; prednisolone sodium succinate 10-30 mg/kg.

tachycardia, and anxiety). Individually, the clinical signs do not prove hypoxemia, but together they suggest hypoxemia. There are several methods of oxygen therapy. The method selected depends on the expected duration of therapy, the patient's demeanor, and equipment availability. Available methods include the face mask, oxygen bag (hood) or oxygen cage, transtracheal administration, and nasal insufflation. The ultimate goal of oxygen therapy is to provide adequate oxygen to the blood using the lowest possible inspired oxygen concentrations.

Venous Access

The appropriate vein to catheterize depends on several factors such as the size and species of the animal, the skill of the operator placing the catheter, therapeutic goals, and the animal's injury or disease. Any vessel that is visible or palpable is a candidate for percutaneous catheterization. The cephalic and saphenous veins are easily accessible routes that can be catheterized quickly. The maximum fluid flow rate of a catheter is determined primarily by the internal diameter and length of the catheter and the height of the fluid bag above the patient (Table 11-2).

A short, large-gauge catheter is needed if fluids are to be administered rapidly. It is also advisable to keep administration tubing short. Avoid using excessive extension tubing and unnecessary connectors, which reduce flow rates.

If vascular access cannot be obtained, establishing an intraosseous line (Figure 11-4) is a reasonable alternative. Fluid or drugs administered by this route are taken up rapidly into the circulatory system.

Fluid Resuscitation

The most effective way to improve oxygen delivery is to increase cardiac output by optimizing preload with fluid administration.

Crystalloids. Isotonic crystalloids that have concentrations of electrolytes (sodium, chloride, potassium, and bicarbonate-like anions) similar to those of extracellular fluid often are used to treat hypovolemic shock. These fluids freely and rapidly distribute between the intravascular and interstitial compartments. After 30 minutes, 98% of the volume of fluids infused into the intravascular compartment shifts into the interstitial compartment. Examples of commonly used crystalloids include lactated Ringer's solution, normal saline, Normosol-R (Abbott Laboratories, North Chicago, Illinois), and Plasmalyte 148 (Baxter Healthcare, Deerfield, Illinois). A commonly cited fluid dosage goal of isotonic crystalloids is 80 to 90 ml/kg/hr for

Table 11-2 Fluid Flow Rates Based on Catheter Gauge and Height of Fluid Bag

	Flow rate (ml/min)	
Catheter Gauge	Height 3 ft	Height 6 ft
16	88	152
18	75	114
20	45	75

From Fulton RB, Hauptman JG: In vitro and in vivo rates of fluid flow through catheters in peripheral veins of dogs, *J Am Vet Med Assoc* 198(9):1473, 1991.

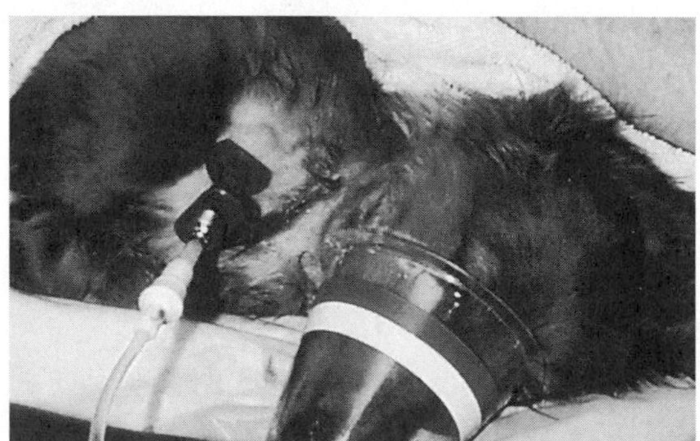

Figure 11-4
Fluid administration via intraosseous catheter.

the dog and 50 to 55 ml/kg/hr for the cat (equivalent to one blood volume). Individual animal requirements vary, so it may be necessary to administer 0.5 to 1.5 times the usual volume to resuscitate the patient. The patient's condition must be reassessed frequently (i.e., about every 10 to 15 minutes) during large-volume or rapid fluid administration.

Hypertonic crystalloids such as 7.5% saline are recommended for use in shock therapy when it is difficult to administer large volumes of fluids rapidly enough to resuscitate the patient. Hypertonic saline causes fluid shifts from the intracellular space to the extracellular (including intravascular) space, improving venous return and cardiac output. Hypertonic saline also causes vasodilation and improves tissue perfusion. The recommended dosage range is 4 to 6 ml/kg over 5 minutes. Dextran 70 has been added to hypertonic saline to potentiate and sustain vascular volume augmentation. Because of the fluid steal that occurs, isotonic crystalloids should be administered at 40% to 60% of the shock dosage of fluids.

Hypotonic fluids such as 5% dextrose in water, half-strength saline, and half-strength lactated Ringer's should not be used to treat hypovolemic shock. These fluids contain too much free water and distribute excessively to the intracellular compartment.

Colloids. Colloids are high-molecular-weight solutions that do not cross capillary membranes readily. Colloids are better blood volume expanders than are isotonic crystalloids; 50% to 80% of the infused volume remains in the intravascular space. Colloids should be administered when crystalloids are not improving or maintaining blood volume restoration. Intravascular colloid oncotic pressure (COP) is important in maintaining intravascular volume. Large volumes of crystalloids decrease COP, whereas colloids increase COP. Colloids should be administered when the total protein or albumin decreases below 4.0 g/dl or 1.5 g/dl, respectively. Colloids include plasma, blood, Oxyglobin® (Biopure, Cambridge, Massachusetts) and the synthetics, dextran 70 (Gentran 70, Baxter Healthcare, Deerfield, Illinois), and hetastarch (Hespan, DuPont, Wilmington, Delaware). Plasma provides albumin, immunoglobulins, platelets, and clotting factors. The approximate plasma dosage is 10 to 40 ml/kg, but it should be administered to effect. Large volumes of plasma may be needed to affect total protein or albumin concentrations.

Hemoglobin must be available in sufficient concentrations to ensure adequate oxygen content. If hemoglobin decreases from 15 g/dl to 10 g/dl, oxygen content is reduced by one third; cardiac output must increase to maintain adequate oxygen delivery (see Figure 11-1). In the absence of hemoglobin measurements, hemoglobin can be estimated from the microhematocrit. The hemoglobin usually is about one third the hematocrit value. The hematocrit should be maintained around 30%. Oxygen delivery is limited when the hematocrit decreases below 20%. Whole blood and packed red blood cells are administered at 10 to 30 ml/kg and 5 to 15 ml/kg, respectively; again, these must be administered to effect. These dosages increase the hematocrit approximately 5% to 15%.

As an alternative to plasma, synthetic colloids may be administered. If the patient is a cat or suspected or known to have closed-cavity hemorrhage, head trauma, pulmonary contusions, or cardiogenic shock, fluid therapy should be conservative; the colloid should be administered no faster than 5 ml/kg over 15 to 20 minutes. The 5-ml/kg boluses are titrated to effect. It has been reported that rapid colloid administration can cause nausea in cats. Otherwise, dextran and hetastarch can be given as a bolus of 10 to 40 ml/kg to effect. Because the synthetic colloids only replace intravascular volume, crystalloids still must be given to replace interstitial fluid deficits. Crystalloids administered with colloids are given at 40% to 60% of the dosage of crystalloids used alone.

Dextran and hetastarch can interfere with platelet function and can prolong coagulation parameters more than can be attributed to simple hemodilution. Blood products and oxypolygelatins can cause allergic reactions.

Dosage (μg/kg/min) × (kg)(body weight) = Drug (mg) to place in 250 ml/fluids

Administer at 15 ml/hr

Figure 11-5

Quick formula for calculating μg/kg/min constant-rate infusions.

STEROIDS

The efficacy of steroids in treating hypovolemic shock remains controversial. Initial animal research studies indicated that steroids are beneficial in shock; large human clinical studies show no beneficial effect reducing mortality. Steroids can stabilize cell and organelle membranes, improve oxygen delivery to the tissues, and improve intermediary metabolism, but they also can reduce resistance to infection. If steroids are to be used, they should be administered early. Suggested shock dosages are dexamethasone sodium phosphate 4 to 8 mg/kg and prednisolone sodium succinate (Solu Delta Cortef, Pharmacia and Upjohn, Kalamazoo, Michigan) 10 to 30 mg/kg.

SYMPATHOMIMETICS

Sympathomimetics such as dopamine (Abbot Laboratories, North Chicago, Illinois) and dobutamine (Dobutrex, Eli Lilly, Indianapolis, Indiana) are indicated when the patient is unresponsive to vigorous fluid therapy and arterial blood pressure, vasomotor tone, and tissue perfusion have not returned to acceptable levels. These drugs support myocardial contractility and blood pressure with minimal vasoconstriction. Blood pressure monitoring is recommended. Dopamine, a precursor of norepinephrine, has dose-dependent effects. At 0.5 to 3 μg/kg/min, dilation of renal, mesenteric, and coronary vascular beds occurs because of its dopaminergic effect. Heart rate and contractility increase at a dosage of 3 to 7.5 μg/kg/min; this is a result of β_1 activity. At dosages greater than 7.5 μg/kg/min, α- receptor stimulation and vasoconstriction occur. Dobutamine has primarily β activity. It increases contractility and has minimal effect on heart rate and peripheral vascular resistance except at higher dosages. The dosage range is 5 to 15 μg/kg/min. Sympathomimetics should not be a substitute for adequate volume restoration. Fluid resuscitation remains the cornerstone of shock therapy. The technician should be able to calculate constant-rate infusions (CRI) using the formula in Figure 11-5.

MONITORING

Many of the signs associated with shock are related to the compensatory mechanism the body invokes to maintain life. Clinical signs must be assessed frequently because the hemodynamic and metabolic sequelae of shock change continually. Monitoring begins with the physical assessment and is integrated with physiologic monitoring and evaluation of cellular function (acid-base balance and other laboratory values).

PHYSICAL PARAMETERS

Respiratory. Can the patient meet its ventilation and oxygenation requirements? Are the rate and tidal volume adequate, is the breathing effort smooth and easy, and is the breathing pattern regular? Are breath sounds normal? Abnormal breath sounds could be described as crackles, wheezes, squeaks, muffled, and quiet.

Cardiovascular. Cardiovascular system assessment may begin with the heart rate. There are several causes of tachycardia and bradycardia. If arrhythmias are auscultated, then an electrocardiogram (ECG) is indicated. Indicators of peripheral perfusion include mucous membrane color, CRT, urine output, and appendage temperature.

Normal mucous membrane color is pink. Pale mucous membranes may indicate anemia or vasoconstriction. Brick red or hyperemic mucous membranes may indicate vasodilation and is seen in the early phases of septic shock. Normal capillary refill is 1 to 2 seconds. Prolonged CRT is associated with decreased peripheral perfusion. Normal urine production is 1 to 2 ml/kg/hr; it decreases when perfusion is decreased or when mean arterial pressure is less than 60 mm Hg. Appendage temperature decreases as a result of vasoconstriction and poor peripheral perfusion. A strong pulse indicates a good pulse pressure and stroke volume, and a weak pulse indicates decreased stroke volume.

Physiologic Monitoring Parameters

Oxygen Saturation. *Spo*$_2$ is commonly used to refer to oxygen saturation readings obtained with a pulse oximeter. Pulse oximetry provides noninvasive and continuous information about the percent oxygen bound to hemoglobin. Normal Spo_2 is greater than 95%. The patient is seriously hypoxemic when the Spo_2 is 90% or less. Caution should be exercised when interpreting Spo_2 values of animals breathing 100% oxygen. Animals with a Pao_2 of 500 mm Hg still have an Spo_2 of 98% to 99%.

Arterial Blood Pressure. Arterial blood pressure is measured by indirect and direct methods. Arterial blood pressure is the product of cardiac output, vascular capacity, and blood volume. The three determinants work in concert to maintain blood pressure. If one of the three becomes subnormal, the other two should compensate. Normal systolic, diastolic, and mean blood pressures are approximately 100 to 160, 60 to 100, and 80 to 120 mm Hg, respectively. Systolic and mean blood pressures below 80 mm Hg and 60 mm Hg, respectively, warrant therapy. Causes of hypotension include hypovolemia, peripheral vasodilation, and decreased cardiac output. Hypertension can be caused by chronic renal failure, an adrenal tumor (pheochromocytoma), or any other factor that increases cardiac output.

Central Venous Pressure. Central venous pressure (CVP) is the blood pressure in the intrathoracic anterior vena cava compared to a column of water in a plastic manometer or a pressure transducer and oscilloscope. Changes in pressure in the thorax produce fluctuations in the water manometer or waveforms on the oscilloscope. CVP is a measure of the heart's ability to pump fluids returned to it and is also an estimate of the relationship of blood volume to blood volume capacity. CVP should be measured when heart failure is suspected or as an aid in determining the endpoint of aggressive fluid therapy. A reasonable preload has been achieved when the CVP approaches 10 cm H_2O (7.5 mm Hg). If cardiac output, pulse quality, blood pressure, or perfusion parameters (CRT, mucous membrane color, urine output, and appendage temperature) are acceptable, effective blood volume restoration probably has been accomplished. If not, it can be assumed that the heart cannot handle the venous return.

Laboratory Parameters

Hematocrit and Total Solids. Hematocrit (Hct) and total solids (TS) can be used to gauge fluid therapy, estimate hemoglobin concentration, and, to a certain degree, assess blood loss. The two tests should be interpreted together to minimize errors in interpretation. An increase in both Hct and TS indicates dehydration; a decrease in both Hct and TS suggests recent blood loss or clear fluid administration. An increase in TS and normal Hct may indicate anemia with dehydration. Both Hct and TS may be normal in peracute blood loss. TS may decrease with reduced albumin levels; albumin is a contributor to oncotic pressure.

Electrolytes. Electrolytes play a major role in maintaining intercompartmental water balance and cell function. Baseline electrolytes should be obtained and monitoring continued as therapy progresses. Fluid therapy can alter various serum electrolyte concentrations, and it may be necessary to adjust the electrolyte composition in the fluids being administered. Commonly measured electrolytes include serum potassium, sodium, chloride, magnesium, and ionized calcium.

Arterial pH and Blood Gases. Monitoring of arterial blood gases is an excellent way to assess ventilation and oxygenation. $Paco_2$ tells how well the patient is ventilating. A $Paco_2$ less than 35 mm Hg or greater than 45 mm Hg indicates hyperventilation or hypoventilation, respectively. Pao_2 indicates how well the patient is oxygenating. A Pao_2 less than 80 mm Hg is considered hypoxemia, although the patient may not be given treatment until it approaches 60 mm Hg. The pH combined with bicarbonate or base balance indicates the patient's metabolic status. Normal pH is 7.35 to 7.45, a pH less than 7.35 is called acidemia, and a pH greater than 7.45 is called alkalemia. A patient has metabolic acidosis if the bicarbonate is less than 18 mmol/L or base deficit is more negative than –4. Alkalosis is identified by a bicarbonate greater than 27 mmol/L and a base excess greater than +4.

Jugular venous Po_2 samples below 30 mm Hg or greater than 60 mm Hg may be caused by decreased oxygen delivery to the tissues and reduced oxygen uptake by the tissues, respectively. Venous Po_2 and arterial Po_2 are not correlated.

Colloid Oncotic Pressure. COP can be measured and used to guide fluid therapy. COP is a force created by large plasma proteins that do not move freely across capillaries. The presence of colloids in the vascular space pulls water from the interstitium into the vascular space. The goal is to maintain a COP greater than 18 mm Hg.

Lactate. When perfusion decreases and oxygen delivery is reduced, the body shifts from aerobic to anaerobic metabolism, resulting in lactate formation. Elevated blood lactate (greater than 2 mmol/L) has been proposed as an indicator of inadequate tissue oxygenation. Although elevated blood lactate levels often signify generalized tissue hypoxia, a normal value does not rule out regional lactate production.

CONCLUSION

Shock is a dynamic and complex syndrome; the focus of therapy and monitoring is oxygen delivery. To improve the oxygen content component of oxygen delivery, oxygen or hemoglobin can be administered in the form of packed red blood cells or whole blood. To improve the cardiac output component, fluids can be administered in the form of crystalloids or colloids, which improves preload. Drug therapy also may be needed to improve contractility and heart rate and in some cases reduce afterload. Improving cardiac output and systemic vascular resistance also improves the patient's blood pressure. Understanding the pathophysiologic and compensatory mechanisms of this complex syndrome will aid the veterinary technician in meeting therapeutic and monitoring goals.

BIBLIOGRAPHY

Chandler CF, Waxman K: Monitoring. In Shoemaker WC et al, eds: *Pocket companion to textbook of critical care,* Philadelphia, 1996, WB Saunders.

Franklin CM, Darovic GO, Dan BB: Monitoring the patient in shock. In Darovic GO, ed: *Hemodynamic monitoring: invasive and noninvasive clinical application,* Philadelphia, 1995, WB Saunders.

Fulton RB, Hauptman JG: In vitro and in vivo rates of fluid flow through catheters in peripheral veins of dogs, *J Am Vet Med Assoc* 198(9):1473, 1991.

Kirby RR: Colloids: those magic fluids. Scientific proceedings of the 23rd annual meeting, San Antonio, Texas, 1997, Veterinary Emergency and Critical Care Society.

Lohrman JM: Clinical aspects of oxygen delivery and consumption. Proceedings from Pathophysiology of Shock, Lewisville, Texas, 1997, Barbara Clark Mims Associates.

Marino PL: Hemodynamic drugs. In *The ICU Book,* Baltimore, 1998, Williams & Wilkins.

Rudloff E, Kirby RR: Hypovolemic shock and resuscitation, *Vet Clin North Am Small Anim Pract* 24:1015, 1994.

Chapter 12

Cardiopulmonary Cerebrovascular Resuscitation

Cardiopulmonary arrest (CPA) is the sudden cessation of spontaneous and effective ventilation and systemic perfusion (circulation). CPA may result from any disease process carried to its extreme that disrupts cardiac or pulmonary homeostasis. Potential causes of CPA include hypoxia, metabolic disorders, trauma, vagal stimulation, anesthetic or other drugs, and environmental influences (hypothermia or hyperthermia). In one study the most common conditions leading to cardiac arrest in young dogs (up to 1.5 years) were infections (gastroenteritis and pneumonia) and trauma. Conditions leading to CPA in older dogs (between 6 and 10 years) were more chronic, such as primary heart disease, autoimmune disease, and malignancy. In the same study, the most common medical condition preceding CPA in cats was trauma, with infectious diseases being the next most common condition.

More than 35 years have elapsed since the combined techniques of mechanical ventilation, external precordial compression, and defibrillation were introduced in human medicine. Today, we know these combined techniques as cardiopulmonary cerebrovascular resuscitation (CPCR). We are fortunate that much of the CPCR research conducted has been carried out in animal subjects. Many of the techniques or procedures used in human medicine also are used in veterinary medicine. The goal of CPCR is to provide adequate ventilatory and circulatory support until spontaneous functions return. CPCR has three phases: basic life support, advanced life support, and prolonged life support. This chapter covers preparation for this ultimate emergency, recognition of CPA, and the three phases of CPCR.

Equipment List

- Defibrillator
- Electrocardiograph
- Crash cart supplies
- Pharmaceutical
  - Atropine
  - Epinephrine
  - 2% Lidocaine (without epinephrine)
  - Dexamethasone sodium phosphate
  - Sodium bicarbonate
  - Calcium chloride or gluconate
  - Lactated Ringer's solution (or hypertonic saline, dextran 70, or hetastarch)
- Airway access
  - Laryngoscope and blades
  - Endotracheal tubes (variety of sizes)
  - Lubricating jelly
  - Roll gauze
- Venous access
  - Butterfly catheters (variety of sizes)
  - IV catheters (variety of sizes)
  - IV drip sets
  - Bone marrow needles
  - Syringes (variety of sizes)
  - Hypodermic needles (variety of sizes)

- Adhesive tape
- Tourniquet

Miscellaneous
- Gauze (3- by 3-inch)
- Stethoscope
- Minor surgery pack
- Suture material
- Scalpel blade
- Surgical gloves

PREPARATION

STAFF

A team approach to CPA management is essential. The ideal number of participants in a resuscitation attempt is three to five. Several CPCR responsibilities (Table 12-1) must be met. Each member of the hospital staff (including receptionist and kennel help) should be trained to carry out one or more of these responsibilities. The team leader usually is the veterinarian; if the veterinarian is not available, then the person with the most experience in performing CPCR should lead the team. Team members must provide ventilation, compress the chest, establish IV lines, administer drugs, attach monitoring equipment, record the resuscitation effort, and monitor the team's effectiveness. Regular practice drills should be held. The benefits are tremendous when the staff can respond quickly and efficiently. A stuffed animal can be used as the patient during these drills. Each person should understand his or her responsibilities during an arrest. After each practice session or true resuscitation, a self-evaluation should be performed.

TABLE 12-1 Cardiopulmonary Cerebrovascular Resuscitation Responsibilities and Tasks

Responsibility	Tasks
Airway management	Establish airway. Ventilate.
Cardiovascular management	Compress chest.
Venous access	Place IV lines. Start IV fluids.
Effectiveness monitoring	Attach ECG. Check pulse. Check mucous membrane color. Check Doppler flow. Check end-tidal CO_2.
Drug administration	Administer drugs. Document drugs given and response.

FACILITIES

The area where the resuscitation effort takes place should be large enough for a CPCR team and equipment. An oxygen source should be readily available. Good lighting is needed; it facilitates endotracheal intubation and visualization of veins, and if open chest massage is attempted, it allows visualization of internal structures. If CPCR is to be performed on a table, then the height of the table should be adjustable. If a table is too tall, it is difficult to perform chest compressions effectively. If the height of the table is not adjustable, then a footstool should be made available or CPCR should be performed on the floor. Avoid grated surgical prep tables if possible. They have too much give, which can be counterproductive during chest compressions. If you have no choice and must use a prep table, then put a board on or below the grate to provide extra support. The table must have a solid surface. If some form of crash cart is not used, then the drugs, electrocardiograph (ECG), suction machine, and defibrillator should be in close proximity. A shelf and a few drawers should be set aside for emergency supplies.

EQUIPMENT

The use of a crash cart or kit makes resuscitation more efficient by keeping the necessary supplies readily available. The crash cart or kit may be as simple as a fishing tackle box or as elaborate as a mobile tool chest (Figure 12-1). If a cart is used, additional equipment such as the suction machine, ECG, and defibrillator can be stored on the cart. The crash cart or kit should be checked at the beginning of each shift and restocked immediately after each use.

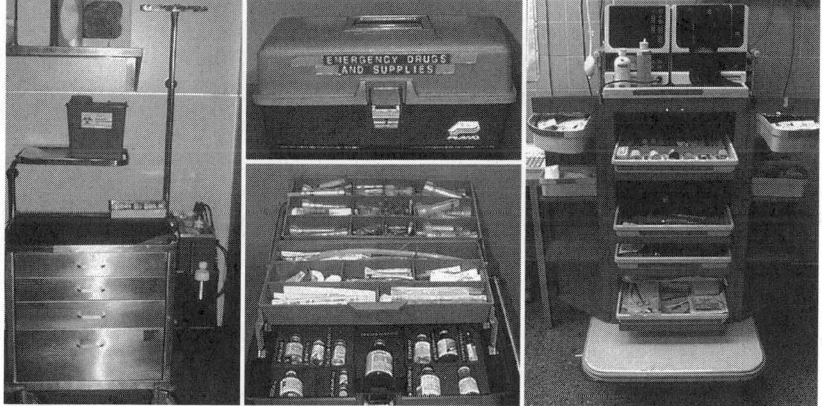

Figure 12-1

Examples of an emergency kit and crash cart.

RECOGNITION

Veterinary technicians are often in a position to recognize impending problems such as CPA. The technician's efforts should be directed toward determining which patients are at risk for developing CPA. The technician should look for decreasing mentation or lack of response; change in respiratory rate, depth, and pattern; change in pulse rate, rhythm, or quality; abnormal ECG rhythms; or unexplained changes in anesthetic depth. If the patient's condition begins to deteriorate, medical and nursing interventions are needed. It is often easier to prevent an arrest than to treat an arrest. CPCR should be initiated if the patient is apneic, the pulse is absent, or the heart cannot be auscultated. Pupils may become dilated within 20 to 40 seconds after arrest. Knowledge of recent medications administered should be used when assessing pupils; drugs such as atropine and epinephrine can cause the pupils to dilate. If there is any question whether the patient is in CPA, CPCR should be initiated until proven otherwise.

BASIC LIFE SUPPORT

The primary objective of basic life support (BLS) is to temporarily support the patient's oxygenation, ventilation, and circulation. This is accomplished by administering manual artificial ventilation and external chest compressions. Remembering the mnemonic ABC (Box 12-1) helps the resuscitation team focus on the priorities of BLS.

AIRWAY

The first priority for BLS is to establish an airway. Usually an endotracheal tube is inserted to ensure a patent airway. On occasion, a tracheostomy tube may be indicated if there is an upper airway obstruction. If tracheostomy tubes are not available and the patient has an upper airway obstruction, an endotracheal tube can be used as a tracheostomy tube. A variety of endotracheal and tracheostomy tubes and the associated airway management supplies (laryngoscopes, stylets, roll gauze, and syringes) should be readily available. In addition, suction should be available to remove blood, mucus, pulmonary edema fluid, and vomitus from the oral cavity and trachea. The endotracheal tube must be placed properly. Proper placement is confirmed by visualization; chest auscultation for breath sounds also is helpful.

BREATHING

The second priority is to initiate artificial ventilation. The patient is attached to a breathing source that delivers 100% oxygen, such as an AMBU bag

Box 12-1 Mnemonic for Key Steps in Basic Life Support

Airway: establish airway.
Breathing: once every 3-5 sec.
Circulation: 80-120 compressions/min.

or anesthetic machine. Initially, the patient is given two quick breaths of 1 to 1.5 seconds in duration and then ventilated once every 3 to 5 seconds, interspersed with chest compressions. Artificial ventilation should provide moderate hyperventilation to offset any developing metabolic acidosis. Effective ventilation also helps to remove carbon dioxide that is generated with sodium bicarbonate administration. Arterial blood gases can be used to gauge the effectiveness of the artificial ventilation.

Circulation

The final priority of BLS is to initiate artificial circulation. This can be accomplished through external or internal cardiac compression. The effectiveness of cardiac compression depends on the transmission of force to the heart and intrathoracic vessels.

External Cardiac Compression. External cardiac compression can be carried out with the patient in lateral or dorsal recumbency. With the patient in lateral recumbency, one or both hands are placed on the lateral thoracic wall over the area of the heart (fourth to fifth intercostal space, at the costochondral junction). In larger patients (5 kg or greater), the arms should be kept extended and locked. The compressive force is applied by bending at the waist (Figure 12-2). Do not compress the chest by bending the elbows because it will be difficult to generate an appropriate force to effect perfusion. In patients weighing less than 5 kg, the thumb and first two index fingers can be used to compress the chest. It has been suggested that the compressions be delivered with enough force to displace the thorax by 25% to 33% of its diameter. The rate of compressions ranges from 80 to 120 per minute. Some researchers suggest placing patients in dorsal recumbency if they weigh more than 15 kg or if they have barrel chest, as long as the patient can be stabilized. Placing the patient in dorsal recumbency and compressing the sternum increase intrathoracic pressure and subsequent forward blood flow.

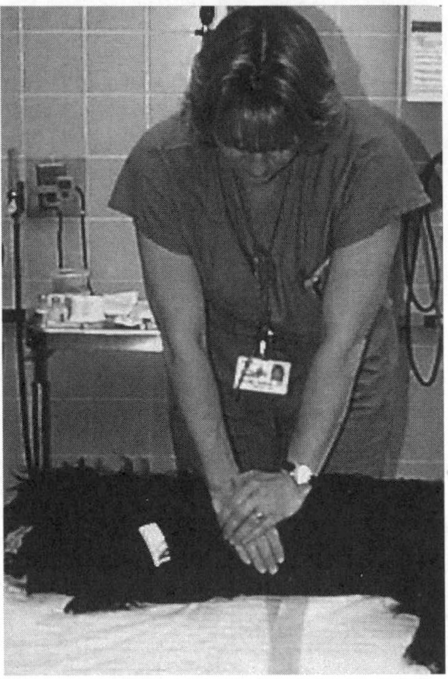

Figure 12-2
Proper technique for applying chest compressions. Note that the arms are extended and the technician is bending at the waist.

Internal Compression. Internal or direct cardiac compression has been shown to be more effective than external chest compression. The advantages over external compressions include greater cardiac output and blood pressure; better cerebral, myocardial, and peripheral tissue perfusion; and higher survival rate with improved neurologic recovery. Other advantages include the ability to assess ventricular filling between compressions or the ability to determine what type of cardiac arrest is present in the absence of an ECG monitor. With the chest open, the descending aorta can be compressed to force blood to the brain and coronary circulation. It has been suggested that a pericardectomy be performed to prevent cardiac tamponade.

Immediate internal compression is indicated if the patient has rib fractures, pleural effusion, pneumothorax, or cardiac tamponade. Otherwise, internal cardiac compression should be performed if effective artificial circulation and tissue perfusion are not evident within 5 minutes of cardiac arrest. The thoracotomy also is performed if effective spontaneous rhythm has not commenced after 10 minutes.

The patient is placed in left lateral recumbency for an emergency thoracotomy. Time is not wasted performing a surgical prep, but the coat is clipped in long-haired dogs enough to see the rib spaces. An incision is made at the fourth or fifth intercostal space from just below the dorsal epaxial muscles down to 2 cm short of the sternum but not through the pleura. The person ventilating the patient should stop while the chest cavity is entered with a pair of curved Mayo scissors. The scissors are then opened slightly and slid along the cranial edge of the caudal rib to enlarge the opening. A gloved hand is inserted into the chest and the heart compressed between the fingers and the palm of the hand. Small hearts can be compressed between two fingers. Internal cardiac compression is performed rhythmically. Care should be taken not to puncture the heart with fingertips or twist the heart. If spontaneous beating returns and the patient is stable, the chest cavity is irrigated with sterile saline; a sterile surgical skin prep is performed, and the chest cavity is closed.

Mechanism of Blood Flow. Two theories explain mechanisms of forward blood flow during CPCR. The classic theory is the cardiac pump theory. The heart is compressed between the two thoracic walls, forcing blood out of the heart and into the arterial circulation. This is equivalent to the systolic phase of a normal heartbeat. Atrioventricular valves prevent retrograde blood flow. Chest relaxation creates subatmospheric intrathoracic pressure and allows venous return and heart filling, similar to the normal diastolic phase.

The thoracic pump mechanism of blood flow is a newer theory that was recognized more than 20 years ago. It is hypothesized that chest compressions cause a rise in intrathoracic pressure, which is transmitted to the intrathoracic vasculature; intrathoracic structures are compressed. There is also collapse of venous structures in the thorax, which prevents retrograde venous blood flow. Intrathoracic pressure falls when chest compressions are relaxed, allowing return of venous blood from the periphery into the thoracic venous system. It is hard to say which mechanism predominates during CPR; the mechanism may depend on several factors, including patient size, chest compliance, the presence or absence of pleural filling defects, and cardiomegaly. It may be best to try to maximize the effects of both mechanisms.

Assessing Effectiveness. The effectiveness of the team's efforts must be monitored frequently. Improvement in mucous membrane color and the presence of a palpable pulse during CPCR have been used for assessing effectiveness. However, even in the best circumstances palpating a pulse can be difficult. Placing a Doppler flat probe on the cornea is a more reliable method of assessing blood flow through the common carotid artery than using the Doppler at peripheral sites.

Monitoring peripheral pulses with quantitative Doppler techniques has shown that the pulse generated during compression is from venous flow, not arterial flow. If a direct arterial line is in place, arterial pressure waveforms and pressures can be used to assess effectiveness of therapy, providing a compression-to-compression assessment of the technique. The goal is to achieve a diastolic pressure of 40 mm Hg or greater. In the research laboratory, some investigators have shown that when aortic diastolic pressure was raised above 40 mm Hg, usually with α-adrenergic drugs or other special maneuvers, dogs could be resuscitated successfully from CPA. End-tidal CO_2 ($ETCO_2$) has been suggested as a way to assess resuscitation efforts noninvasively. Studies have shown that $ETCO_2$ varies directly with cardiac output during cardiac arrest. Dramatic decreases in $ETCO_2$ occur during cardiac arrest; with CPCR a dramatic increase is seen, and an even more dramatic increase or overshoot is seen when spontaneous circulation returns. In humans, the initial $ETco_2$ measurement obtained at the outset of CPCR is very low (11 to 12 mm Hg), compared with a normal $ETco_2$ of 40 to 45 mm Hg. If resuscitation efforts are not effective, the resuscitation techniques must be changed. It may be necessary to increase or decrease the rate, duration, and depth of compression, change the hand or patient position, change the person performing compressions, or use alternative or augmenting techniques.

Alternative Techniques to Improve Blood Flow. If one technique is not working, move on to another technique. First, try ventilating with every second or third chest compression. This has been shown to increase intrathoracic pressure and to improve cerebral, but not myocardial blood flow. Second, in larger breed dogs, compress the chest where it is widest to maximize the thoracic pump mechanism of blood flow. Third, intermittent abdominal compression, alternating with external chest compression, improves venous return to the chest and has been reported to improve arterial blood pressure and cerebral and myocardial perfusion. Finally, for abdominal counterpressure, a sandbag or a hand is used to apply steady pressure over the midabdomen; this prevents posterior displacement of the diaphragm when the chest is compressed. This technique increases intrathoracic pressure and improves cerebral blood flow.

Additional techniques that might be used to enhance circulation include antishock trousers and an abdominal tourniquet. Antishock trousers can be made of elastic bandage material. The patient's hind legs and caudal abdomen are wrapped with elastic bandage material. Starting from the toes, wrap both hind legs and the tail; wrap up to the caudal abdomen. Be careful not to wrap too far forward on the abdomen because this may cause anterior displacement of the abdominal organs. The bandaging material may improve systemic blood pressure and organ perfusion by preventing the runoff of central blood volume into the periphery. A single abdominal tourniquet also can be used to prevent peripheral runoff of blood. Ten to twenty minutes after the heart restarts and the hemodynamics have had a chance to stabilize, the wraps and tourniquets are removed slowly. Caution should be exercised in removing the wraps and tourniquets. Rapid removal may result in excessive hypotension.

ADVANCED LIFE SUPPORT

Once BLS objectives have been achieved, they must be maintained, and a shift is made to advanced life support (ALS). During ALS, drugs and countershock are administered, based on ECG and clinical findings. A *D* and *E* can be added to the ABC mnemonic (Box 12-2). Drug therapy during CPA is dictated by the type of cardiac arrest present, so ECG monitoring is needed.

DRUGS

Fluids. CPA is a rapidly vasodilating disease process, so crystalloid fluids such as lactated Ringer's are indicated. Dextrose solutions have been implicated in increased morbidity and mortality in association with cardiac arrest and should not be used. The initial dosage of fluids in the dog is 40 ml/kg; in the cat it is 20 ml/kg. The fluids should be given rapidly intravenously, in aliquots sufficient to maintain effective circulating volume. When anemia or hypoproteinemia is present, whole blood, plasma, hetastarch, or dextran 70 may be indicated.

Atropine. Atropine has predominant parasympatholytic effects. Its use in cardiac arrest is based on its vagolytic action. It plays a central role in

Box 12-2 Mnemonic for Key Steps in Advanced Life Support

Airway: establish airway.
B reathing reathin: once every 3-5 sec.
Circulation: 80-120 compressions/min.
Drugs: administer drugs.
Electrical: defibrillate.

preventing and managing CPA associated with intense vagal stimulation. Atropine is indicated in the treatment of ventricular asystole and slow sinus or idioventricular rhythms. The recommended dosage is 0.02 to 0.04 mg/kg.

Epinephrine. Epinephrine has both α- and β-adrenergic properties. Epinephrine's strong α-adrenergic properties cause arterial vasoconstriction. Diastolic blood pressure is increased, which results in augmented coronary and cerebral blood flow. Aortic diastolic pressure is the critical determinant of success or failure of resuscitative efforts in animals and humans. The drug also causes constriction of large veins, which displace blood out of the venous capacitance vessels. It has been reported that a higher dosage of epinephrine (0.2 mg/kg) may be more effective than the previously recommended dosages (0.02 mg/kg). The higher dosage tends to improve cerebral blood flow but also predisposes the patient to ventricular fibrillation. Initial dosages of epinephrine should be low and titrated upward until the desired effect is achieved.

2% Lidocaine. Lidocaine is a class 1 antiarrhythmic agent. Lidocaine is most commonly used to treat ventricular arrhythmias (i.e., premature ventricular contractions or ventricular tachycardia). Lidocaine can be used to supplement treatment of refractory ventricular fibrillation. It is used as a background drug to raise the fibrillatory threshold. Studies suggest that lidocaine increases the energy requirements for defibrillation. The dosage is 0.5 to 1.0 mg/kg in cats and 1 to 2 mg/kg in dogs.

Magnesium Sulfate or Chloride. Hypomagnesemia has been reported in critically ill dogs and can contribute to the development of lethal ventricular arrhythmias such as ventricular tachycardia and fibrillation. Magnesium has been used to treat such arrhythmias. The exact mechanism of action is not clear. It is not known whether magnesium is effective because it repletes an intracellular or extracellular deficit or because of some intrinsic antiarrhythmic property irrespective of magnesium level. It has been suggested that magnesium therapy be considered for patients with refractory ventricular fibrillation. The dosage is 1 to 2 g given over 2 minutes.

Sodium Bicarbonate. The use of sodium bicarbonate ($NaHCO_3$) has been deemphasized. It was one of the primary drugs used to treat cardiac arrest. The premise for its use was that it corrected metabolic acidosis generated by anaerobic metabolism in hypoxic tissues. It was felt that the metabolic acidosis was associated with decreased cardiac function and a lowered ventricular fibrillation threshold. Intracellular pH, not blood pH, determines cardiac viability and the likelihood of resuscitation. Ideally $NaHCO_3$ administration should be guided by venous blood gas results, but in the absence of blood gases, $NaHCO_3$ can be given empirically at a conservative dosage of 0.5 mEq/kg per 5 minutes of cardiac arrest after the first 5 to 10 minutes unless the patient is known to have preexisting metabolic acidosis. Moderate hyperventilation helps offset a developing respiratory acidosis or is necessary as a result of CO_2 development when $NaHCO_3$ is administered.

Bretylium Tosylate. Bretylium is an antiarrhythmic drug that has been used to treat refractory ventricular fibrillation or pulseless ventricular tachycardia if defibrillation has not been previously successful. Delayed hypotension is a side effect of bretylium administration and should not become a factor during resuscitation. The dosage of bretylium is 5 to 10 mg/kg.

10% Calcium. Calcium is not currently recommended for routine cardiac arrest treatment. Calcium has been used routinely during CPCR to augment cardiac contractility. However, excessive intracellular calcium concentrations cause sustained muscular contraction ("stone heart") and myocardial and cerebral vasoconstriction. Calcium has also been implicated in reperfusion injury. Reperfusion injury occurs when ischemic tissue is reperfused or reoxygenated, leading to cellular damage. It remains to be seen whether calcium is beneficial in patients with prolonged arrest. Calcium is indicated when the patient is hyperkalemic or hypocalcemic or has calcium channel blocker toxicity. The calcium dosage is 0.2 ml/kg 10% calcium chloride or 0.6 ml/kg 10% calcium gluconate.

Route of Drug Administration. Site selection for drug administration during CPCR involves the following considerations: speed with which venous access can be obtained, technical abilities of the person attempting venous access, difficulties encountered in obtaining venous access, rate of drug delivery to the central circulation, and the duration of effective drug levels after injection. Several options (Box 12-3) are available for delivering drugs during CPA. Drug circulation time depends on the cardiac output generated during CPCR. It appears that the central or jugular vein is the most desirable because drugs are deposited near the heart. Drugs administered at the central venous site provide higher drug concentrations in a shorter period of time.

Aside from patient movement during CPCR, it is easy to place a jugular catheter in a patient with CPA because the jugular vein usually is palpable. Peripheral venous drug administration tends to deliver the drug to the heart in a lower blood concentration and at a slower rate than central venous administration. Experimental studies in animals demonstrate that drug delivery after peripheral injection is enhanced by following the injection with 10- to 30-ml saline flushes and elevating the extremity. The circulation time is shorter and the peak concentration is higher. In one study a 0.5-ml/kg flush solution permitted a peripherally administered model drug to reach the central circulation as quickly as and in a concentration equivalent to that of a centrally administered drug during CPCR in dogs.

Few studies have examined the intraosseous (IO) route for delivering drugs during CPCR, but it remains an option. The IO route has been used in human medicine for treating pediatric CPA. An intramedullary cannula is inserted into the femur, humerus, wing of the ilium, or tibial crest. Shock treatment volumes of fluids and drugs can be injected into the medullary canal, and rapid uptake results from the abundant endosteum-medullary blood supply.

A limited number of drugs (Box 12-4) can be administered by the intratracheal route. The intratracheal route has been advocated for drug administration when venous access is not accessible, but peak concentrations are lower than those obtained by other routes. Some studies have indicated that drug uptake from the tracheal surface during resuscitation is sporadic, undependable, and delayed. If this route is to be used, double the intravenous dosage of the drug, dilute with 5 to 10 ml of saline if needed to provide enough volume, and inject it via a long catheter placed through the endotracheal tube to the carina. Finally, hyperventilate the patient a few breaths to help disperse the drug.

Several years ago the American Heart Association deemphasized the use of intracardiac injections. Chest compressions must be stopped while the injection is made. In addition, several potential complications are associated with this procedure: myocardial trauma, lacerated coronary arteries, pericardial effusion, and refractory ventricular fibrillation if the heart muscle is injected with epinephrine. As a result, this route should be used

Box 12-3 Methods of Drug Delivery

Jugular venous
Peripheral venous (cephalic)
Intraosseous
Intratracheal
Intracardiac

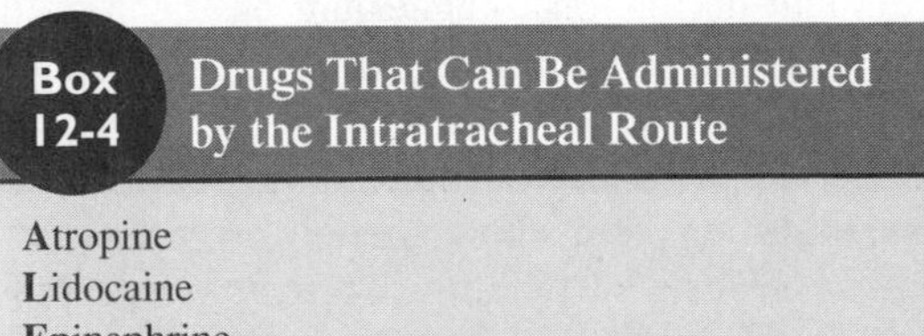
Box 12-4 Drugs That Can Be Administered by the Intratracheal Route

Atropine
Lidocaine
Epinephrine

only as a last resort after all other methods have failed, if at all.

Regardless of the drug administration route, effective chest compressions must be maintained throughout the CPCR endeavor so that the drug can circulate.

DEFIBRILLATION

The purpose of defibrillation is to eliminate the chaotic asynchronous electrical activity of the fibrillating heart. This is accomplished by passing an electrical current through the heart, causing the cardiac cells to depolarize and repolarize in a uniform manner, with resumption of organized and coordinated electrical and contractile activity. Defibrillation stands a better chance of being successful if performed early in the CPCR endeavor. There are two methods of defibrillation: direct current and chemical. Direct current defibrillation is performed using a defibrillator. The defibrillator paddles are placed firmly over the heart on each side of the chest after a contact gel has been applied. The person performing the defibrillation should yell "clear" and make sure that nobody is in contact with the patient or anything associated with the patient immediately before discharging the defibrillator. An energy level is set and the defibrillator is discharged. The energy necessary for external defibrillation is at least 3 J/kg. The internal defibrillation energy level is at least 0.2 J/kg. Excessive energy levels and repeated defibrillation can cause myocardial damage, so it is best to start at the lower energy levels and increase as needed.

Although not as effective, chemical defibrillation or a precordial thump can be tried when a defibrillator is not available. The dosage for chemical defibrillation is 1 mEq/kg potassium chloride followed by 0.2 ml/kg 10% calcium chloride or 0.6 ml/kg calcium gluconate. The precordial thump is a sharp blow over the precordium.

CARDIAC RHYTHMS

In a study, the three types of rhythms noted during CPA were electromechanical dissociation or pulseless (23.3%), asystole (22.8%), and ventricular fibrillation (19.8%). Additional rhythms encountered during CPA include sinus bradycardia, sinus tachycardia, and ventricular tachycardia. Early recognition of the cardiac rhythm dictates the type of therapy needed. A focused and directed approach is needed to treat CPA. An algorithm or flow sheet helps the CPCR team make therapeutic decisions. An algorithm of the three most common types of rhythms is included in this section. It is important to remember that if the patient's rhythm changes, the CPCR team must use a different algorithm. For example, if the patient goes from asystolic rhythm to ventricular fibrillation, the team must switch from the asystole algorithm to the ventricular fibrillation algorithm.

Electromechanical Dissociation or Pulseless Rhythm. The electrical pattern in pulseless rhythms may be almost normal in appearance, or the QRS complexes may appear wide and bizarre (Figure 12-3). There is no detectable pulse or

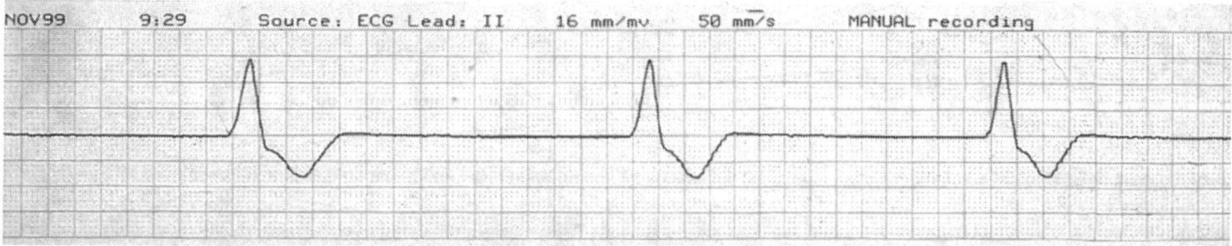

Figure 12-3
Electrocardiogram of pulseless rhythm.

Box 12-5 Pulseless Rhythm Algorithm

- Continue effective CPR.
- Epinephrine 0.02-0.2 mg/kg.
  - Increase to high dosage if nonresponsive.
- Search for treatable causes:
  - Hypoxia.
  - Acidosis.
  - Hyperkalemia.
  - Hypovolemia.
  - Cardiac tamponade.
  - Tension pneumothorax.
- Consider
  - Fluid challenge:
    - Cat: 20 ml/kg bolus.
    - Dog: 40 ml/kg bolus.
  - Atropine 0.04 mg/kg (if heart rate is slow).
  - Dexamethason $NaPO_4$ 2-4 mg/kg.
  - Sodium bicarbonate 0.5 mEq/kg/5 min.
    - If preexisting metabolic acidosis, start at 0 time.
    - If no preexisting metabolic acidosis, start at 5 min into arrest.

Box 12-6 Algorithm for Asystole

- Continue effective CPR.
- Epinephrine 0.02-0.2 mg/kg q 3 min.
  - Increase dosage by 0.02 mg/kg every 3-5 min.
- Atropine 0.04 mg/kg.
- If uncertain, check other ECG leads and evaluate for ventricular fibrillation (if ventricular fibrillation, go to appropriate protocol).
- Consider
  - Fluid challenge:
    - Cats 20 ml/kg bolus.
    - Dogs 40 ml/kg bolus.
  - Sodium bicarbonate 0.5 mEq/kg/5 min.
    - If preexisting metabolic acidosis, start at 0 time.
    - If no preexisting metabolic acidosis, start at 5 min into arrest.
  - Pacemaker.
  - 10% Calcium gluconate 60 mg/kg.
    - Only if:
      - Hyperkalemia.
      - Hypocalcemia.
      - Calcium channel.
      - Blocker toxicity.

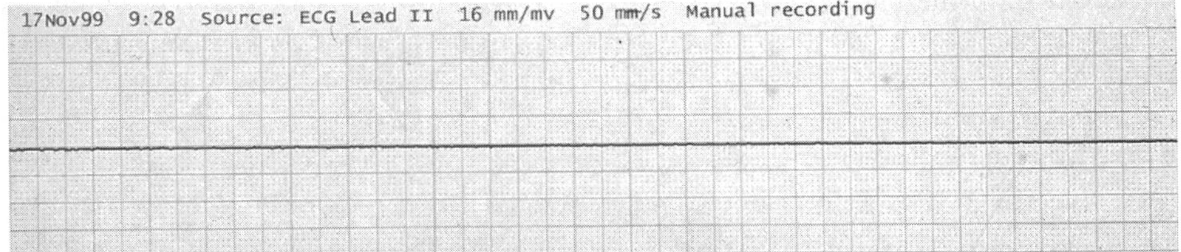

Figure 12-4

Electrocardiogram of asystole.

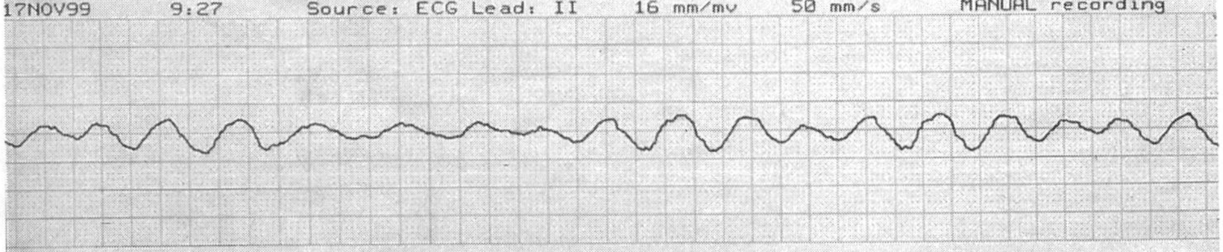

Figure 12-5

Electrocardiogram of ventricular fibrillation.

heartbeat. Therapy (Box 12-5) should be aimed at determining the underlying cause, such as hypoxia, acidosis, hyperkalemia, hypovolemia, cardiac tamponade, or tension pneumothorax. Epinephrine is indicated, and fluid bolus, atropine, steroids, sodium bicarbonate should be considered.

Asystole. Asystole is characterized by no electrical activity (a flat line on the ECG) or mechanical activity (Figure 12-4). This type of arrest may be caused by end-stage cardiac or pulmonary disease or increased vagal tone. There is no detectable pulse or heartbeat and there is no heart movement. Epinephrine and atropine are the primary drugs (Box 12-6) used to treat this rhythm. Fluid bolus, sodium bicarbonate, pacemaker, and calcium therapy should be considered.

Ventricular Fibrillation. Ventricular fibrillation is characterized by chaotic electrical activity (Figure 12-5) and no mechanical activity. The ECG display shows no definable pattern and marked irregularity in rhythm, and P waves and QRS complexes are unidentifiable. There also is no detectable pulse or heartbeat. The heart resembles a quivering bag of worms. Defibrillation is the treatment of choice (Box 12-7).

Box 12-7 Algorithm for Ventricular Fibrillation

Continue effective CPR.
Defibrillate:
- 3 J/kg external.
- 0.2 J/kg internal.

Defibrillate:
- 4 J/kg external.
- 0.3 J/kg internal.

Defibrillate:
- 5 J/kg external.
- 0.4 J/kg internal.

Epinephrine 0.02-0.2 mg/kg.
Defibrillate:
- Previous setting.

2% Lidocaine:
- Dogs: 2-4 mg/kg.
- Cats: 0.2 mg/kg.

Defibrillate:
- Previous setting.

Search for treatable causes:
- Metabolic disturbances.
- Hypothermia.
- Hypovolemia.

Increase epinephrine from previous dosage.
Consider
- Sodium bicarbonate 0.5 mEq/kg.
- Second dose of lidocaine (half of the previous dose).

Defibrillate:
- 3-5 J/kg external as needed.
- 0.2-0.4 J/kg internal as needed.

Consider
- Magnesium sulfate or chloride 1-2 g/kg over 2 min if fibrillation refractory to other therapy.
  or
- Bretylium 5-10 mg/kg.

If ventricular fibrillation persists, repeat epinephrine in increasing doses and defibrillate as needed.

PROLONGED LIFE SUPPORT

Once the heart is beating spontaneously, the patient should be monitored closely. Special attention should be paid to the cardiovascular, pulmonary, and central nervous systems. It is helpful to monitor as many parameters as possible for each system; this gives you a clear overview of the patient status.

Check the heart rate and rhythm. If arrhythmias are present, antiarrhythmic drugs, correction of electrolyte abnormalities, or oxygen therapy may be indicated. The blood pressure, central venous pressure, and pulse pressure are indications of the heart's mechanical activity. The patient's mucous membrane color, capillary refill, urine output, and toe web temperature are indications of the peripheral perfusion. What is the patient's respiratory rate and character of breathing? Does the patient seem to be taking adequate breaths? Can you auscultate airway sounds? If airway sounds cannot be heard, pleural filling defects must be ruled out. What is the patient's mental status? Is its condition improving or deteriorating? Mannitol, corticosteroids, or diuretics may be indicated.

CONCLUSION

The clinician should know the owner's wishes with regard to CPCR if the animal arrests. Does the owner want an emergency thoracotomy, closed chest CPCR, or no resuscitation? Many factors come into play when deciding whether CPCR is to be attempted: the patient's current condition, the prognosis for recovery, the patient's age, and the financial limitations of the owner. Animals that survive CPCR often are those that were young and healthy before the arrest or those who had a drug reaction. The survival and hospital discharge rates of patients who experience cardiac arrest are low. A University of California at Davis study reported that 3.8% of dogs and 2.3% of cats were still alive at 1 week. A Colorado State study reported that the hospital discharge rates were 4.1% for dogs and 9.6% for cats. Even with the dismal survival rates, if a resuscitation is to be undertaken it must be managed aggressively and the veterinary team must have a plan for CPA management. An informed, prepared, and efficient CPCR team is necessary for successful resuscitation.

BIBLIOGRAPHY

Crowe DT: Evaluation of a Doppler flow detector probe on the eye for determining effectiveness of blood flow generation with cardiac massage in dogs, *Proceedings of the Third International Veterinary Emergency and Critical Care Symposium* 3:837, 1992.

D'alecy L et al: Dextrose-containing intravenous fluid impairs outcome and increases death after eight minutes of cardiac arrest and resuscitation in dogs, *Surgery* 100:505, 1986.

Gaddis GM, Dolister M, Gaddis ML: Mock drug delivery to the proximal aorta during cardiopulmonary resuscitation: central vs peripheral intravenous infusion with varying flush volumes, *Acad Emerg Med* 2(12):1027, 1995.

Gonzalez ER: Pharmacologic controversies in CPR, *Ann Emerg Med* 22(2):317, 1993.

Grauer K, Cavallaro D: Sudden cardiac death: the role of electrolytes in cardiac arrest. In *ACLSA comprehensive review,* vol 2, St Louis, 1993, Mosby.

Hackett TB, Van Pelt DR: Cardiopulmonary resuscitation. In Bonagura JD, ed: *Current veterinary therapy,* ed 12, Philadelphia, 1995, WB Saunders.

Haskins SC: Cardiopulmonary resuscitation. In Kirk RW, ed: *Current veterinary therapy,* ed 10, Philadelphia, 1989, WB Saunders.

Haskins SC: Internal cardiac compression, *J Am Vet Med Assoc* 200:1945, 1992.

Henik RA: Basic life support and external cardiac compression in dogs and cats, *J Am Vet Med Assoc* 200:1925, 1992.

Jaffe AS: Cardiovascular pharmacology I. *Circulation* 74(Suppl IV):70, 1986.

Kass PH, Haskins SC: Survival following cardiopulmonary resuscitation in dogs and cats, *J Vet Emer Crit Care* 2:57, 1992.

Kayser SR, Callaham ML: A critical reappraisal of the pharmacologic management of cardiac arrest, *Pharm Ther Forum* 33:6, 1985.

Kern KB, Niemann JT: Perfusion pressure. In Paradis NA, Halperin HR, Nowak RM, eds: *Cardiac arrest: the science and practice of resuscitation medicine,* Baltimore, 1996, Williams & Wilkins.

Kerz T, Dick W: Routes for drug administration during cardiopulmonary resuscitation, *Anaesthetist* 45(6): 550, 1996.

Marino PL: Cardiac arrest. In *The ICU book,* Baltimore, 1998, Williams & Wilkins.

Martin LG, Matteson VL, Wingfield WE, et al: Abnormalities of serum magnesium in critically ill dogs: incidence and implications, *J Vet Emerg Crit Care* 4:15, 1994.

Martin LG, Wingfield WE, Van Pelt DR, et al: Magnesium in the 1990s: implications for veterinary critical care, *J Vet Emerg Crit Care* 3:105, 1994.

McGeorge F: Diagnosis during cardiac arrest real time monitoring. In Paradis NA, Halperin HR, Nowak RM, eds: *Cardiac arrest: the science and practice of resuscitation medicine,* Baltimore, 1996, Williams & Wilkins.

Rebello CD, Crowe DT: Cardiopulmonary resuscitation: current recommendations, *Vet Clin North Am* 19:1127, 1989.

Rush JE, Wingfield WE: Recognition and frequency of dysrhythmias during cardiopulmonary arrest, *J Am Vet Med Assoc* 200:1932, 1992.

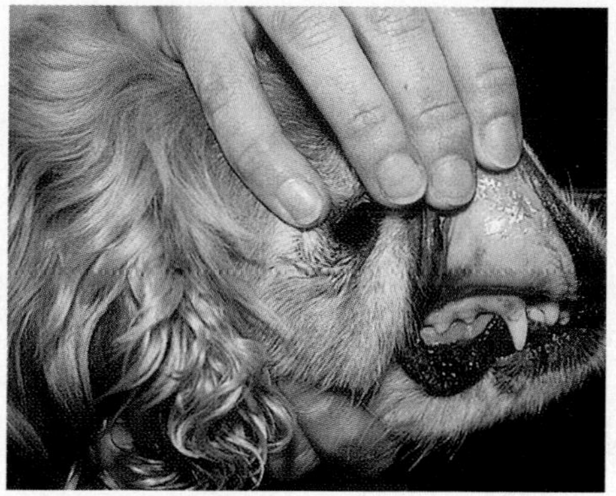

Color Plate 1

Icterus mucous membrane color in a cocker spaniel with liver disease.

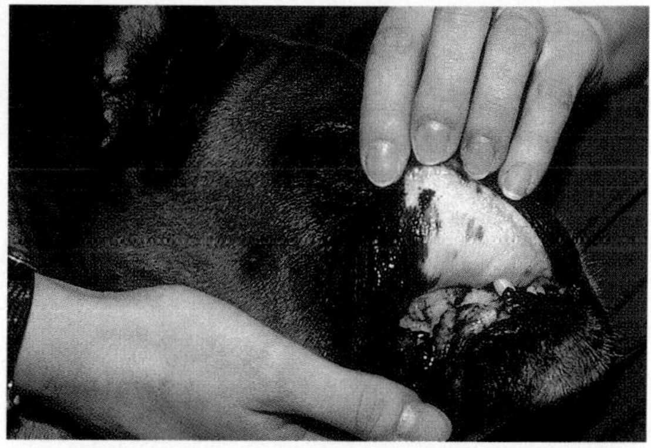

Color Plate 2

Pale mucous membrane color in a boxer with a packed cell volume of 13%.

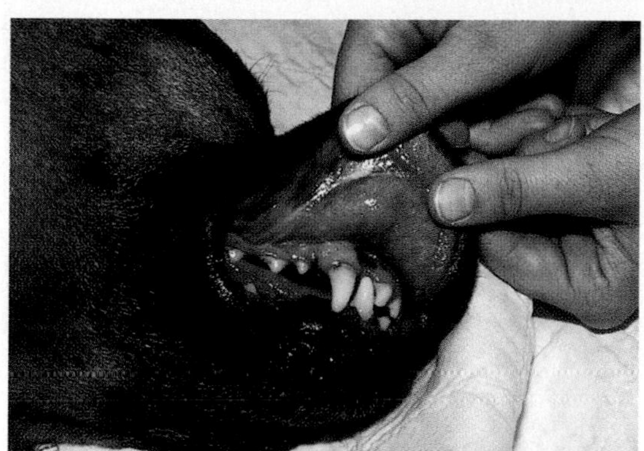

Color Plate 3

Brick red mucous membranes in a mongrel with septic shock.

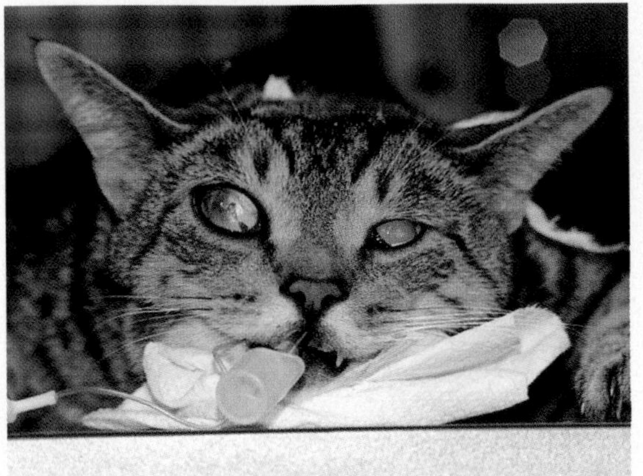

Color Plate 4

A cat with buthalmia (enlargement and distention of the globe) in the right eye caused by glaucoma.

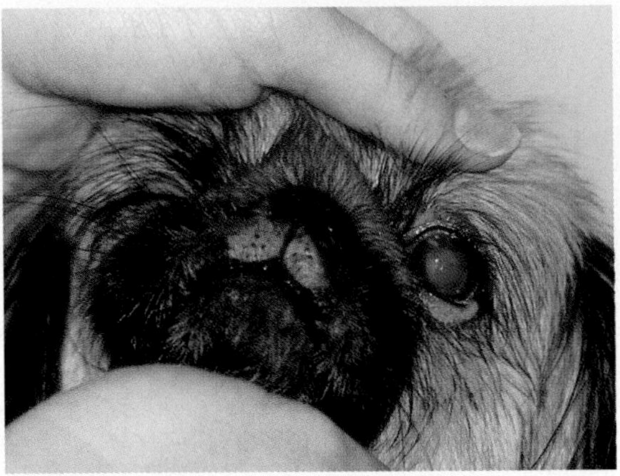

Color Plate 5

A Pekinese with conjunctival hyperemia, with mucopurulent discharge in the left eye caused by a corneal ulcer.

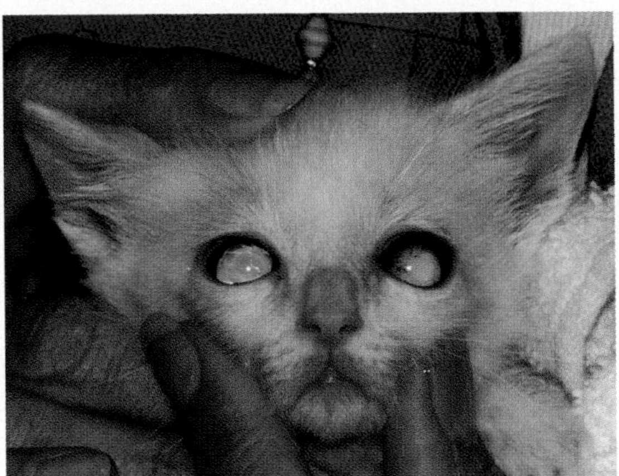

Color Plate 6

A kitten with congenital cataracts in both eyes.

Tomaselli GF: Etiology, electrophysiology, and mechanics of ventricular fibrillation. In Paradis NA, Halperin HR, Nowak RM, eds: *Cardiac arrest: the science and practice of resuscitation medicine,* Baltimore, 1996, Williams & Wilkins.

Weil MH, Tang W: Wolf Creek Conference IV on Cardiopulmonary Resuscitation: addressing the scientific basis of reanimation, *New Horizons: The Science and Practice of Acute Medicine* 5:97, 1997.

Wingfield WE: Cardiopulmonary arrest and resuscitation in small animals. In part 1: basic life support, *Emerging Sci Technol Adv Vet Med* 2:21, 1996.

Wingfield WE: Controversial issues in cardiopulmonary resuscitation. In *Scientific Proceedings, 23rd annual meeting of the Veterinary Emergency & Critical Care Society,* 1997.

Wingfield WE, Van Pelt DR: Respiratory and cardiopulmonary arrest in dogs and cats: 265 cases (1986-1991), *J Am Vet Med Assoc* 200:1993, 1992.

Zaritsky AL: Resuscitation pharmacology. In Chernow B, ed: *Essentials of critical care pharmacology,* Baltimore, 1994, William & Wilkins.

Chapter 

Trauma

A well-equipped hospital with a well-trained team of doctors, technicians, and receptionists is essential for treating the seriously injured patient. The team must be prepared to address both the medical needs of the patient and the emotional needs of the family. Medical skills go hand in hand with caring and compassion. Although this chapter deals primarily with the medical management of trauma, taking care of the distraught owner can be as important as taking care of the medical needs of the animal.

Survival of the injured patient depends on many factors, including the type and severity of the injury and the medical treatment provided. Recognition, assessment, action, and reassessment are the four essential components of effective trauma management. Technicians and veterinarians must be able to recognize critical injuries quickly because the outcome of very severe injury often is determined within the first few minutes. Technicians usually have the first contact with patients in the hospital. Therefore they must be able to assess the patient rapidly and determine whether potentially life-threatening injuries are present. The veterinary team must be able to act immediately and treat the problems in order of priority. Resuscitation may entail multiple invasive procedures, laboratory tests, advanced diagnostic tests including contrast radiographic studies and ultrasound examination, and emergency surgery, often during the first hour after the injury. Therefore the hospital must be equipped and the team trained to deal with all possible emergencies.

Initially, it should be assumed that the patient has a serious injury. By anticipating the worst, the team is more likely to recognize injuries and their secondary effects. All patients should be evaluated in the same stepwise fashion, starting with the ABCs of airway, breathing, and circulation. A patient with a distal forelimb fracture sustained during a fall may also have a pneumothorax, which can be overlooked easily if a complete assessment is not performed.

Once the patient has been resuscitated, aggressive monitoring is vital. Tracking changes in vital signs and other physiologic parameters allows technicians and doctors to determine whether the patient's status is deteriorating. Detailed flow sheets and treatment sheets must be used. Because injured patients are at serious risk for secondary complications such as pneumonia, delayed healing, and the systemic inflammatory response syndrome (SIRS), intensive monitoring and treatment may help prevent some of these complications (Table 13-1 and Figure 13-1).

Equipment List

Saline bowls (small and large)
Scalpel handle and no. 10 and no. 11 blades
Towel clamps (minimum 8)
Mayo scissors, curved
Metzenbaum scissors, curved
Sharp, blunt scissors
Kelly hemostatic forceps, curved (8)
Halsted mosquito forceps, curved (8)
Rochester-Carmalt hemostatic forceps, curved (6)
Sponge forceps, curved
Allis tissue forceps (4)

TABLE 13-1 Trauma Management Responsibilities of the Veterinary Technician

- Preparing emergency room and operating room
- Receiving phone calls
- Providing first aid instructions
- Securing patient's airway (O_2, intubation if indicated)
- Managing positive-pressure ventilation with positive end-expiratory pressure (if needed)
- Establishing intravenous access
- Setting up and interpreting monitoring devices
- Assessing and managing pain
- Maintaining charts
- Communicating with veterinarians and families

Right-angle forceps (small and large)
Debakey or Cooley tissue forceps (short and long)
Russian thumb forceps
Brown-Adson tissue forceps
Serrefine forceps (bulldog clamps, 2)
Balfour retractor (small and large)
Mayo-Hegar needle holders (small and large)
Yankauer, Poole, and Frasier suction tips
Silastic tubing
Bulb syringe
Laparotomy pads (8)
Rommel tourniquet (umbilical tape, silastic or red rubber tubing, and orthopedic wire)
Cotton towels (4 small and 4 large)

READINESS

READY AREA AND CRASH CART

Each hospital should have a ready area. The ready area is where all emergency patients requiring immediate care are brought for examination and treatment (see Figure 13-2). This should be the same area where in-hospital emergencies are treated. Usually it is a central location such as the main treatment room, although it can be the surgical prep area. It should be near the operating room because seriously injured trauma patients may need surgery as part of their resuscitation. The ready area must have all the necessary equipment

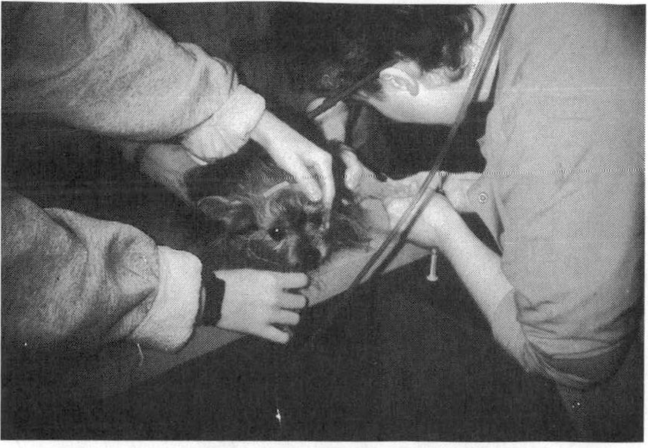

Figure 13-1

Flow-by oxygen is administered immediately upon presentation and while other procedures are performed.

for full resuscitation, including open chest cardiopulmonary resuscitation. Oxygen, airway and vascular access devices, fluids (crystalloids and colloids), suction, monitoring equipment, and basic bandaging supplies must be readily available. A crash cart with multiple drawers should be outfitted with all the necessary supplies. The crash cart should be checked once or twice daily to ensure that all the necessary supplies are present and equipment is in working condition. A piece of tape placed diagonally across the cart can be used to indicate whether materials have been removed. When the cart is used the tape is taken off and not replaced until the missing supplies have been replaced. The tape also can be dated and initialed after each check so that other members of the team can be certain that the cart has all the necessary equipment.

Monitoring equipment should be kept on the top of the crash cart. This should include suction and equipment to continuously monitor electrocardiograms, blood pressure, capnography, and pulse oximetry. All equipment should be checked once or twice daily to ensure that it is plugged in and in good working condition. Several sizes of blood pressure cuffs should be available (usually 2- to 5-cm widths). Good overhead lighting is essential. Both a wide-beam dish light and a focusing high-intensity cool beam light should be available. Direct light sources that can be worn, such as a

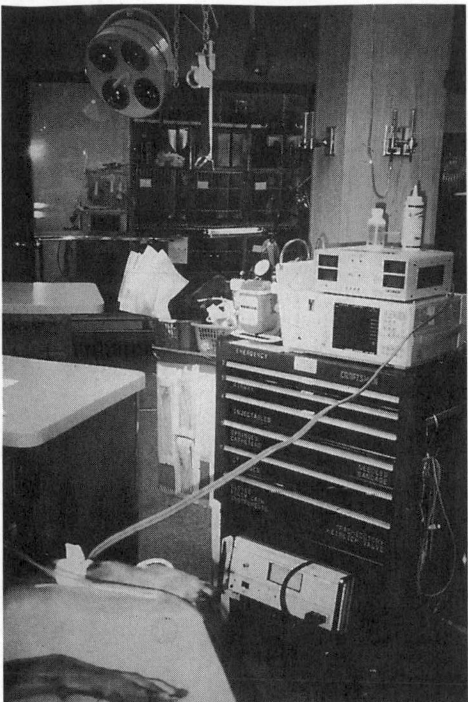

Figure 13-2

A ready area must be available for quick and successful resuscitation.

head loupe or inexpensive head lamps, or snake lights (available from hardware stores), allow close assessment of the airway, oral cavity, and wounds while freeing both hands.

Sterile surgical supplies should be kept with the crash cart. These should include scalpel blades, curved Mayo scissors, curved hemostats, and various sizes of polypropylene suture material (sizes from 2-0 to 5-0) for vascular suturing, tracheotomy, or resuscitative thoracotomy. Polypropylene suture can be autoclaved multiple times without losing strength. Satinsky forceps, although expensive, are invaluable as vascular forceps for controlling hemorrhage from large vessels such as the vena cava or the aorta. Ideally, a pair of Balfour retractors or Finochietto rib retractors should also be available. Laparotomy pads and towels should be sterilized and available. Both can be used to cover and protect open wounds from infection and to apply pressure to bleeding wounds. If a resuscitative thoracotomy is needed, they also can be used to pack bleeding areas. Red rubber tubes are effective vascular occlusive devices. When wrapped around a vessel and pulled tight with hemostats, a red rubber tube acts as an atraumatic Rommel tourniquet.

Suction Equipment

Suction equipment should be capable of generating effective pressures. Electronic suction devices are ideal; however, hand-held suction devices (Mityvac) are an inexpensive but effective alternative. A suction trap should be placed between the suction tip and the tubing. This will help prevent clogging of the tubing. Several different types of suction tips should be available. A Yankauer suction tip is useful for removing oral and pharyngeal secretions. A dental tip can be used to remove vomitus and clots from the rima glottis and trachea. Tracheal whistle-tip catheters can be used to remove frothy secretions, vomit, and blood from the trachea. Suction also can be attached directly to the end of the endotracheal tube if the patient is intubated and fluid or exudate is obstructing the tube. The suction device should always be ready for immediate use. This means that the suction tip should be attached to the tubing and the tubing should be attached to the suction unit. If an electric unit is being used, the machine should be plugged in.

Fluids

Trauma patients often need large volumes of intravenous fluids. Balanced electrolyte solutions that are buffered are the preferred crystalloid solutions. This includes lactated Ringer's solution, Normosol-R, and Plasmalyte-A. Because patients may need blood products, a crystalloid that does not contain calcium is preferred. The calcium binds the citrate in blood products, and simultaneous infusion of blood- and calcium-containing fluids through the same catheter is contraindicated. Because 75% to 80% of crystalloids infused will have left the intravascular space within 1 hour, most patients need colloids to help maintain euvolemia. Both synthetic and biologic colloids should be readily available. Synthetic colloids include dextran 70 and hetastarch. Biologic colloids include whole blood, packed red blood cells, and fresh frozen plasma. Because injured patients are at risk for developing coagulopathies secondary to loss of clotting factors and platelets, fresh whole blood and fresh frozen plasma often are indicated in the severely hemorrhaging patient.

Autotransfusion

Autotransfusion equipment should be available. If large volumes of blood are present in the thoracic or abdominal cavity, the blood can be collected into sterile containers and reinfused as an autotransfusion. When using a suction unit to collect the blood, care should be taken to avoid suctioning air simultaneously. Commercial autotransfusion systems are available, but the cost may be prohibitive for most veterinary hospitals. A simple but effective way to administer autotransfusions is to use a bag designed for delivering liquid enteral nutrition as the transfusion bag. These bags have a large opening at the top with a cap. The cap is removed and the blood is poured into the bag. Blood administration sets can be attached to the food bags and then can be gas sterilized as a unit. A simpler method is to use a sterile 1 L intravenous fluid bag. The top is cut along approximately 30% of the front panel. In this way, the bag can be hung and blood can be poured into the bag through this hole. Blood is collected from the patient and placed into the transfusion bag. Ideally this blood should be administered through a filter, but in an emergency a filter is not essential. It is often more important that the patient receive the blood rapidly, and filters decrease the infusion rate.

Radiology and Ultrasound

High-quality radiographs are a necessary part of evaluating injured patients. A 300- to 500-mA x-ray machine and an automatic processor that can develop films within several minutes are needed. Accurate technique charts should be available for taking the standard lateral and ventrodorsal views as well as horizontal beam radiographs. Horizontal beam radiography causes much less stress to the patient, especially if the patient is showing signs of respiratory distress. It is an effective way to detect free fluid in the chest or abdominal cavity. Radiograph plate holders should be available for this purpose. The technician should be trained to perform contrast radiographic studies such as nonselective angiography, intravenous urography, double-contrast cystography, peritoneography, and barium series. Contrast dyes, tubes, and catheters should be stocked in radiology for these studies. Both positioning charts and protocols for contrast studies should be posted or readily available.

Injured patients that are nonambulatory or unconscious should be secured to Plexiglas or wood spinal boards and radiographed through the boards. Trauma films or survey radiographs of the animal from nose to tail looking for obvious injuries can be taken effectively through wood or Plexiglas boards. A variety of positioning devices should be available to help decrease staff exposure to radiation. This includes things such as V trays, foam pads, and cushions filled with beads.

Ultrasound is an emerging diagnostic test of choice for rapid evaluation of the internally hemorrhaging patient. Free fluid can be visualized rapidly in the abdominal or thoracic cavities or the pericardial sac. Depending on the skill of the ultrasonographer, it can also be used to determine injuries to liver, spleen, kidneys, and bladder. An ultrasound survey can be completed in 5 to 10 minutes.

Laboratory

Basic laboratory equipment ideally includes a centrifuge for spinning packed cell volumes and separating serum, a refractometer for blood, urine, and fluid analysis, and equipment for running basic chemistries and a white blood cell count. A good microscope is essential for performing manual differentials and evaluating urine and fluid cytology. Tubes and a heating block for measuring activated clotting times should be available. Being able to evaluate acid-base status and blood gas variables can make a significant difference in developing trauma treatment plans. New point-of-care devices are fairly inexpensive and allow rapid (2 minutes) assessment of blood gas, acid-base status, and electrolytes using very small volumes of whole blood (0.05 ml). In addition, the ability to measure lactate levels can be very useful for assessing the effectiveness of resuscitation. The only accurate way to determine the need for synthetic colloid infusion is to measure colloid osmotic pressures. An instrument is available for this purpose.

SURGERY

Many seriously injured patients need surgery as part of their resuscitation. Because time is of the essence for many of these patients, the anesthesia machine must be set up and the operating room kept ready. A major surgical pack and gowns should be ready to be opened at a moment's notice. The suction unit must be functional and ready to receive suction tubing from the surgeon. Electrocautery equipment should be plugged in and the ground plate should be in place. A surgical headlight greatly enhances visualization of bleeding and traumatized tissues and vessels and should be a standard part of the operating room equipment. Trauma surgical packs should contain the basic equipment for an exploratory laparotomy or thoracotomy. In addition, towels and laparotomy pads for packing large bleeding wounds and red rubber tubes for use as vascular occlusion devices should be sterilized. Many injured patients are hypothermic or develop hypothermia during resuscitation and surgery, and a means of warming the patient should be available.

WARMING DEVICES

Keeping a patient normothermic is very important because hypothermia interferes with normal metabolic functions. This can lead to problems such as vasodilation, cardiac dysfunction, and impaired coagulation. When rewarming a hypothermic patient in hemorrhagic shock, care should be taken to warm the body core first. Warming the periphery leads to vasodilation and can worsen both core hypothermia and shock.

Warm water circulating blankets are an effective way to keep patients warm while avoiding burns. However, the nonmobile patient always should be monitored closely because any warming device can cause burns. Artificial warming devices and hot water bottles should not come in direct contact with the patient's skin but should be wrapped or covered in a towel first. A blanket warmer is handy for keeping towels and blankets warm. Warm water bottles can be kept in an incubator or be microwaved. If intravenous fluid bags are being used as warm water bottles, food coloring should be added to the bags so that they can be identified easily for reuse and not used inadvertently for parenteral fluids. Homemade warming bags can be made from fabric sacks filled with rolled oats. These can be microwaved and are reusable. Commercially available devices that circulate hot air are very effective for keeping patients warm in the operating room. Bubble wrap can be warmed in the microwave (in a bowl of water) and wrapped around the patient. The air cells retain heat well. Bubble wrap or plastic food wrap can be sterilized and used in the operating room to help prevent hypothermia. Intravenous fluids should be kept warm in an incubator or warmed in a microwave oven. Fluids administered rapidly at room temperature can lower the patient's temperature significantly.

Commercially available infant isolettes and tables can be purchased at reasonable cost through used hospital equipment suppliers. Heat lamps can be purchased or made from an exposed light bulb to provide additional external heat. These can overheat the patient, and close monitoring is needed. Temperatures should never exceed 110° F.

THE TEAM

The veterinary team—technicians, doctors, and receptionists—must be mentally and physically ready to perform the necessary tasks. All team members must be dedicated and trained to do their jobs. Technicians must be familiar with the location and operation of all the equipment needed for diagnosis and treatment. They must know how to place intravenous catheters, bandage wounds, and perform anesthesia. They must understand various procedures so that they can prepare instruments and equipment and assist when indicated. Familiarity with the techniques, tests, procedures, and treatments enables the technician to monitor for complications and efficacy.

Drills are the most effective way to prepare the team for emergencies. These drills can be performed on stuffed animals or cadavers. This encourages teamwork and allows the staff to practice psychomotor skills. It allows each person to know exactly what his or her responsibility is during an emergency. Through practice sessions, recognition, assessment, and treatment become more automatic during a real emergency.

Protocols

It has been shown in human hospitals that implementing treatment protocols significantly decreases morbidity and mortality. These protocols should be readily available for everyone to use. Drug dosage for cardiopulmonary resuscitation should be posted in a visible location. Resuscitation algorithms should be posted so that under the stress of the emergency, resuscitation is performed in an orderly fashion and important treatments are not overlooked.

FIRST AID AND SAFETY

Initial treatment often begins at the scene of the accident. Prehospital care may significantly influence outcome. Safety and first aid information can be provided to the owner during the initial telephone contact that can help them at the scene and en route to the hospital. Most owners will be stressed and frightened because a family member has just been hurt. Calming the owner is important to gain accurate information so that appropriate first aid instructions can be given. A calm owner also is much more capable of following instructions. The tone of voice that the technician uses may be as important as the information dispensed. If the owner has not had any previous first aid experience, it may be best to advise him or her to confine the patient to a box, strap to a board, or otherwise limit movement and transport the animal as rapidly as possible.

Several basic rules should always be followed. The first step is to ensure that the scene is safe. This means watching for other vehicles, broken glass, spilled chemicals, and other hazards. The second step is to ensure the safety of the owner or staff while working directly with the animal. Blood on the patient may be human blood. To avoid contagious diseases such as hepatitis and human immunodeficiency virus, direct contact with blood should be minimized and ideally avoided until the source of the blood is determined. At the scene this means towels or clothing should be used to apply direct pressure on wounds. In the hospital this means gloves should always be worn before handling animals with blood on their fur. Injured animals often are frightened and in pain. Appropriate precautions for restraint should be used. Muzzles should be placed when available. Plastic muzzles that cover the entire nose and mouth and contain multiple holes to enable breathing and drainage of oral secretions often are easier to place and more comfortable for the patient than standard muzzles, which fit tightly over the bridge of the nose. If a muzzle is not available, a tie or belt can be wrapped around the muzzle of a dog. If there is facial hemorrhage or if making a muzzle is not possible, a blanket or large jacket can be used to cover the patient's head.

Movement of the patient should be minimized until the full extent of the injuries is known. The pet should be transported on a board or in a box if it is nonambulatory. If it is ambulatory, it should not be allowed to jump in and out of the vehicle, and walking should be kept to a minimum to avoid aggravating the patient's injuries. For instance, a partial body wall hernia may become a complete hernia if the animal jumps. Direct pressure should be applied to wounds with a clean cloth whenever possible. Alternatively, with bleeding from extremities, hands can encircle and squeeze the limb or tail proximal to the wound to help control hemorrhage. Newspapers, large sticks, or pieces of wood can be used as splints for lower limb injuries.

PATIENT ASSESSMENT

TRIAGE

Triage is the sorting of patients according to the severity of their injury or illness to ensure that the most critical problems are treated first. Triage usually is done by the technician, who quickly evaluates each patient upon arrival and determines how rapidly each needs to be treated. Patients that have been involved in serious accidents should be triaged immediately to the ready area of the hospital for evaluation.

PRIMARY AND SECONDARY SURVEY

When the patient arrives at the hospital, gloves should be worn, animals should be muzzled, and patient movement should be kept to a minimum. The animal should be approached from the rostral direction and surveyed quickly for breathing effort and respiratory pattern, abnormal body or limb posture, the presence of blood or other materials in or around the patient, and any other gross abnormalities. The patient should be brought to the ready area immediately for assessment. A primary survey should be completed within 60 seconds. The primary survey assesses level of consciousness and the ABCs. The level of consciousness is evaluated rapidly using a simple scoring system such as AVPU (alert [A], verbally responsive [V], responsive to painful stimuli [P], or unresponsive [U]. If the animal is unconscious, the head and neck should be extended to help provide a clear airway. The airway is checked for patency by visual examination. Take appropriate precautions when examining a patient's oral cavity and oropharynx to avoid being bitten.

Once the level of consciousness has been evaluated the patient's airway is assessed by looking, listening, and feeling. If the patient shows signs of an exaggerated inspiratory effort, the airway may not be patent. Increased respiratory effort, paradoxical chest wall movement, abdominal wall movement with respiration, nasal flare, open mouth, extended head and neck, abducted elbows, and cyanosis all are indicators of respiratory distress that warrant immediate treatment. This is followed immediately by breathing assessment, which is done by watching chest wall motion and listening to tracheal and lung sounds bilaterally. It is important to assess lung sounds bilaterally because the animal may have a significant unilateral pneumothorax or hemothorax. It is also important to listen to lung sounds before listening to heart tones because the ear is much less sensitive to softer sounds once it has adjusted to louder sounds. The thorax and abdomen should be percussed (Table 13-2). Circulation is assessed by checking mucous membrane color and capillary refill time and auscultating heart tones while palpating central (femoral) pulses. Finally, a very rapid assessment and palpation of the abdomen, flank, pelvis, spine, and limbs are performed.

Vital signs are taken after the primary survey is completed. Vital signs include heart rate, pulse rate and strength, respiratory rate, mucous membrane color, capillary refill time, and temperature. Tem-

TABLE 13-2 Percussion: Method and Interpretation

Method

1. Lay hand on chest wall or body surface being examined.
2. Tap firmly on the middle finger of hand on patient with middle and ring finger of opposite hand.
3. Strike or tap several times until strength of tap is consistent and sound generated can be interpreted.

Interpretation

- Very low-pitched, resonant sound (hollow sound) indicates air-filled structure under body wall.
- Moderate pitch with slight resonance (solid sound) indicates fluid- or tissue-filled structure under body wall.
- High-pitched sound with significant resonance indicates solid structure, possibly under pressure, or fluid-filled structure under pressure under body wall.

perature should always be checked last for several reasons. Patients with extremely slow heart rates can have a vagally induced arrest with stimulation of the rectum. In these patients an axillary or ear temperature should be taken. In addition, in most patients the respiratory and heart rates increase when a cold thermometer is placed in the rectum.

Blood pressure measurement is very important in all trauma patients. For example, a high heart rate and high blood pressure indicates pain. A high heart rate and low blood pressure indicates hypovolemic shock. Jugular veins should be clipped and assessed for distention, filling time, and relaxation time. A mildly distended jugular vein will be noted when the animal is in lateral recumbency. A highly distended jugular vein or one that is distended with the animal standing or in sternal recumbency indicates a high central venous pressure, usually associated with a severe pneumothorax or pericardial effusion in the patient in shock. A flat jugular vein is consistent with hypovolemia, as is a jugular vein that takes a long time to fill (more than 4 seconds) when pressure is placed at the thoracic inlet to occlude the vein (as if one were doing a jugular venipuncture). A vein that has normal distention but slow relaxation time (longer than 2 seconds) indicates that the right side of the heart may be overloaded (indicating chronic right heart failure, chronic liver disease, or acute heart failure). Peripheral vein distention often can be assessed in dogs. With the patient in lateral recumbency, normally there should be mild distention of the cephalic and lateral saphenous veins if the vein is below the level of the right atrium. Raising the limb should cause the vein to flatten. The difference in height of the leg from when the vein is distended and when it becomes flat can be measured. This can be used to assess improvement in venous volume during resuscitation.

Cyanosis can be difficult to detect in patients with severe hemorrhage because 5 g/dl hemoglobin (equivalent to a hematocrit of 15%) is needed to produce visible cyanosis. Fluorescent lights also interfere with accurate evaluation of mucous membrane color in the face of pallor.

Once vital signs are measured, baseline data can be collected. This includes a lead 2 electrocardiogram and baseline laboratory work. A minimum laboratory database should include packed cell volume, total solids, blood urea nitrogen via Azostix, and blood glucose. The blood sample can be collected by hematocrit tubes from the hub of the catheter stylet. A drop of blood can be placed on a slide at this time for a blood smear to evaluate red cells, white cells, and platelets. A more extended database should include electrolytes, venous blood gas, serum albumin, activated clotting time, and platelet estimate or count. A complete database includes a complete blood cell count, chemistry panel, urinalysis, arterial blood gas, and a coagulation profile, including an antithrombin level if possible. Usually the minimum or extended database is collected initially, and further tests are considered once the patient has been fully examined and resuscitation has been started. Treatment for arrhythmias or laboratory abnormalities should be instituted as indicated.

Resuscitation is started as the primary survey is being completed. Analgesics should be given to the patient once airway and circulatory resuscitation has been initiated. If the primary survey indicates severe abnormalities such as an inadequate airway, then the airway is immediately established before the physical examination is completed and any diagnostics or other treatments are performed.

Hemorrhage also is controlled at this time. Sterile gauze, sterile laparotomy pads, and sterile towels can be used as pressure bandages. If strikethrough occurs, the initial dressing should not be removed; a second dressing should be placed over the first one. In some cases bleeding can be controlled by applying digital pressure to superficial major arteries supplying the hemorrhaging area. Pressure to the deep area adjacent and ventral to the mandible controls maxillary artery flow and controls hemorrhage to the head. Pressure to the axillary area controls brachial artery blood flow, and pressure applied to the inguinal and femoral canal region controls femoral artery blood flow. In smaller animals pressure can be placed on the caudal abdomen, thus occluding external iliac blood flow. If there is significant bleeding from a distal extremity, blood pressure cuffs can be placed proximal to the wound and inflated to 20 to

40 mm Hg above systolic pressure. This will effectively control most serious hemorrhaging while more definitive treatment is being instituted. Tourniquets should be avoided whenever possible because they can cause permanent neurologic and vascular damage within minutes.

In cases of severe hemorrhagic shock or ongoing significant abdominal or pelvic hemorrhage, limited external counterpressure using a wrap incorporating the hindlimbs, pelvis, and abdomen probably will be needed. External counterpressure places pressure indirectly on blood vessels under the bandage. Because flow is proportional to the radius of the vessel to the fourth power, any decrease in the radius of the vessel significantly decreases flow (and hemorrhage) through that vessel. If the hindlimbs are not included in the bandage, blood may pool in the hindlimbs. The wrap can be made of towels and duct tape or roll cotton and a full bandage. Towels are placed between the hindlimbs. The hindlimbs and abdomen are wrapped in a spiral fashion using large towels, and the towels are held in place with duct tape. If the wrap incorporates the cranial abdomen, diaphragm movement will be compromised. For this reason, respiration must be monitored closely. The wrap must not be too tight; two fingers should fit easily under the wrap when it is completed. If desired, a blood pressure cuff can be partially inflated and incorporated into the bandage. The wrap is then secured placing approximately 30 mm Hg pressure on the abdomen. Higher pressures can lead to serious compromise of the circulation to the gastrointestinal tract and the kidney and can lead to irreversible damage. Urine output in these patients should be monitored closely.

The wrap is left in place until the patient is hemodynamically stable. When the wrap is removed, it is unwrapped slowly, moving caudally. Blood pressure is monitored closely during removal, and if systolic blood pressure drops by more than 5 mm Hg, removal is stopped and fluids infused. If pressure continues to drop, the wrap is replaced. If pressures remain stable, the wrap is removed slowly.

Once the primary survey is completed and an initial database has been collected, a secondary survey usually is completed. This entails a complete examination of the patient in a systematic fashion from the nose to the tail (Figure 13-3).

HISTORY

Once the secondary survey is completed, the history is taken. If the patient is stable, a capsule history can be taken when the patient arrives at the hospital. A useful mnemonic is *AMPLE:*

Allergies: Does the animal have any known allergies?
Medications: Is the animal on any medications? If so, what types and dosages?
Past history: Has the animal had any past medical problems?
Lasts: When were the animal's last meal, defecation, urination, and medication?
Events: What is the problem now? Give details.

Certain details relating to the injury are particularly important. These include the time elapsed since the injury, the cause of the injury (fall, hit by car, gunshot), the speed of the car if the animal was hit, evidence of loss of consciousness at the scene, approximate amount of blood lost at the scene, and deterioration or improvement in the patient since the time of injury. It is also important to know whether the patient has other underlying medical

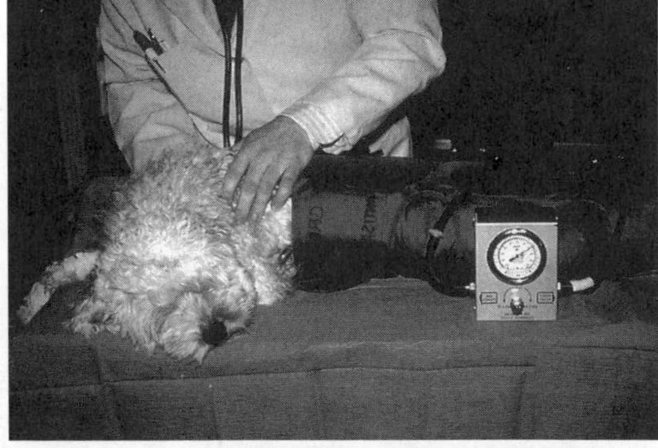

Figure 13-3

A wrap made of towels and tape or shock trousers can be used to control hemorrhage.

diseases or is being treated with any medication. Having the owner fill out a history sheet helps provide complete information on the pet and gives the owner something to do while the preliminary evaluation and resuscitation are being performed.

ADDITIONAL DIAGNOSTIC TESTS

Once the patient has been examined completely, a history has been taken, and resuscitation has been initiated, further tests may be indicated. Trauma radiographs are survey radiographs taken of the entire body. If the patient is on a wooden or Plexiglas board, the radiographs should be taken through the board and the patient should not be moved into dorsal recumbency until spinal injury has been ruled out. If the patient is stable, lateral and ventrodorsal views should be taken. Survey radiographs should be taken and assessed before extremities or other localized sites are radiographed. Once again, treatment should be instituted as abnormalities are detected. Contrast studies may be indicated.

If abdominal hemorrhage or rupture of an abdominal viscus (e.g., urinary bladder, bowel) is suspected, ultrasound and ultrasound-guided abdominocentesis should be performed. Four-quadrant abdominocentesis can be performed, but there is a high incidence of false-negative results if only small amounts of abdominal fluid are present. If ultrasound is not available, diagnostic peritoneal lavage or diagnostic peritoneal irrigation should be performed. Diagnostic peritoneal lavage requires a multiholed catheter, warm crystalloids (0.9% saline or lactated Ringer's solution), and a collection bag. The patient is placed in left lateral recumbency, and the ventral midline of the abdomen is surgically prepped. Local anesthetic is infused, and the catheter is inserted approximately 2 cm caudal to the umbilicus on the midline or just lateral to the midline. Fluids are infused into the abdomen (20 ml/kg), the abdomen is massaged gently to mix the fluid, and a sample is collected. Fluid is analyzed for packed cell volume, total solids, potassium and creatinine (if a ruptured urinary bladder is suspected), and cytology. The catheter can be left in and the packed cell volume reassessed at 5- to 10-minute intervals for signs of ongoing hemorrhage. Performing diagnostic peritoneal irrigation is more simple. It can be done with the patient in any position. Two 18-gauge hypodermic needles are inserted into the abdominal cavity. One needle is placed in a more dorsal location and crystalloids are infused. The second needle is placed in a dependent or ventral position. Fluid is infused until it starts to drip from the second needle. Again a fluid sample is collected and analyzed, as for diagnostic peritoneal lavage.

RESUSCITATION

GOALS OF RESUSCITATION

The signs of shock include increased respiratory rate and effort, tachycardia with weak or bounding pulses, pale or muddy mucous membranes, delayed capillary refill, and low body temperature.

The goal of resuscitation is to reverse the signs of shock and provide effective oxygen delivery to the cells. This means that oxygen must be delivered to the alveoli and that once there it must be taken up by the pulmonary circulation. There must be adequate hemoglobin to transport the oxygen because the content of oxygen in the blood is far more dependent on hemoglobin than on dissolved oxygen. Once the oxygen is taken into the blood it must be transported to the peripheral tissues. This requires adequate circulating volume and a heart that can pump effectively. Preload, or the amount of venous volume that returns to fill the heart, should be maximized. Treatment is aimed at restoring oxygen levels and blood flow to all tissues.

OXYGEN

Oxygen should be provided immediately at high flow rates by flow-by, mask, baggie, or oxygen collar. An unconscious patient without a good gag reflex should be intubated immediately and oxygen provided via the endotracheal tube. Nasal oxygen provides an inspired oxygen fraction of 0.4 to 0.5, whereas oxygen collars and baggies provide an inspired oxygen fraction of 0.8 to 0.9. Therefore nasal oxygen may not be the ideal initial means of providing oxygen. Oxygen cages should not be used because the patient cannot be monitored adequately; every time the door to the cage is opened, there will be significant fluctuations in inspired oxygen concentration, and most new oxygen cages do not allow the inspired oxygen fraction to exceed 0.4.

If the respiratory rate and effort and mucous membrane color are not improving with oxygen supplementation, either the patient has an injury that is interfering with ventilation or there is inadequate pulmonary circulation. Injuries leading to impaired ventilation include pneumothorax, hemothorax, fractured ribs causing hypoventilation from pain, diaphragmatic hernia, or severe pulmonary contusions. Thoracentesis is indicated if lung sounds are dull and hemothorax or pneumothorax is suspected. Thoracentesis should always be performed in the patient with suspected pneumothorax before radiographs are taken. The distress caused by positioning for radiographs may cause the patient to arrest. If negative suction is not obtained during thoracentesis, a chest tube must be placed immediately. If the patient is suspected of having significant intrapulmonic hemorrhage and the side of the hemorrhage is known, the patient should be placed in lateral recumbency with the affected side down. This allows more effective ventilation of the more normal side. If the patient has severe pulmonary contusions and is decompensating despite oxygen supplementation, the patient may need to be rapidly anesthetized, intubated, and started on positive-pressure ventilation. Some of these patients need ventilatory support for several days until the contusions heal.

Patients needing intubation should be left in lateral recumbency. Technicians should be able to intubate patients in both lateral and dorsal recumbency and to use a laryngoscope. If a patient is significantly hypotensive, raising the head may cause a sufficient decrease in cerebral blood flow to induce cardiac arrest. Laryngeal stimulation that can occur with blind intubation can cause a vagal response leading to cardiac arrest in the severely hypotensive or bradycardic patient. Once the patient is intubated, the lungs should be auscultated bilaterally to ensure that the trachea has been intubated and that the tube is not in a bronchus. If lung sounds cannot be auscultated, the esophagus may have been intubated or the patient may have an airway obstruction or disruption. If the patient cannot be intubated orotracheally because of oral, pharyngeal, or laryngeal injuries, a tracheotomy is indicated.

Fluids

Intravenous fluids must be provided to the patient in shock as oxygen is being supplemented. One or more large-bore intravenous catheters must be placed. A vascular cutdown may be needed for patients in severe shock. Because flow is directly proportional to the radius to the fourth power and inversely proportional to the length of the catheter, a short, large-bore catheter is more effective for rapid fluid administration than a long, small-bore catheter. Peripheral catheters are suitable in most cases. Ideally a jugular catheter should be placed if large volumes of fluids are to be administered because this allows measurement of central venous pressure. This is the only way to measure preload.

A combination of crystalloids and colloids should be delivered at whatever rate is needed to improve the patient's hemodynamic status. A patient with severe hypovolemic shock needs fluids administered at a much faster rate than does a patient with mild shock. Patients in shock need intravascular volume resuscitation, not interstitial resuscitation. Crystalloids are administered in 20- to 30-ml/kg increments. To maintain an adequate intravascular volume, colloids should be infused. For patients with signs of mild shock, crystalloids usually are sufficient. For patients with signs of moderate to severe shock, colloids are needed. Synthetic colloids such as dextran 70 or hetastarch should be administered in 5-ml/kg increments to a maximum volume of 20 ml/kg. Synthetic colloids can be bolused to dogs. Cats may vasodilate in response to boluses of hetastarch, and colloids should be administered over 20 to 25 minutes in cats to avoid worsening the hypotension. Because many of these patients are in shock from blood loss, the most effective colloid for resuscitation is whole blood. Blood products should be infused as indicated to maintain a packed cell volume between 25% and 30% and an albumin greater than 2.0 g/dl.

Because the goal of intravenous fluid therapy is to restore adequate circulating volume, fluids should be administered incrementally until hemodynamic parameters have normalized. This can be most effectively monitored by ensuring that the heart rate returns to a more normal level and that blood pressure is at least 100 mm Hg systolic.

Patients that are not responding to fluid therapy may have serious internal abdominal hemorrhage. Serious intraabdominal hemorrhage can come from blunt liver trauma, which leads to liver fractures, splenic lacerations, and renal avulsions. These patients may need hypotensive resuscitation or limited external counterpressure. Alternatively, surgery may be needed as part of the resuscitation.

Resuscitating the Patient with Severe Hemorrhage

Hypotensive resuscitation is reserved for patients in whom it is thought that hemorrhage will worsen if blood pressure is restored to normal. In these patients it may be appropriate to restrict fluid resuscitation until the source of the hemorrhage is controlled. Fluids are infused to reach a blood pressure of 85 to 100 mm Hg systolic. Elevations in blood pressure are controlled in an effort to avoid disrupting soft clots that are starting to form. In addition, decreasing the amount of fluids administered reduces the chance that the patient will develop dilutional coagulopathy. For patients with severe intraabdominal hemorrhage, limited external counterpressure also is needed.

BANDAGES AND SPLINTS

As problems are discovered during the secondary survey, specific treatments may be needed. This includes controlling external hemorrhage with direct pressure, placing splints, and keeping the patient warm. Most wound infections occur after the patient enters the hospital. Hospital bacteria and bacteria from human hands often are the cause. Whenever possible, sterile dressings (sterile bandage material, laparotomy pads, or towels) should be placed initially to help prevent secondary complications. Ideally, wounds should be clipped and cleaned before dressings are placed. It is most important to keep the wound moist and protected from further injury, contamination, and infection. When time permits, the wounds can be cleaned and treated properly.

All wounds should be clipped and cleaned once resuscitation is complete. Sterile water-soluble jelly (KY) should be placed in wounds before clipping. This helps prevent hair from getting lodged in the wound and prevents desiccation. Wounds should be cleaned with dilute povidone-iodine or chlorhexidine solution. Wounds should not be irrigated in the awake patient that has not received analgesia because this is painful. Irrigation with a 35-cc syringe and an 18-gauge needle is an effective way to clean wounds. Puncture wounds should not be flushed under pressure because this may force dirt and debris deeper into the wound.

Once the wound has been cleaned, a sterile dressing is placed. Wet-to-dry dressings are used if there is residual contamination or necrotic tissue. In some cases sterile water-soluble jelly or sterile antibiotic ointment is placed in the wound and the wound is covered with a nonadherent dressing such as a Telfa pad. The wound dressing is then covered with a padded layer followed by cling and a water-repellent outer wrap. Bandages must be kept clean and dry. If they are soiled, they must be changed immediately. This is especially important if urine gets into the bandage, because urine is very caustic to tissues. Bandages must be changed as soon as there is strikethrough to prevent wicking of external contaminants and bacteria into the wound through the wet bandage. To prevent infection, gloves should be worn whenever dressings on an open wound are changed.

Effective temporary splints can be placed on distal extremity injuries before radiographs are taken. Splinting can prevent a closed fracture from becoming an open fracture. It also helps stabilize fractures, preventing further injury by bone fragments, which can create shearing injury to the soft tissue, and promotes patient comfort by immobilizing the injury. Splints can be placed using newspaper and white porous tape or duct tape. Bubble wrap also makes a very effective lightweight splint.

A properly placed splint stabilizes the joint above and below the fracture. Bandages should always be placed from the digits proximally and should incorporate the lateral two digits. Toes must be monitored to ensure that they stay warm and do not start to swell. If coolness or swelling is noticed, circulation to the foot is being compromised and the splint or bandage should be removed immediately.

SURGICAL RESUSCITATION

Surgery may be needed to stabilize a patient. It may not be possible to stabilize these patients' respiratory or cardiovascular status until surgery has been performed. Examples of patients to whom this applies include those with severe external hemorrhage (such as a lacerated artery), severe ongoing internal hemorrhage, and diaphragmatic hernias. Anesthesia in these patients can be challenging. A dedicated anesthetist is essential. The severely hemorrhaging patient will need large volumes of warmed fluids and blood products intraoperatively.

BASIC MONITORING

The patient should be monitored closely during resuscitation, during any intraoperative period, and in the intensive care unit after resuscitation. The frequency of monitoring depends on the severity of the patient's condition. Monitoring may be needed as often as every 15 minutes or only every 4 to 6 hours if the patient is stable. Trends often are more important than exact numbers. Basic monitoring includes measuring the level of consciousness, respiratory rate and effort, heart rate, pulse rate and pulse strength, and temperature. Monitoring the difference between rectal and toe web temperature can help assess peripheral perfusion. The temperature difference under normal circumstances should be no more than 7° F. Jugular venous distention, jugular filling time, and jugular relaxation time are crude monitors of central venous pressure. Variation in pulse quality or detection of pulse deficits is consistent with ventricular premature contractions or potential pericardial effusion. The lungs should be auscultated frequently (every 2 to 4 hours) to check for the presence of pneumothorax, hemothorax, or pulmonary contusions. Urine output should be kept at 0.5 ml/kg/hr or higher to ensure adequate renal perfusion. Fluid intake and output should be monitored and fluids adjusted every 4 to 6 hours as indicated. Analgesics should be administered based on whether the animal appears to be in pain rather than on a set schedule. Pain is physiologically and psychologically detrimental and should be controlled as well as possible (Table 13-3).

Basic monitoring in the injured patient should include frequent blood pressure measurement until the patient is hemodynamically stable. Blood pressure should remain as close to 120/80 mm Hg as possible unless the patient's blood pressure is being kept deliberately low, as in hypotensive resuscitation.

There are three main methods for monitoring blood pressure: direct, oscillometric, and Doppler. Direct blood pressure monitoring is ideal but is rarely done in emergencies because of the time needed to place an arterial catheter and the necessary monitoring equipment. For accurate monitoring of the critically injured patient in the intensive care unit, an indwelling arterial catheter should be placed whenever possible. A Doppler blood pressure monitor is preferred in most injured patients because both blood pressure and flow to distal extremities can be assessed. Arrhythmias such as ventricular premature contractions also can be heard once the operator's ear has been trained to listen for irregularities in the flow signal.

TABLE 13-3 Goals for Measured Parameters for Injured Patients

Parameter	Goal
Respiratory rate	18-36/min
Heart rate	60-130/min
Heart rhythm	Sinus If ventricular premature contractions, unifocal, no significant pulse deficits, heart rate <160/min, no R on T arrhythmia
Temperature	Normal: ΔT <7° F
Blood pressure	Systolic 90-130 mm Hg Diastolic 60-100 mm Hg
Blood flow	Doppler sounds good
Central venous pressure	4-8 cm H_2O
Urine output	>0.5 ml/kg/hr
Pulse oximetry	>94%
Packed cell volume	25%-45%
Total solids	4.5-7.5 g/dl
Albumin	>2.0 g/dl
Platelet estimate	>5-8/high-power field
Activated clotting time	<120 sec (180 sec if received hetastarch)

ΔT, Difference between rectal and axillary or rectal and toe web temperature.

Basic laboratory monitoring also should include measuring the packed cell volume, total solids, glucose, and blood urea nitrogen by Azostix.

ADVANCED MONITORING

More advanced monitoring includes the use of electrocardiography, pulse oximetry, and central venous pressure. Ventricular premature contractions and ventricular tachycardia are the most common arrhythmias seen in injured patients. Ventricular premature contractions should be treated if they are multifocal, they are affecting perfusion (significant pulse deficits), the heart rate is elevated (usually above 160 bpm), or there is evidence of R on T phenomenon. Treatment includes using supplemental oxygen, maximizing tissue perfusion, and administering a constant-rate infusion of antiarrhythmics (lidocaine or procainamide).

Pulse oximetry can be monitored on the awake patient; however, measurements are subject to technical errors. If perfusion is poor, the oximeter may not detect adequate flow to get an accurate reading. Strong ambient light, pigmented skin, and motion can cause artifacts. Oxygen saturation should read about 94% to 95% on room air. If the patient has oxygen saturation readings of 90% to 92% on supplemental oxygen, arterial blood gas should be checked because this patient may need mechanical ventilation.

Central venous pressure monitoring should be performed in all patients in whom fluid overload is a potential complication. Monitoring trends may be more important than exact numbers. Ideally, the central venous pressure should be kept between 4 and 8 cm Hg. Central venous pressure readings are inaccurate as an indicator of circulating volume if there is a pneumothorax, abdominal counterpressure wrap, or right heart failure. If central venous pressure is normal (and none of the preceding conditions exists), but blood pressure is still low, cardiac function probably is inadequate and positive inotropic support may be indicated.

Laboratory monitoring includes regular assessment of electrolytes and blood gas parameters. Venous blood gases can be used for accurate assessment of pH and acid-base status, but arterial blood gases are needed to monitor oxygenation. Albumin levels, coagulation parameters, and platelet numbers also should be assessed. If the patient has an indwelling urinary catheter, daily urine sediments should be evaluated because urinary tract infections are a common complication of indwelling catheters. The frequency of laboratory monitoring depends on how critical the patient's condition is. In cases of suspected active hemorrhage, the packed cell volume should be monitored every 30 minutes. If the patient is stable, blood work can be checked twice daily.

POSTRESUSCITATION CARE: THE FIRST 24 HOURS

The severely traumatized patient is at risk for developing the systemic inflammatory response syndrome. Respiratory and cardiovascular parameters must be maintained as normal as possible. Laboratory parameters should be monitored and values kept as close to normal as possible.

Patients with significant blood loss obviously have lost a significant amount of endogenous clotting factors. In addition, tissue trauma can activate the coagulation cascade and, if left uncontrolled, can lead to disseminated intravascular coagulation. Patients in shock often are hypothermic and acidotic, which can cause dysfunction of the coagulation system. Infusing large volumes of crystalloids or synthetic colloids can dilute the remaining coagulation factors, leading to dilutional coagulopathy.

Many of these patients have multiple tubes in place. All tubes should be labeled carefully to ensure that oxygen is not delivered into a nasogastric tube and enteral feedings are not infused intravenously. If nasal tubes are in place, the patient should be monitored for signs of skin irritation at the suture site and signs of rhinitis. If adhesive tape gets wet, it can lead to a moist dermatitis. Both complications usually are mild and self-limiting; however, if the patient is experiencing discomfort the tube may need to be switched to the other nostril or removed. Bandages on feeding tubes such as esophagostomy, gastrostomy, and jejunostomy tubes should be changed daily or twice daily during the initial healing period (3 to 5 days). Ostomy sites should be examined visually for signs of inflammation or discharge and should be palpated for signs of pain. Any abnormalities should be reported because infection may be present.

Bandages on chest tubes also should be changed daily or twice daily, with visualization and palpation of the chest tube exit site. The site should be cleaned with an antibacterial solution (dilute chlorhexidine or povidone iodine) and a sterile dressing placed. Triple-antibiotic ointment should be used in generous quantities at the exit site to help form a seal. The entire area should be covered with a thoracic bandage. Patients should wear Elizabethan collars as needed to prevent them from chewing or removing the tubes. The suture sites for urinary catheters should be examined closely for signs of irritation. Closed collection systems, such as intravenous fluid administration systems, should be replaced every 48 to 72 hours.

Many of these patients are inactive or have trouble ambulating. Patient comfort is very important. Analgesics should be administered as often and at as high a dosage as necessary to keep the patient comfortable. Uncontrolled pain can cause harmful physiologic effects such as tachycardia, vasoconstriction, and compromised ventilation. Pain should never be used to limit an animal's movement. For instance, if a patient has a suspected soft tissue injury to a limb, it is better to control the pain and support the limb in a padded bandage or splint than to keep the animal immobile through pain. Analgesics ideally should be administered parenterally or locally. Epidural catheters are a very effective way to minimize pain. Fentanyl patches also are effective; however, in some severely injured patients the sedation and cardiovascular depression caused by the fentanyl can be excessive, in which case the patch should be removed.

Patients should be kept on padded bedding and turned every 2 to 4 hours. Larger patients should be monitored closely for the development of decubital ulcers. Gentle physiotherapy should be performed on all limbs possible when the patient is recumbent. Not only does this improve patient comfort but it stimulates circulation, and once the patient can ambulate it allows the pet to ambulate more rapidly. This becomes especially important in older animals or animals with arthritis (Table 13-4).

NUTRITION

Nutritional support is vital to injured patients because they are in a hypermetabolic state. Patient morbidity can be reduced significantly if enteral nutritional support is provided within the first 12 to 24 hours. Enteral nutrition is preferred over

TABLE 13-4 Intensive Care Unit List of Concerns

Airways, lungs, ventilation (work of breathing, dead space, SpO_2, $ETCO_2$, PCO_2)
Cardiac contractility, relaxation and rhythm (ECG, CO)
Vascular volume, flow, pressure (arterial and central venous), and tone
Oxygen delivery, including Hgb and PaO_2
Substrate delivery and use (glucose)
Fluid balance (water, albumin, colloid osmotic pressure)
Electrolyte balance (Na, K, Cl, Ca, Mg, P)
Acid-base balance (pH, HCO_3, BE)
Renal function, urine output, urine specific gravity, sediment
Energy-protein balance (enteral and parenteral nutrition)
Mentation, LOC, cranial and peripheral nerves
Pain and anxiety control
Gastrointestinal function, motility, and integrity
Skin, muscle, and joint care
Immune function (WBCs, small and large proteins)
Coagulation (platelets, BT, ACT, FDPs, coagulation panels)
Drugs (dosages, metabolism, compatibility, and route)
Catheter and tube sites
Surgical incisions, bandages, splints
General nursing care (physical therapy, mobility)
Assurance and communication (patient and owner)
Charting complete

SPO_2, Oxygen saturation by pulse oximetry; *$ETCO_2$*, end-tidal carbon dioxide; *PCO_2*, carbon dioxide pressure; *ECG*, electrocardiogram; *CO*, cardiac output; *Hgb*, hemoglobin; *PaO_2*, arterial oxygen pressure; *BE*, base excess; *LOC*, level of consciousness; *WBCs*, white blood cells; *BT*, bleeding time; *ACT*, activated clotting time; *FDPs*, fibrin degradation products.

parenteral nutrition because enteral nutrition helps preserve the gastrointestinal barrier, thus decreasing bacterial translocation. It also helps preserve immune function and normal intestinal, pancreatic, and biliary secretions.

Enteral nutritional support can be provided most easily by tube feeding if the patient will not eat. Nasoesophageal and nasogastric tubes are placed easily. If longer-term nutritional support is anticipated, an esophagostomy or gastrostomy tube may be indicated. Feeding tubes can be placed easily at the time of exploratory celiotomy for use postoperatively. Microenteral nutrition, or providing small amounts of glucose and a balanced electrolyte solution, may be beneficial. This is usually provided at rates of 0.1 to 0.5 ml/kg body weight per hour. If the patient cannot tolerate full enteral nutrition, this can be increased slowly and liquid enteral diets can be added to the infusion. This can be delivered by constant-rate infusion or as intermittent boluses. Parenteral nutrition should be supplemented if enteral access is not available and it is anticipated that the patient will not be eating for 2 to 3 days. Caloric intake should be at resting energy requirements to 1.5 times resting energy requirements. Overfeeding the patient with respiratory difficulties should be avoided because excess carbon dioxide will be produced. This excess carbon dioxide must be offset by an increase in respiratory rate.

ASSESSMENT AND MANAGEMENT OF SPECIFIC INJURIES

The degree of tissue trauma varies with the type of trauma and the velocity and mass of the impact. Force is equal to the mass multiplied by the velocity squared ($F = MV^2$). The greater the force, the more significant the tissue trauma. For instance, a dog hit in the head with a baseball bat will sustain a very different injury from a dog shot in the head. And a dog hit by a bicycle will sustain a much milder injury than one hit by a car.

Trauma generally is divided into two types: blunt and penetrating. Blunt trauma, which involves crushing force, usually results from collision with an object. This can occur if the animal falls, is stepped on, or is hit by an object such as a car or baseball bat. Penetrating injuries generally are those inflicted by knives, arrows, and bullets and impalements with objects such as sticks or metal rods. Bite wounds can cause both penetrating and blunt trauma. Significant shearing forces can be applied after penetration, especially with bite wounds. The seriousness of the injury often depends on what is penetrated. A better understanding of the mechanism of injury allows greater appreciation of possible internal injuries, which can enable the team to minimize patient morbidity and mortality.

Several types of traumatic injury can lead to death rapidly if the injury is not assessed accurately and treated immediately. These are airway disruptions or obstructions, tension pneumothorax, severe pulmonary contusions, and massive internal thoracic or abdominal hemorrhage. A high index of suspicion should be maintained for these injuries.

In this section injuries are grouped by anatomic location. These injuries can be caused by the animal being hit by a car, colliding with a solid object (such as jumping off a balcony), being bitten by another animal, being bitten and shaken, being hit by a penetrating missile (gunshot, arrow), or being impaled. A description of how to assess, manage, and monitor these patients during the resuscitation period is provided. In all cases it is assumed that oxygen will be provided as well as intravenous fluid support and analgesics. It is also assumed that basic diagnostics and monitoring are being performed. This section is not all inclusive but provides an overview of the more common injuries seen by an emergency service. No impaling object should be removed until the wound tract is explored. The object may have passed through or may be lodged in the heart or the abdominal aorta. Premature removal may lead to rapid exsanguination. The only exception to this rule is any object that is thought to be compromising respiration to the point of impending arrest (generally through obstruction).

Head and Facial Trauma

Assessment. Patients with head trauma present with varying levels of consciousness, from normal mentation to coma. Head trauma can lead to traumatic brain injury. Trauma to the brain stem is life threatening and can lead to alterations in respiratory pattern and cardiovascular derangement. Facial fractures can lead to intraoral and intranasal hemorrhage and subsequent respiratory difficulty. Blood can pool in the oropharynx, obstructing the airway.

Management. A clear airway is the first priority. The airway should be cleared of as much of the blood, vomitus, or other secretions as possible; however, extreme care should be taken to ensure that no one is bitten. A gagging response should be avoided in the patient with traumatic brain injury because this will elevate intracranial pressure and decrease cerebral blood flow. Suction using a Yankauer suction tip may be necessary. If patients are unconscious on presentation with no gag reflex, they must be intubated rapidly. This should be done without lifting the head because the decrease in blood flow to the brain caused by this maneuver can lead to a cardiac arrest. A laryngoscope should be used because excessive manipulation of the larynx can cause a vagally mediated bradycardia with subsequent hypotension and even arrest. Nasal tubes should be avoided because sneezing can elevate intracranial pressure.

The second priority is to ensure adequate cerebral blood flow. The intracranial volume comprises the brain tissue, the cerebrospinal fluid, and the blood vessels. Because the brain is contained by the skull, any change in one of the compartments affects the other two. Pressure on the jugular veins during venipuncture or catheter placement should be avoided because this may raise intracranial pressure and decrease perfusion to the brain. Fluids should be administered to maintain normal blood pressure. These patients must not be volume overloaded or allowed to become hypertensive because this can exacerbate intracranial hemorrhage; however, hypotension is even more detrimental. Sedatives may be needed if the patient is severely disoriented or hypertensive. The use of medications such as corticosteroids, furosemide, and mannitol is controversial. If there is a compressed skull fracture or the patient's neurologic status is worsening, intracranial pressure monitoring and emergency surgery for a decompressive craniotomy may be necessary. Hyperbaric oxygen therapy delivered within 2 to

6 hours of the head injury has been shown to be effective in ameliorating ongoing secondary neuronal ischemia caused by edema and swelling and to decrease ongoing hypoxic injury to the brain. Recumbent patients should be kept in a horizontal position and turned every 2 to 4 hours. When placing the patient in a cage, care must be taken to ensure that the neck is not flexed, which can compromise the airway and venous outflow via the jugular veins, increasing intracranial pressure. Mild elevation of the head up to 30 degrees is acceptable, but the neck must not be flexed. Elevating the head slightly may decrease the risk of silent regurgitation and aspiration.

Severe epistaxis may necessitate the use of intranasal epinephrine or nasal packing. Definitive surgery may or may not be necessary, depending on the type of injury. These animals must be kept very quiet and often need sedation. Sneezing and hypertension worsen epistaxis. Acepromazine may interfere with platelet action, but this rarely is a clinical problem.

Monitoring. Level of consciousness, pupil size and symmetry, respiratory pattern, heart rate, mucous membrane color, blood pressure, central venous pressure, packed cell volume, and total solids should be monitored. Blood gases and electrocardiogram readings should be evaluated as indicated. Platelet numbers, a buccal mucosal bleeding time to check for platelet dysfunction, and a coagulation screen are indicated.

Cervical Soft Tissue Injury

Assessment. Cervical trauma can lead to airway avulsion, airway obstruction from hemorrhage or swelling, and laceration of major vessels. These animals can present with varying degrees of respiratory distress. Blood loss can be highly variable. Injury to other soft tissues including muscle, subcutaneous tissue, and skin also is highly variable.

Management. The animal's respiratory rate and pattern should be observed closely. Any animal that has noisy breathing has a compromised airway and must be monitored closely because an obstruction may develop. Exaggerated chest movement without airway sounds is a hallmark of airway obstruction. The animal that is struggling to breathe and has pronounced respiratory efforts may have an avulsed larynx or trachea. These patients need immediate anesthesia and intubation or an awake tracheostomy. Transtracheal or nasotracheal oxygen may help in the interim. The trachea should be auscultated. The entire area should be carefully palpated and clipped thoroughly to evaluate the extent of hemorrhage and swelling. Any wound should be cleaned and a sterile bandage placed. Extreme care should be taken when placing a cervical bandage because patient movement often tightens these bandages.

If there is any concern about associated spinal injury, the patient must not be moved until the injury is stabilized. Cervical spinal injuries at or above the level of C4 can lead to loss of diaphragm function and subsequent respiratory compromise.

Monitoring. Mucous membrane color, respiratory rate and effort, heart rate, blood pressure, and pulse oximetry should be monitored. The hematocrit and total solids, blood gases, and electrocardiogram should be evaluated as indicated. Neck bandages should be checked every 4 to 6 hours for tightness and loosened as needed.

Chest Injury

Assessment. Chest trauma can lead to musculoskeletal injuries such as fractured ribs, lacerated muscles, and bruising. Intrathoracic trauma most commonly leads to pneumothorax, hemothorax, and pulmonary contusions. These patients present with varying degrees of respiratory distress. Hypoventilation caused by pain from fractured ribs is a significant concern.

Management. Oxygen should be provided immediately if a chest injury is suspected. Respiratory rate and effort should be assessed rapidly. Rapid, shallow ventilation often indicates pain from fractured ribs and intrapleural disease (pneumothorax or pneumohemothorax). Tension pneumothorax should be suspected if the patient has shallow, rapid respiration, an expanded thorax, limited movement of the chest wall with ventilation, and distended jugular veins. Deep, gasping breaths often indicate severe pulmonary contusions. Auscultation and percussion of the thorax should be performed. Dull lung sounds and dull or hyperresonant areas on percussion are consistent with intrapleural disease, and thoracentesis is indicated. Thoracentesis should be done bilaterally (because the mediastinum is complete in dogs) and should precede radiographs. A chest tube may be indicated. Analgesia should be provided early during the course of treatment with opioids and local anesthetics. All wounds should be clipped and cleaned, and sterile dressings should be placed. The exception may be a large wound in the pleural space. If this is sealed, tension pneumothorax may result. A chest tube may need to be placed through this hole or an occlusive dressing placed that is sealed on three sides only, with the fourth side acting as a pop-off valve. If the patient has a suspected flail chest and the animal is in lateral recumbency, the flail side should be placed down. A flail chest is a segment of chest wall that moves paradoxically with each breath (in when the patient inhales and out when the patient exhales). This is caused by three or more adjacent ribs being fractured in more than one location, creating a free-floating segment of chest wall. Fluids should be administered to maintain normal blood pressure. In the case of severe intrathoracic hemorrhage, hypotensive resuscitation may be indicated until surgery to control the hemorrhage definitively can be performed.

Patients with fractured ribs or other significant chest trauma need effective analgesia. This can be given via epidural, intrapleural, or local intercostal nerve blocks or frequent parenteral injections.

Monitoring. Patients with chest injuries must be monitored continuously until they are stable. Vital signs including respiratory rate and effort, mucous membrane color, heart rate, and blood pressure should be assessed frequently. In the severely hypoxic patient, rectal temperatures can cause vagally mediated bradycardia and hypotension, and axillary temperatures should be monitored instead. Blood gas measurements are ideal but can stress the patient excessively. In this case, pulse oximetry should be performed continuously if possible. Patients with chest trauma often develop ventricular premature contractions and ventricular tachycardia secondary to traumatic myocarditis. These patients should have continuous electrocardiogram monitoring and pulses should be palpated routinely for deficits. In most patients with chest tubes, continuous underwater suction is indicated. If the patient is on continuous underwater suctioning, the tubing should be stripped every 4 to 6 hours and intermittent hand aspiration should be done. Chest tube sites should be cleaned twice daily and sterile dressings placed. Connections should be checked frequently for signs of loosening or dislodgment.

Chest dressings must be changed once or twice daily initially. If the wounds have a large volume of exudate, more frequent dressing changes may be indicated. Bandages that are placed too tightly can lead to compromised ventilation and should be checked every 4 to 8 hours. Two fingers should fit underneath the bandage easily. If the bandage is on too tight, it can be cut along the dorsum until the outer layers no longer spread and the edges can be taped together using elastic tape. Most opioids cause some respiratory depression, and respiration should be monitored closely. However, analgesics should not be withheld because the pain associated with injuries to the chest significantly decreases the effectiveness of ventilation.

Abdominal Injury

Assessment. Intraabdominal injury can lead to significant hemorrhage from solid visci (e.g., liver, spleen), vascular injury to major vessels, and lacerations to the bowel, leading to peritonitis. Persistent vomiting, increasing abdominal pain, and abdominal distention all are indicators of a significant intraabdominal injury. Percussion may indicate areas of dullness, fluid waves, or areas of resonance, suggesting intraabdominal air accumulations. Splenic injuries can be associated with ventricular premature contractions. Retroperitoneal injuries can be more difficult to diagnose, but if the patient is becoming more anemic and there is no other known source of blood loss, then the bleeding may be coming from the retroperitoneal space.

Management. Patients with abdominal injuries often present with multiple injuries, and the airway and breathing should be assessed and managed before abdominal injuries are treated. Nasogastric decompression is important to decrease vomiting from gastric distention (from aerophagia or fluid) and to encourage the stomach to return to normal motility. This is especially important if the patient has had surgery for abdominal injuries or has an open abdomen. Pharmacologic control of vomiting may be needed. Vomitus should be checked for frank blood or digested blood ("coffee grounds") using an occult blood test if it is not grossly apparent. Urine should be assessed for the presence of hemorrhage grossly, using a dipstick test, and microscopically. If the patient is not producing urine within the first 4 hours of hospitalization, the possibility of a ruptured urinary bladder should be entertained. The stool should be monitored for signs of hemorrhage and melena. The hair covering the ventral and lateral aspects of the abdomen and caudal rib cage should be clipped and examined for the presence of wounds or bruising.

Monitoring. All vital signs must be monitored, including mucous membrane color, respiratory rate and effort, heart rate, and blood pressure. Ongoing hemorrhage is always a concern; therefore serial packed cell volumes and total solids should be assessed. The abdomen should be monitored closely for signs of distention or excessive bruising. Serial circumferential measurements of the abdomen using a tape measure is more sensitive than direct observation. Urine output should be monitored hourly during initial resuscitation, then every 4 hours.

Musculoskeletal Injury

Assessment. All suspected areas of trauma should be relieved of weight bearing and should be immobilized until the injury has been evaluated completely. This can be done by keeping the animal in lateral recumbency or confining it to a small space. Some musculoskeletal injuries are readily apparent because of the soft tissue trauma surrounding the injury. Non–weight-bearing lameness usually indicates luxation, fracture, or severe ligament injury. Partial weight bearing usually indicates a less severe injury. Severe hemorrhage into muscle compartments can lead to compartment syndrome. This occurs when the pressure rises when the muscle fascia is intact and the patient hemorrhages into the muscle belly to the point that circulation to the affected area is obstructed. Because this rapidly leads to tissue necrosis, it is important to recognize the condition early. Clinical signs can include severe swelling, signs that the affected area is becoming more painful than would be expected, decreased temperature of the toes of the affected limb in comparison to a normal limb, and increasing loss of movement or sensation. Fractures can lead to laceration of underlying soft tissue. For instance, rib fractures can be associated with a lacerated lung and pneumothorax. Femoral fractures can lead to laceration of major femoral vessels. Pubic fractures can lacerate the urethra. Patients with suspected spinal fractures should be immobilized to a board by taping them with duct tape or similar material. These patients must be radiographed before they are allowed to move, because movement may cause a significant worsening of the injury.

Management. All distal limb fractures should be splinted before radiographs are taken or the patient is moved, and patients should be kept as immobile as possible until the full extent of the injuries is known. Pain should not be used to immobilize patients, and analgesics should always be administered. Wounds should be protected with sterile dressings or covered with sterile towels. If it is suspected that compartment syndrome is present, pressure must be released immediately. This is done by performing fasciotomies in the operating room under aseptic conditions.

Monitoring. The patient should be monitored closely for evidence of soft tissue injury under fracture sites (i.e., monitor for urination with pubic fractures, pneumothorax with rib fractures, and compartment syndrome with long bone fractures).

COMMUNICATION

Communication with the owner is one of the technician's most important responsibilities. When the critically injured patient arrives and the doctor cannot leave the patient, the technician often can relay basic information on patient status, reassure the owner, and gain permission for procedures or treatment. Because technicians work with the patients more closely than the doctors, often they are much more informed about the nuances of the patient's condition. Therefore the technician can provide important information about the patient's comfort, urination and defecation habits, appetite, and water intake to the owner. Owners need to feel that their pet is being treated well, not just from a medical perspective but also from a psychological and emotional perspective. The veterinary technician is the patient's advocate as well as the owner's advocate. If any part of the patient's care is not being addressed adequately, it is the technician's responsibility to inform the veterinarian and make recommendations to resolve the issues.

CONCLUSION

The injured patient's survival depends on a well-equipped facility and a highly educated staff. An organized trauma work station must be established. The trauma team should review their roles to be prepared for the arrival of this type of an emergency.

Patient assessment begins with triage. This evaluation is performed quickly to determine the severity of the injury. It is also the time to determine which patient should be seen first if more than one is waiting.

The primary survey is used for the initial examination, which includes vital sign readings, the collection of samples for laboratory analysis, hemorrhage control, and any other immediate needs. Once resuscitation has begun the secondary survey can begin. This is the complete examination of the patient from head to tail.

Many forms of trauma can occur. The veterinary technician must fully understand the equipment available and techniques used to stabilize these patients.

BIBLIOGRAPHY

Alverdy J, Chi HS, Sheldon GF: The effect of parenteral nutrition on gastrointestinal immunity. The importance of enteral stimulation, *Ann Surg* 205:681, 1985.

Bagley RS: Intracranial pressure in dogs and cats, *Compend Contin Educ Pract Vet* 18:605, 1996.

Bickell WH, Wall MJ, Pepe PE, et al: Immediate versus delayed resuscitation for hypotensive patients with penetrating torso injuries, *N Engl J Med* 331:1105, 1994.

Bongard F, Pianim N, Dubecz S, et al: Adverse consequences of increased intra-abdominal pressure on bowel tissue oxygenation, *J Trauma* 39:519, 1995.

Clifton GL: Hypothermia and hyperbaric oxygen as treatment modalities for severe head injury, *New Horiz* 3:474, 1995.

Crowe DT: Diagnostic abdominal paracentesis techniques: clinical evaluation in 129 dogs and cats, *J Am Anim Hosp Assoc* 20:225, 1984.

Crowe DT: Performing life-saving cardiovascular surgery, *Vet Med* 84:77, 1989.

Crowe DT, Devey JJ: Assessment and management of the hemorrhaging patient, *Vet Clin North Am* 24:1095, 1994.

Crowe DT, Devey JJ: Nasal, nasopharyngeal, nasotracheal, nasoesophageal, nasogastric and nasoenteric tubes: insertion and use. In Bojrab MJ, Ellison G, Slocum B eds: *Current techniques in small animal surgery,* ed 4, Baltimore, 1998, Williams & Wilkins.

Crowe DT, Devey JJ: Thoracic drainage. In Bojrab MJ, Ellison G, Slocum B, eds: *Current techniques in small animal surgery,* ed 4, Baltimore, 1998, Williams & Wilkins.

Dawson RB: Transfusion: volume expansion, oxygen transport, hemostasis, transfusion reactions, autotransfusion. In Cowely RA, Conn A, Dunham CM, eds: *Trauma care,* vol 2: *Medical management,* Philadelphia, 1987, JB Lippincott.

Dewey CW, Budsberg SC, Oliver JE: Principles of head trauma management in dogs and cats. 1, *Compend Contin Educ Pract Vet* 14:199, 1992.

Kirby R, Rudloff E: The critical need for colloids: maintaining fluid balance, *Compend Contin Educ Pract Vet* 19:705, 1997.

Kowalenko T, Stern S, Dronen S, et al: Improved outcome with hypotensive resuscitation of uncontrolled hemorrhagic shock in a swine model, *J Trauma* 33:349, 1992.

Moore EE, Moore FA: Immediate enteral nutrition following multisystem trauma: a decade perspective, *J Am Coll Nutr* 10:633, 1991.

Rainey TG, Read CA: Pharmacology of colloids and crystalloids. In Chernow B, ed: *The pharmacologic approach to the critically ill patient,* Baltimore, 1994, Williams & Wilkins.

Zornow MH, Prough DS: Fluid management in patients with traumatic brain injury, *New Horiz* 3:488, 1995.

Chapter 14

Hematologic Emergencies

If an animal presents with anemia or a bleeding disorder, a thorough history must be taken, the animal assessed, and the appropriate tests performed to determine the cause of the disorder. This chapter covers the types of anemia and bleeding disorders, the most common causes, and how to care for each disorder.

Equipment List

- Intravenous catheters of different lengths and gauges
- Intravenous fluids (colloids and crystalloids)
- Oxygen and delivery devices
- Items for quick assessment tests
  - Capillary tubes
  - Blood glucose test strips
  - Azo strips
  - Refractometer
- Oral vitamin K
- Injectable vitamin K
- Access to blood components
- Simplate II (disposable template with two spring-loaded blades)
- Activated clotting time tubes with diatomaceous earth

ANEMIA DEFINITION AND CAUSES

Anemia, a reduction in the number of circulating red blood cells (RBCs), is confirmed by a decrease in the RBC count, hemoglobin, or packed cell volume (PCV). Rarely a primary disease, anemia usually results from a generalized disease process. Anemia may be suggested by the patient's clinical signs and presenting history. Once anemia is confirmed, its cause should be investigated thoroughly to determine proper therapeutic management.

Causes of anemia include increased RBC loss (i.e., hemorrhage), increased destruction (i.e., intravascular or extravascular hemolysis), or decreased production (i.e., selective or generalized hypoplasia or aplasia of the bone marrow). This classification scheme includes possible mechanisms of anemia and thereby suggests appropriate therapy. Anemia from blood loss generally results from external loss of RBCs and plasma proteins. Hemolytic anemia is characterized by the destruction of circulating RBCs. Hypoproliferative anemia results from ineffective erythropoiesis of various causes. (The red cell life span usually is normal in blood loss anemias and hypoproliferative anemias but is characteristically reduced in hemolytic anemias.)

Based on the erythropoietic response seen in peripheral blood, anemias also can be classified as regenerative or nonregenerative. This is helpful in differentiating blood loss and hemolytic anemias (generally responsive) from depression anemias (generally nonresponsive). Nonregenerative anemias can result from diminished erythropoietin production, inadequate bone marrow response to appropriate cell production stimuli, or ineffective erythropoiesis.

HEMORRHAGE

A significant loss of blood over minutes to hours results in hypovolemia and potential cardiovascular collapse. The therapeutic goal in treating acute hemorrhagic hypovolemia is to stop hemorrhage and support the cardiovascular system. Aggressive, rapid restoration of vascular volume must be instituted while preventing further blood loss if possible. In cases of external hemorrhage, direct pressure can be applied to the bleeding site. There is concern of continued blood loss from uncontrolled sites after intravascular volume resuscitation. Although internal hemorrhage may not be evident on presentation, it should be suspected if shock occurs after trauma.

In choosing resuscitation fluid for vascular space replacement, volume and composition are critical in determining the effectiveness of volume expansion and duration of its effect. After blood loss, the intravascular space is depleted, and only later does interstitial fluid shift from the extravascular into the intravascular space, providing needed volume. Early in the hemorrhagic emergency, replenishing intravascular space losses is a priority. This can be accomplished easily using crystalloid fluid solutions. Crystalloid solutions also enter the extravascular space, so it is necessary to administer two to three times the volume lost. Risk of fluid overload is of concern when a large volume of crystalloids is administered, especially in older patients or those with cardiovascular compromise. Colloid solutions should be considered when there is a need to maintain intravascular oncotic pressure without administering large volumes of fluid. Crystalloid solutions are recommended initially for treating acute blood loss. If blood loss continues and a substantial portion of the blood volume is depleted, colloid solutions can be added.

The symptoms that occur after hemorrhage are a result of blood volume depletion, not a decrease in red blood cell mass. Unfortunately, volume expansion further dilutes hemoglobin remaining within the circulation. Although intravascular volume expansion improves tissue perfusion, patient assessment (e.g., physical examination, history, laboratory tests) will help determine whether enough hemoglobin is present to provide oxygen to vital organs. The need for transfusion should be based on clinical assessment of the signs of anemia because there is no magic laboratory value at which a patient must be transfused. Red cell replacement is not necessary during initial therapy for acute blood loss. The appropriate level of therapy depends on the volume of blood lost, the rate at which it was lost, and the patient's condition.

HEMOLYSIS

Hemolytic anemia is accelerated destruction of RBCs resulting in decreased total red blood cell mass. Whether hemolysis occurs in the intravascular space or, more commonly, in the extravascular space depends on several factors, including the cause and severity of the disease process. Immune-mediated hemolytic anemia (IMHA) may be a primary disease process, also known as idiopathic or autoimmune hemolytic anemia (AIHA), or secondary to infection, drugs, vaccines, toxins, or neoplasia. Reports of AIHA in cats are rare and often associated with feline leukemia virus (FeLV) infection. Therefore this discussion focuses on immune-mediated disease in the dog.

AIHA is a consequence of RBC destruction mediated by autologous anti-RBC antibodies. The specific stimulus causing an animal to develop antibodies to its own tissue remains unidentified. It is hypothesized that a change in antigenicity of the red cells or in individual immune status may cause the immune system to attack its own RBCs.

A secondary immune response directed toward a foreign antigen may lead to inadvertent damage to normal patient cells. Causes of secondary IMHA include neoplasia, infectious disease (parasitic, viral, bacterial, rickettsial, or fungal), toxin exposure, and drug therapy. Neoplasia is the most common cause of secondary IMHA.

Although IMHA is the most common cause of hemolytic disease in dogs, other important causes of hemolysis exist. Differentiation of the cause of hemolysis is important because of the wide variability between therapy and prognosis. Additionally, immunosuppressive drugs used to treat IMHA can be associated with significant side effects.

Hereditary hemolytic disorders resulting from increased RBC fragility have been documented in a number of canine breeds. Phosphofructokinase (PFK) deficiency in English springer spaniels is well documented, and pyruvate kinase (PK) deficiency has been observed in Basenjis, Beagles, and West Highland White Terriers. PK deficiency usually is more severe, with myelofibrosis, osteosclerosis, and death occurring before age 4. PFK deficiency tends to be associated with mild to moderate intermittent intravascular hemolysis, frequently exacerbated by exercise. Dogs with PFK deficiency often show signs of hemoglobinemia or hemoglobinuria during an acute crisis. Both disorders exhibit marked reticulocytosis associated with chronic hemolytic disease. Hereditary RBC disorders should be included as a differential for any dog belonging to an affected breed presenting with markedly regenerative anemia and even mild signs of hemolytic disease. Definitive diagnosis of PFK and PK deficiency can be achieved with specialized testing.

Client education about onion ingestion by pets is warranted because the oxidizing agent *N*-propyl disulfide, found in onions, may cause hemolysis. Oxidation results in structural changes to the RBC, leading to hemolysis that may range from subclinical to severe. Precise toxic ingestion quantity is unknown. One study produced marked hemolysis and anemia in dogs after feeding 5.5 g/kg body weight of dehydrated onions. Heinz bodies and eccentrocytes (RBCs with hemoglobin shifted to one side) appear within 24 hours after onion ingestion. When stained with new methylene blue, Heinz bodies appear as blue to purple refractile bodies on the periphery of the RBC. Because hemolysis associated with onion ingestion is not immune-mediated, patients are Coombs negative. The key to diagnosing onion-induced hemolytic disease in dogs rests on suggestive or conclusive history of onion ingestion, negative Coombs test, and detection of RBC Heinz bodies or eccentrocytes on a peripheral blood smear.

Zinc toxicosis in dogs often is associated with a hemolytic crisis of rapid onset. Zinc-induced hemolytic disease in dogs occurs most commonly after ingestion of zinc-containing foreign bodies. All pennies minted in the United States since 1983 contain 96% zinc and are the most common source of zinc intoxication in dogs. Zinc-containing nuts and bolts also are an important risk factor for zinc intoxication. Signalment and history help establish an index of suspicion of zinc intoxication; many of these dogs are young and have a history of repeated foreign body ingestion. Although the exact mechanism of zinc-induced hemolysis is unknown, intravascular hemolysis often occurs, thereby causing hemoglobinemia and hemoglobinuria.

Both *Ehrlichia canis,* a rickettsial parasite of white blood cells, and *Babesia canis,* a protozoal parasite of RBCs, can induce hemolysis in dogs. Coombs test can be positive in both conditions, thus making them difficult to distinguish from primary IMHA.

Various forms of microangiopathic diseases, including disseminated intravascular coagulation (DIC), hemangiosarcoma, and heartworm infestation, can result in direct RBC damage occurring in the microvasculature, causing clinical signs of hemolysis.

INEFFECTIVE ERYTHROPOIESIS

Anemia caused by ineffective or reduced erythropoiesis may result from nutritional deficiencies (e.g., iron, B_{12}, gastrointestinal malabsorption), drugs, infection (e.g., FeLV, feline immunodeficiency virus), chronic disease (e.g., inflammatory disease), bone marrow infiltration (e.g., leukemia, multiple myeloma), and organ disorders (e.g., renal disease, hypoadrenocorticism). These anemias are chronic and generally nonregenerative or poorly regenerative.

CLINICAL ASSESSMENT

An accurate history, thorough physical examination, and appropriate laboratory tests must be performed to evaluate an anemic patient, determine a diagnosis, and define a therapeutic plan.

History

All pertinent information must be gathered from the owners. Obtaining and assessing a detailed history will help define the nature, severity, and duration of clinical signs and aid in making a correct diagnosis. This attention to detail allows the clinician to establish probability for each possible differential early in the diagnostic process. For example, an anemic English springer spaniel presenting with port wine–colored urine, especially after physical exertion, should alert the clinician to the possibility of PFK deficiency. When a puppy presents with signs of hemolytic disease, the owner should be questioned about the possibility of foreign body ingestion of certain zinc-containing metallic objects.

Complete vaccination history should not be overlooked, because a relationship between recent vaccination and onset of IMHA has been demonstrated. One study showed that 25% of all patients with IMHA were vaccinated within 1 month of presentation and that this complication occurred independent of the type of vaccine used.

The animal's environmental history may suggest possible exposure to toxic and organic substances that create hemolytic conditions (e.g., onions, zinc). Tick exposure also should be investigated. Information about previously diagnosed diseases and any recently or currently administered medication is very important. Additionally, the presence of a previous immune-mediated disease heightens suspicion for the presence of an immune-mediated mechanism. Many drugs have potentially harmful or complicating side effects, resulting in a toxic effect on RBCs (drug-induced IMHA), white blood cells, and platelets.

Physical Examination

A complete physical examination and multiple monitoring procedures may be needed to assess the patient in an anemic crisis. Optimal assessment cannot be based on the result of a single parameter but is based on the results of several physical findings and monitored parameters that should always be evaluated in relation to one another.

The development and progression of clinical signs depend on the rapidity of onset, degree, and cause of anemia in conjunction with the animal's physical activity. Common physical findings are those associated with a decrease in RBC mass: lethargy, weakness, pale mucous membranes, tachycardia, tachypnea, and bounding pulses. The cardiovascular and respiratory system should be evaluated carefully. Perfusion assessment is based on mucous membrane color, capillary refill time (CRT), heart rate, and pulse rate, strength, and character. In a severe anemic state, a low-grade systolic flow murmur may occur secondary to decreased blood viscosity. Mucous membrane color can be used to monitor the patient's response to therapy or indicate the development of a problem. Prolonged CRT suggests compromised tissue perfusion and shock but may be difficult to assess in an anemic patient. Weak and rapid pulses suggest severe dehydration and poor perfusion; bounding pulses suggest anemia. Respiratory rate and effort assessment and careful auscultation help differentiate between decreased oxygen-carrying capability and pulmonary thromboembolism.

Patients should be evaluated for signs of underlying or concurrent disease. Dogs with IMHA should be examined carefully for signs of other immune-mediated disease, such as concurrent immune-mediated thrombocytopenia (IMT + IMHA = Evans syndrome). If petechiation is present, IMT or other coagulopathies, such as liver disease or DIC, should be investigated. Other common physical findings in dogs presenting with hemolytic disease are those relating to accumulation of bilirubin or hemoglobin in blood, urine, and soft tissue. As a result of extravascular RBC destruction, increased quantities of bilirubin are presented to the liver for conjugation and excretion. Bilirubin begins to accumulate in blood, urine, and soft tissue when the quantity of bilirubin present exceeds the liver's capacity to excrete it in the bile. Consequently, dogs with severe extravascular hemolysis present with icterus and pigmenturia, caused by the presence of bilirubin or hemoglobin in the urine. Given the low threshold for urinary excretion of conjugated bilirubin in dogs, bilirubinuria develops early in the disease process and precedes hyperbilirubinemia and icterus. If questioned, owners may remark on presence of pigmenturia. Icterus is easily recognized on all skin surfaces when severe. When more subtle, icterus is best recognized on the gingiva, sclera, conjunctiva, and inner pinnae. If intravascular hemolysis occurs, hemoglobinemia with or without hemoglobinuria may be present.

Splenomegaly or hepatomegaly may be discovered on abdominal palpation. They result from increased RBC clearance by the monocyte phagocytic system in these organs, extramedullary hematopoiesis, and hemosiderosis (accumulation of iron in the liver). Dogs with IMHA may also develop hepatopathy, particularly after glucocorticosteroid therapy. Pyrexia is an inconsistent finding in hemolytic patients, suggesting an immune-mediated or infectious cause, but it may be the result of an underlying disease process.

Laboratory Tests

Although information obtained from the history and specific clinical signs can suggest a diagnosis, certain laboratory tests are necessary for a definitive diagnosis.

Anemia is suggested when one or more of the red cell parameters are below normal for the patient's age, sex, and breed. Of these three parameters, PCV provides a simple, quick, and accurate means of detecting anemia and classifying it as mild, moderate, or severe. Dehydration and splenic contraction may mask anemia, whereas hemodilution may cause a temporary reduction in RBC parameters. Evaluating both PCV and total plasma protein (TPP) levels may help in differentiating these variables. Dehydration is associated with increases in both PCV and TPP, whereas with splenic contraction only PCV elevation is seen. Decreases in both PCV and TPP are associated with hemodilution after acute blood loss or fluid therapy, whereas a reduction in PCV only usually is associated with hemolytic anemias. TPP usually is normal in anemia secondary to decreased production or increased destruction of erythrocytes. In blood loss, both PCV and TPP may be decreased by loss of erythrocytes and plasma proteins and by a compensatory shift of fluid from the interstitial space to the intravascular compartment. The degree of anemia varies with the nature, extent, and duration of the disease process.

Reticulocyte Count

Reticulocyte count is the best indicator of the effectiveness of bone marrow activity. The reticulocyte count during regenerative anemia generally varies with the degree of anemia. The greater the stimulation of marrow erythropoiesis, the greater the reticulocytosis. This is not the case with nonregenerative anemias. Therefore the degree of reticulocytosis must be viewed in concert with the degree of anemia. This may be done by calculating a corrected reticulocyte count (%) or an absolute reticulocyte count (per microliter of blood). The absolute reticulocyte count is calculated by multiplying the percentage of reticulocytes by the RBC count. Alternatively, the percentage of reticulocytes can be corrected for the degree of anemia by using the following formula: corrected reticulocytes percentage = (observed reticulocyte count) × (PCV of patient/mean normal PCV for species). The mean normal PCV is 45% and 37% for dogs and cats, respectively. A corrected reticulocyte count greater than 1% in the dog and cat indicates a regenerative anemia. An absolute reticulocyte count of more than 60,000/μl of blood in the dog is evidence of a regenerative response.

The degree of reticulocytosis generally is greater in hemolytic anemia and is evidenced earlier than in blood loss anemia. Usually, it takes about 3 or 4 days for a significant reticulocytosis to be found in blood after an acute hemolytic or hemorrhagic episode, and a maximal response may take 1 to 2 weeks or longer. Thus reticulocytosis in an anemic patient may indicate increased RBC destruction or blood loss. Conversely, the absence of reticulocytosis in an anemic patient suggests reduced erythropoietin production, marrow depression or failure, defective iron use, or ineffective erythropoiesis. Bone marrow evaluation is necessary to assess RBC production in these patients.

Complete Blood Cell Count/ Blood Film

Much information can be gathered from a complete blood cell count (CBC) (e.g., microhematocrit, hemoglobin concentration, cell counts, RBC indices). Upon careful microscopic examination of a stained blood film, RBC indices and morphology may help characterize an anemia. The mean corpuscular volume (MCV), which represents average RBC size, classifies erythrocytes as normocytic (normal), macrocytic (larger than normal), or microcytic (smaller than normal). For example, an increased MCV may result from cells being released from the bone marrow before reaching full maturity. This is called macrocytic anemia. The mean corpuscular hemoglobin concentration (MCHC) is represented by the terms normochromic (normal hemoglobin content) and hypochromic (less than normal hemoglobin content). For example, a decreased MCHC may result from increased numbers of circulating immature RBCs. This is called hypochromic anemia. The blood smear also may show morphologic features, such as spherocytosis (indicative of IMHA), polychromasia, and anisocytosis.

IMHA and IMT may occur concurrently and are differentiated by a platelet count. If thrombocytopenia is present, then a diagnostic workup for IMT should be performed and appropriate treatment instituted. With any clinical evidence of bleeding, other coagulation studies should be performed to rule out concurrent thrombocytopenia, DIC, or other coagulopathies.

RBC autoagglutination strongly suggests IMHA. Agglutination appears as grapelike clustering of erythrocytes in the blood smear. Agglutination can be distinguished from rouleaux formation on a wet mount preparation of a blood sample. Mix one drop of blood with one drop isotonic saline on a clean microscope slide, cover with a coverslip, and examine under the microscope. Rouleaux, unlike agglutination, should be dispersed by the addition of saline. This test is not infallible because weak agglutinins may cause false negative results. Blood also can be evaluated for presence of macroagglutination (in the tube).

With IMHA, the leukocyte count often is elevated, with a slight to marked neutrophilia and left shift as a result of maximal bone marrow stimulation. A patient in hemolytic crisis may exhibit a marked neutrophilia (60,000 to 70,000 with increase in banded neutrophils) in the absence of infection, so one must evaluate the clinical presentation of each patient and look for other signs that might support infection, along with the white blood cell count.

Coombs Test

Serologic diagnosis of IMHA is based on demonstration of immune-mediated antibody or complement on the surface of RBCs or in serum via Coombs antiglobulin tests. The direct Coombs' test (DCT) demonstrates presence of antierythrocyte antibody or activated complement components on the surface of the patient's RBCs. The indirect Coombs' test (ICT) reveals the presence of antierythrocyte antibody in patient serum. A suspension of the patient's washed RBCs (DCT) or of normal (control) washed RBCs exposed to the patient's serum (ICT) is allowed to react with species-specific antiglobulin, resulting in visible RBC agglutination. In cases of drug-induced IMHA, the offending drug must be incorporated into the test system, or the test can yield negative results.

Antinuclear Antibody Test and Systemic Lupus Erythematosus

If autoimmune disease is suspected, testing for antinuclear antibody and systemic lupus erythematosus is indicated.

Chemistry Profile and Urinalysis

Serum biochemistry profile and urinalysis evaluation is important in detecting and assessing concurrent metabolic disease (e.g., renal, hepatic). Electrolyte disturbances should be monitored closely. Decreased bilirubin and albumin or globulin levels may indicate blood loss. Elevated bilirubin concentration may suggest hemolysis. RBC destruction must be rapid and significant to result in clinical icterus. Blood sample collection is critical in that hemolysis associated with traumatic venipuncture can cause serum bilirubin to be falsely elevated.

Tick Titers

Serology for *Babesia* and *Ehrlichia* should be performed if tick exposure is suspected. Direct examination of capillary blood smears can reveal *Babesia* organisms, but *Ehrlichia* organisms are difficult to detect on peripheral blood smears.

Miscellaneous

IMHA is an important risk factor for pulmonary thromboembolus (PTE). Acute onset of dyspnea with little or no radiographic evidence of pulmonary disease strongly suggests PTE. PTE may be difficult to distinguish from pneumonia in the absence of nuclear scintigraphy. Arterial blood gas evaluation may be helpful in assessing ventilation, oxygenation, and acid-base status.

TREATMENT AND MANAGEMENT

Anemic animals often present to the emergency room in advanced stages of disease, on the verge of cardiovascular collapse, and in need of immediate therapeutic intervention. Although definitive diagnosis ultimately is important, stabilizing the patient's emergent clinical problems is critical. This may include controlling hemorrhage, replacing lost blood volume with appropriate intravenous fluid solutions or blood components, improving the oxygen-carrying capacity with oxygen and RBC support, and taking all necessary measures to combat shock. Once the patient is stabilized it is important to classify the anemia, proceed with diagnostic evaluation, determine the underlying cause, and begin appropriate therapy.

The patient's clinical signs help determine the severity of the anemia. Animals do not tolerate acute-onset anemia secondary to hemolysis or hemorrhage as well as chronic anemia caused by hemolysis or decreased RBC production. In chronic anemia, compensatory mechanisms (e.g., increase in heart rate and size) allow toleration of a much lower hematocrit.

The primary therapeutic goal is to manage the anemic crisis. The animal should be kept quiet and receive oxygen therapy if necessary. Clinical laboratory tests should be performed immediately and therapy instituted promptly after test samples are obtained. The benefit of transfusion therapy must be weighed against its inherent risks.

HEMOSTASIS

When a patient presents with abnormal bleeding, it is important to determine the cause. Although it is the responsibility of the veterinarian to diagnose the condition and choose an appropriate therapy, the veterinary technician should anticipate the needs of the veterinarian and, most importantly, the patient. This entails a basic understanding of the physiology of hemostasis.

Hemostasis, the body's balancing mechanism that arrests hemorrhage while maintaining blood flow within the vascular compartment, occurs through a complex series of events involving the vessels, platelets, plasma coagulation factors, and fibrinolytic system. The role of each component in hemostasis depends on the size of the vessel and the amount of damage that has occurred. Bleeding in smaller vessels may be controlled by a simple response involving the vasculature and platelets (e.g., normal wear and tear on capillaries), whereas incorporation of the plasma coagulation factors is necessary for controlling hemorrhaging in larger damaged vessels.

The first response to blood vessel injury is vasoconstriction, which allows diversion of blood flow around the injured area. Once the endothelial lining of the vessel is disrupted, the subendothelial connective tissue (i.e., collagen fibers) is exposed. Circulating platelets pool to the area of injury and, with the help of adhesive proteins such as collagen, fibrinogen, fibronectin, and von Willebrand factor (vWF), adhere to the endothelial lining to arrest the initial bleeding. This process is known as platelet adhesion. Once the platelets adhere to the subendothelium, they change shape and secrete certain biochemical substances that enhance platelet layering in the injured area (platelet aggregation). The platelets form a complete but unstable plug. This portion of the hemostatic process, involving the vasculature and platelets, is called primary hemostasis and usually is adequate to stop bleeding in smaller vessels.

With greater damage or larger vessels, secondary hemostasis involving plasma coagulation factors becomes necessary. Plasma coagulation factors are produced in the liver and circulate in the blood in the inactive form. They become activated only when exposed to certain substances (tissues or platelet phospholipids). Initiation of the extrinsic and intrinsic clotting pathways leads to activation of all factors in a cascadelike effect, converging in a common pathway. Tissue thromboplastin, released from the injured vessel wall, initiates the extrinsic clotting pathway. This is an extravascular process in that tissue thromboplastin is not normally found in blood and must gain entry to the vascular system. Clotting via the intrinsic pathway begins when blood comes into contact with a foreign substance or surface (i.e., damaged endothelium). Activated platelets release a phospholipid, allowing coagulation factors in this pathway to activate one another. In the intrinsic pathway, all factors necessary for clot formation are within the circulating blood (intravascular). The result of this clotting cascade is the creation of fibrin, a threadlike protein. The fibrin threads form an insoluble meshwork over the site of the platelet plug, consolidating and stabilizing the clot.

For simplicity, the pathways are reviewed as divided processes here. However, the classic cascade presentation of fibrin formation has many underlying complexities and interrelationships that go beyond the scope of this chapter.

The final step in hemostasis is fibrinolysis. Once the vessel is healed, fibrinolytic enzymes digest the clot that has been formed, restoring normal blood flow. Clot lysis produces small pieces of fibrin, called fibrin split products (FSPs, or fibrin degradation products), which are cleared from circulation by the liver. Small levels of FSPs always appear in the circulation as a result of bleeding and clotting secondary to normal wear and tear on vessels. Another contribution of hemostasis is to keep the body in balance in regard to bleeding and clotting. FSP levels increase during episodes of excessive bleeding with diffuse coagulation (i.e., DIC) and in patients with compromised liver function. After clot digestion, vessel wall endothelium is reestablished and returned to its original state.

DISORDERS OF PRIMARY HEMOSTASIS

VASCULAR ANOMALIES

Vascular integrity must be maintained for uninterrupted blood flow. Congenital or acquired blood vessel abnormalities can lead to irregular flow dynamics or loss of vascular integrity and subsequent activation of clotting mechanisms.

QUANTITATIVE PLATELET DISORDERS

Patients with a low platelet count (thrombocytopenia) experience bleeding when inadequate numbers of platelets are available to form a platelet plug. Causes of low platelet count include massive blood loss, bone marrow neoplasia, chemotherapy, radiation therapy, antibody formation to platelets, and massive consumption in clot formation (i.e., DIC).

Immune-mediated thrombocytopenia is one of the most common causes of platelet destruction and subsequent thrombocytopenia. IMT can be a primary disorder in which no cause of the antiplatelet antibody production can be identified, called idiopathic thrombocytopenia purpura, or a secondary disorder in which antibodies are produced in response to antigenic stimuli (e.g., drugs, vaccines, infections, neoplasia). IMT can be acute, chronic, or recurrent and range from mild to severe.

QUALITATIVE PLATELET DISORDERS

Platelets must have adequate function and number to participate optimally in hemostasis. When the platelet quality is compromised, platelet adhesion or aggregation at the site of endothelial damage may be abnormal. Congenital disorders of platelet function are rare. Some of the more common inherited thrombopathias in veterinary medicine are platelet storage pool disease of the American cocker spaniel, thrombasthenia of the otter hound, Chediak-Higashi syndrome of the Persian cat, and others in the basset hound, spitz, Great Pyrenees, and domestic shorthair cat.

Certain drugs can have a pronounced adverse effect on platelets. Some drugs can induce thrombocytopenia (e.g., heparin), and others inhibit platelet response (e.g., aspirin, nonsteroidal antiinflammatory drugs). Drug-induced hemostatic abnormalities usually resolve when the drug is discontinued. However, after aspirin exposure, platelet inhibition persists throughout the life span of the platelet.

Bleeding abnormalities can be a clinical manifestation of acute or chronic renal failure. Platelet dysfunction secondary to uremia is the primary cause of hemorrhage in these patients. Compromised platelet function also can be seen in patients with chronic liver disease. Additionally, in patients with portal hypertension and associated congestive splenomegaly, thrombocytopenia can occur.

VON WILLEBRAND DISEASE

Von Willebrand disease (vWD) is a common inherited bleeding disorder in Doberman pinschers, rottweilers, German shepherds, golden retrievers, and more than 50 other breeds. These patients lack vWF, a necessary adhesive protein that promotes platelet adhesion and aggregation after vascular injury. Patients with vWD vary in presentation from nonclinical to severe hemorrhage.

DISORDERS OF SECONDARY HEMOSTASIS

When a coagulation factor deficiency is present, fibrin stabilization of the platelet plug cannot occur and hemostasis is impaired. Clotting defects can result from decreased factor synthesis, factor loss or consumption, factor molecular defects interfering with function, and factor inactivation by inhibitors (e.g., warfarin) or antibodies resulting from certain drugs. Coagulation factor protein deficiencies can be inherited or acquired.

Hemophilia

Hemophilia A results from a molecular defect or absence of the procoagulant portion of factor VIII. It is the most common hereditary coagulation disorder in dogs. A sex-linked autosomal-recessive disorder carried on the X chromosome, the disorder is expressed in only males, although females may be asymptomatic carriers. Factor IX (Christmas factor) deficiency, known as hemophilia B, is also a sex-linked autosomal-recessive disorder with similar clinical symptoms. Hemophilia B is less common than hemophilia A.

Liver Disease

All coagulation factors, with the exception of vWF (produced by endothelial cells), are synthesized in the liver. The liver also clears FSPs and activated coagulation factors from the circulation. Chronic liver disease often is associated with hemostatic alterations in hemorrhagic episodes.

Anticoagulant Rodenticide Intoxication

Anticoagulant rodenticides act as antagonists to vitamin K, which is necessary for producing biologically active coagulation factors II, VII, IX, and X. If the patient is deficient in vitamin K, vitamin K–dependent factors are produced by the liver but cannot function normally. Newer anticoagulant rodenticides (e.g., brodifacoum, diphacinone) have much longer half-lives, necessitating a longer treatment time than does warfarin. Removing the toxic substance is key, but patients may need coagulation factor support in the form of fresh frozen plasma or fresh whole blood transfusion to stop hemorrhage. The body does not contain an excessive store of vitamin K, so oral vitamin K_1 must be administered to allow vitamin

K–dependent factors to function. Duration of vitamin K therapy is determined by the type of anticoagulant rodenticide ingested.

Disseminated Intravascular Coagulation

In certain pathologic situations, the coagulation response may become accelerated and the fibrinolytic system overwhelmed. Clot formation begins to appear not only at the site of endothelial damage but randomly throughout the circulation, creating an imbalance between bleeding, coagulation, and fibrinolysis, called DIC. The condition often manifests as diffuse hemorrhage resulting from the consumption of coagulation factors and platelets. Many stimuli may trigger the coagulation cascade in this way (e.g., sepsis, neoplasia, massive trauma, envenomation).

Therapy for DIC is treatment of the underlying disease or process. Replacing blood components (e.g., packed RBCs, fresh frozen plasma, platelet-rich plasma, cryoprecipitate) may be necessary to maintain blood volume and support hemostatic function in patients that are bleeding actively. Using heparin to treat DIC remains controversial. Heparin is thought to slow or stop coagulation by partnering with antithrombin III, thereby inhibiting critical substances of hemostasis. Heparin, an anticoagulant, can increase bleeding. Careful monitoring is necessary when incorporating this controversial treatment modality.

CLINICAL ASSESSMENT

An accurate history, thorough physical examination, and certain laboratory tests must be performed to evaluate a bleeding patient, determine a diagnosis, and define a therapeutic plan.

History

A complete history is critical in beginning a workup for a hemostatic defect. All pertinent information must be gathered from the owners. Questions should be clear and thought-provoking. Devising a list of questions for owners to review can prompt them to remember important details. Does the animal have any previously diagnosed diseases? Is the animal taking any medication? A list of any prescription or over-the-counter medications should be included because many drugs have a toxic effect on platelets, white blood cells, and red blood cells. The animal's environmental history may suggest potential exposure to toxic substances such as anticoagulant rodenticide poisons or lead. Tick exposure also should be considered.

It is vital to evaluate the current bleeding episode. Characterize the bleed as localized or multifocal. Is this the animal's first bleeding episode, or is there a history of bleeding? These facts may help differentiate between an acquired or hereditary disorder. Specific breeds are susceptible to specific coagulopathies. Any information the owner has about breed history could provide helpful clues. Many breeders are learning more about bleeding disorders affecting their particular breeds and family lines.

Physical Examination

Clinical signs found on physical examination can help determine the origin of the bleeding episode. Small surface bleeds (e.g., petechiation, ecchymosis, epistaxis, hematuria) usually suggest platelet or vascular abnormalities. Larger bleeds or bleeding into body cavities (e.g., hematoma formation, hemarthroses, deep muscle hemorrhage) suggest clotting factor deficiencies. A combination of these clinical signs is not uncommon. Mucous membrane color, CRT, pulse rate and quality, and respiratory rate and effort also lend information about bleed severity and potentially life-threatening complications.

Laboratory Tests

Although information obtained from the history and specific clinical signs may suggest a diagnosis, certain laboratory tests are necessary for definitive diagnosis. Much information can be gathered from a CBC alone. Serial hematocrit determinations can help demonstrate progression or stabilization of bleeding because the body takes a certain amount of time to equilibrate after an acute bleeding episode.

Normal platelet count is 150,000 to 400,000/μl. Abnormal bleeding can occur with platelet counts below 40,000/μl, although patients vary and some animals may not exhibit clinical signs associated with bleeding with a platelet count of 2000/μl. The thrombocytopenic patient needs extra care (e.g., extra cage padding, avoidance of central vessels for blood collection, extended application of pressure to venipuncture sites). In an animal exhibiting signs of surface bleeding with a normal platelet count, consideration should be given to platelet quality. Platelet function is as important as platelet number.

Certain tests are available to monitor coagulation in patients with suspected coagulopathies. Prothrombin time (PT) measures extrinsic and common clotting pathway activity, whereas activated partial thromboplastin time (aPTT) measures intrinsic and common pathway activity. Prolongation of PT and aPTT is seen when clotting factors are depleted below 30% of normal. PT and aPTT samples must be collected and processed carefully to avoid potential sample errors. Atraumatic venipuncture and smooth blood flow into collection tubes are necessary to avoid extraneous clotting mechanism activation. Samples should be processed immediately after collection. Samples often are sent to an outside laboratory, necessitating plasma freezing. Individual factor deficiency determinations are assay specific. The PIVKA (Proteins Induced by Vitamin K Antagonism or Absence) test is a screening test similar to PT but is thought to be more useful in diagnosing anticoagulant rodenticide intoxication.

FSP elevation occurs with excessive bleeding and fibrinolysis and in animals with severe liver dysfunction. Interpreted in conjunction with the PT, aPTT, and platelet count, elevated FSP levels are useful as a diagnostic indicator of DIC.

Practical Hemostatic Tests

The following are simple, in-house tests using no specialized equipment. They are quick, inexpensive, practical tests that allow recognition and characterization of hemostatic defects. These tests often are called cage-side tests because they provide results almost immediately.

Platelet Estimation. A quick, reasonably accurate estimation of platelet numbers can be made from a stained blood smear. After routine preparation and staining, the blood smear is scanned to ensure that platelet distribution is even and that there is no evidence of platelet clumping. The average number of platelets in approximately 5 to 10 oil immersion fields is counted to estimate platelet numbers. The count is ranked as very low, low, normal, or high. One platelet per oil immersion field represents approximately 20,000 platelets. Approximately 8 to 12 platelets per oil immersion field is considered normal.

Although platelet estimation helps detect thrombocytopenia in an emergency, a true platelet count is needed to classify the severity of depletion. Ongoing platelet quantitation is helpful in monitoring the course of a disease or patient response to certain therapies.

Bleeding Time Tests. Bleeding time is the time it takes for bleeding to stop after a vessel is severed. The two bleeding time tests used most often in veterinary medicine today are buccal mucosal bleeding time (BMBT) and cuticle bleeding time (CBT).

The BMBT assesses platelet and vascular contribution to hemostasis, thereby evaluating primary hemostasis (Technical Tip Box 14-1). A disposable template with two spring-loaded blades is used to produce standardized incisions in the buccal mucosal surface of the upper lip. The blades create 5-mm long, 1-mm deep incisions. The duration of bleeding from these incisions is monitored.

The BMBT is a screening test. Like any other screening test, it is not 100% sensitive, so it cannot detect all primary hemostatic defects. This test

Box 14-1 Technical Tip: *Buccal Mucosal Bleeding Time*

Materials

Bleeding time device
Gauze strip
Filter paper or gauze sponges
Timing device

Procedure

1. Place animal in lateral recumbency.
2. Expose mucosal surface of upper lip. Position a gauze strip around the maxilla to fold up the upper lip. Tie the strip gently, just tight enough to partially block venous return.
3. The incision site should be void of surface vessels and slightly inclined so that shed blood from the incision can flow freely toward the mouth. Place bleeding time device flush against mucosal surface, applying as little pressure as possible, and press the tab to release the scalpels.
4. Let stab incisions bleed freely, undisturbed, and time until bleeding stops. Excessive blood should be blotted as often as necessary to prevent blood flow into the patient's mouth. Place filter paper or gauze sponge approximately 3 to 4 mm below the incision, taking care not to disturb the incision site and any clot that is forming.
5. The end point is recorded when the edge of the filter paper or sponge does not soak up free-flowing blood. The bleeding time is the mean bleeding time for the two incisions. Normal bleeding time is less than 4 minutes.

also does not differentiate between vascular defects and platelet function defects. The BMBT is prolonged in cases of thrombocytopenia or thrombocytopathia, vWD, uremia, and aspirin therapy. Obviously, one should not perform this test on any patient that is known to be thrombocytopenic. Although it has limitations, there are several advantages to this test. Commercial bleeding time devices are readily available. The templates are standardized, so results are reproducible. It is a simple and quick test to perform, and the results are available almost immediately. Patients seem to tolerate the procedure well. The incisions produced are well above the concentrated pain fibers in the lip. Some animals are startled by the noise the scalpels make when released from the device, but the procedure itself is not painful.

Box 14-2 Technical Tip: *Cuticle Bleeding Time*

Materials

Guillotine-type nail clipper
Timing device

Procedure

1. Place patient in lateral recumbency.
2. Make a clean transection of the nail, just into the quick, using a guillotine-type toenail clipper.
3. Let the nail bleed freely, undisturbed, and time until bleeding stops. the normal bleeding time is less than 5 minutes in the dog and less than 3 minutes in the cat. If the nail starts to rebleed once it has stopped, the bleeding time is considered abnormal.

The CBT is another bleeding time test (Technical Tip Box 14-2). The CBT is useful for evaluating overall hemostasis. It is sensitive to defects in vascular integrity, platelet function, and coagulation.

A prolongation of this bleeding time is seen with primary or secondary hemostatic defects. The CBT has some limitations. It is even less specific than the BMBT in that it does not differentiate between primary and secondary hemostatic compromise. It is very technique dependent and difficult to standardize, but it can become reproducible with practice. It can be somewhat uncomfortable for the patient because a richly innervated and highly vascular area of the nail is being transected. For this reason, the CBT is best performed on anesthetized patients. It is a good test to use for presurgical assessment of bleeding potential in patients at risk based on their history and physical examination.

Activated Clotting Time. The activated clotting time (ACT) is a simple, inexpensive screening test for severe abnormalities in the intrinsic and common pathways of the clotting pathway (Technical Tip Box 14-3). It evaluates the same pathways as aPTT. Some argue that ACT is less sensitive at detecting factor deficiencies than aPTT in that factors must be decreased to less than 5% of normal to prolong ACT, whereas the aPTT is prolonged with factor deficiency less than 30% normal.

ACT prolongation occurs with severe factor deficiency in the intrinsic or common clotting pathway (e.g., hemophilia), in the presence of inhibitors (e.g., heparin, warfarin), or in cases of severe thrombocytopenia caused by the lack of platelet phospholipid (mild prolongation of 10 to 20 seconds). The ACT is inexpensive, easily learned, quick to perform, and reproducible and provides immediate results. It is a very useful measurement of coagulation in emergencies when compared with aPTT. The possibility of technical and laboratory error must be considered. This is not to suggest that one should rely solely on the ACT; in most situations, the ACT should be followed up with an aPTT.

Box 14-3 Technical Tip: *Activated Clotting Time Test*

Materials

Vacutainer sleeve
Vacutainer single collection needle
ACT tube containing diatomaceous earth
37° C electric heat block (can substitute hot water bath or hold in hand)

Procedure

1. Warm ACT tube in heat block to 37° C for approximately 3 minutes.
2. Perform clean venipuncture on an unthrombosed vessel. Discard the first few drops of blood to eliminate tissue thromboplastin, the tissue factor responsible for activating the extrinsic pathway.
3. Puncture the ACT tube with the distal needle and collect approximately 2 ml blood. Begin timing as soon as blood enters the tube.
4. After collection, invert the tube several times to mix with diatomaceous earth and place in heating block.
5. After 30 seconds from start of timing, gently tilt the tube and examine for clot formation. Return tube to heat block and repeat procedure every 10 seconds.
6. The ACT time is the time from collection of blood in the tube to initial clot formation. In the dog, the normal is 60 to 110 seconds. In the cat, the normal is 50 to 75 seconds.

TREATMENT AND MANAGEMENT

The major indication for platelet transfusion is to stop bleeding in patients with decreased platelet number or function. Platelet preparation is difficult because of the large volume needed to increase platelet numbers measurably in large dogs. In some patients, however, bleeding cessation has been achieved after transfusion without a measurable increase in platelet number. In veterinary medicine it is more practical to treat thrombocytopenia and thrombocytopathia with active bleeding with fresh whole blood, from which the patient receives both platelets and RBC support. In cases of platelet destruction, the survival of transfused platelets is a matter of minutes rather than days. If the patient is bleeding acutely into a vital structure (e.g., brain, myocardium, pleural cavity), platelet transfusion may be warranted. In most instances, however, medical management usually is the treatment of choice.

Coagulation factor replacement is achieved by administering plasma products. The whole blood–derived components include fresh frozen plasma, frozen plasma, and cryoprecipitate. Before receiving transfusion support, patients must be evaluated to determine whether they need multiple coagulation factor replacement (e.g., DIC, liver disease) or just an isolated component (e.g., hemophilia, VWD).

CONCLUSION

Hematologic emergencies are common in small animals. The veterinary technician must understand the various disorders that can occur.

Many tests can be performed quickly to determine PCV, clotting time, bleeding time, and other values. The samples for clinical laboratory tests must be drawn immediately before therapy is instituted. These tests provide very important information and assist in determining the type and severity of the disorder. The technician must understand the function of these tests and perform them correctly. Samples must be collected with care.

Continual monitoring is essential. The veterinary technician plays a vital role in ensuring a successful outcome.

BIBLIOGRAPHY

Kirby R, Crowe DT, eds: *The Veterinary Clinics of North America, small animal practice: Emergency medicine.* Philadelphia, 1994, WB Saunders.

Kristensen AT, Feldman BF, eds: *The Veterinary Clinics of North America, small animal practice: Canine and feline transfusion medicine.* Philadelphia, 1995, WB Saunders.

Murtaugh RJ, Kaplan PM, eds: *Veterinary emergency and critical care medicine.* St Louis, 1992, Mosby-YearBook.

Willard MD, Tvedten H, Turnwald GH, eds: *Small animal clinical diagnosis by laboratory methods* (2nd ed). Philadelphia, 1994, WB Saunders.

TABLE 15-3 Common Presenting Signs in Cardiac Emergencies

Sudden death
Cyanosis
Dyspnea
Collapse
Hind limb paresis
Syncope
Tachypnea
Exercise intolerance
Cough
Abdominal distention (ascites)

Vasoconstriction improves blood pressure, but it also tends to increase afterload and reduce cardiac output. Animals with poor myocardial function are very sensitive to changes in afterload; a small change in afterload can lead to a much greater change in cardiac output.

CONTRACTILITY

Contractility is a change in stroke volume that is independent of changes in preload or afterload. Increases in contractility occur when the amount of calcium in the cells of the heart muscle is increased by chemicals produced by the body, such as epinephrine, or by drugs such as digoxin or dobutamine. Contractility is more difficult to evaluate than the other determinants of systolic function, but if preload and afterload remain constant, changes in cardiac output and shortening fraction can be used to assess changes in contractility.

HEART RATE AND RHYTHM

Preload, afterload, and contractility determine stroke volume. The last determinant of systolic function is heart rate. Abnormal heart rhythms can alter the normal sequence and duration of atrial and ventricular contraction (dyssynergy). Changes in heart rate have much more of an effect on the duration of diastole than on the duration of systole. Increases in heart rate usually increase cardiac output. Very fast heart rates can reduce cardiac output by not allowing the ventricle to fill adequately during diastole. Bradycardia also reduces cardiac output. The heart normally maintains adequate cardiac output as the heart rate slows by taking advantage of the increase in preload caused by the extra time the ventricle has to fill in diastole. At some point, however, the heart cannot accept enough blood and cardiac output decreases.

DIASTOLIC FUNCTION

During diastole the ventricle relaxes and fills with blood. Diseases that cause systolic dysfunction often interfere with relaxation and filling, but heart failure caused by diastolic dysfunction can occur even when systolic function is normal. Diastolic dysfunction probably leads to heart failure in many of the cardiac diseases that affect cats, such as hypertrophic cardiomyopathy, hyperthyroidism, and restrictive cardiomyopathy. These diseases can cause the ventricle to become so noncompliant that the filling pressure needed to produce a normal end-diastolic volume may be high enough to cause signs of congestive failure.

HEART FAILURE

The result of many types of heart disease is heart failure. Heart failure can be defined as the inability of the heart to supply adequate blood flow to meet the metabolic needs of the body or to provide adequate blood flow only with excessive increases in ventricular filling pressure. This definition allows heart failure to exist in three forms: forward or low-output failure when perfusion is inadequate, congestive heart failure when filling pressures are excessive, or a combination of forward and congestive failure. Heart failure takes different forms and varies in severity. Commonly used scales for classifying the severity of heart failure, such as the New York Heart Association classification (NYHA), often are based on the level of activity that produces signs of failure. Animals with mild failure can tolerate some exercise without showing signs of failure, and severely affected animals show signs of failure while at rest. Because most pets do not exercise vigorously, many owners do not recognize heart failure until it affects everyday activities (Table 15-4).

Low-Output or Forward Failure

Low-output failure occurs when the heart cannot pump enough oxygenated blood to the tissues. Severe low-output failure, especially when accompanied by hypotension, is called cardiogenic shock. A healthy 30-kg dog has a cardiac output of about 4 L/min at rest, with each liter of blood containing 200 ml oxygen. Twenty-five percent of the oxygen in the blood is consumed by the dog's tissues. If heart disease forces the dog's cardiac output to drop, the volume of oxygen delivered to the tissues will also drop. Because oxygen consumption has not changed, the body must somehow compensate if normal function is to be maintained. If the change in cardiac output is not too severe, the body can compensate by extracting more oxygen from the blood. The limit to this form of compensation usually is reached when cardiac output drops below 2 L/min. Oxygen delivery has now been cut in half and 50% of the oxygen in the blood is consumed by the tissues. When blood flow drops below this limit, cardiac output may not be adequate to meet the metabolic needs of the body, resulting in inadequate oxygen delivery and low-output failure. Exercise increases the body's demand for oxygen. If the heart cannot pump enough blood to supply the increased demand, the animal's ability to exercise is reduced.

Congestive or Backward Failure

Congestive heart failure occurs when increased pulmonary or systemic venous and capillary pressures cause fluid to leak from the capillary beds and accumulate in tissue (edema) or in body cavities (effusions). Congestive heart failure generally is categorized as right or left heart failure according to whether systemic or pulmonary venous pressure is increased by heart disease. Normally the pressure in the venous system is low, about 0 mm Hg in the right atrium and about 2 mm Hg in the left atrium. Right heart failure usually is evident when right atrial pressure reaches 10 mm Hg and left generally occurs when left atrial pressure exceeds 20 mm Hg.

Table 15-4 New York Heart Association Classification

Class I	Signs of heart disease but no signs of failure
Class II	Signs of heart disease and signs of failure with vigorous activity
Class III	Signs of heart disease and signs of failure with minimal activity
Class IV	Signs of heart disease and signs of failure at rest

When a disease increases venous pressure equally on both sides of the heart, as in pericardial effusion, right heart failure develops first. This is because signs of congestive failure occur at lower pressure on the right side. Left heart failure develops more quickly than right heart failure. This is because the systemic veins can hold much more blood than the pulmonary veins.

The Relationship Between Hemodynamic Measurements and Clinical Signs of Heart Failure

Cardiac output and right atrial or left atrial pressure indicate whether heart function is adequate or whether heart failure exists. Patients who are not in failure should have a cardiac output that is greater than 2 $L/min/m^2$ and right and left atrial pressures less than 5 and 12 mm Hg, respectively. Forward failure would exist if the patient's cardiac output was less than 2 $L/min/m^2$ at rest. Congestive failure should be present if the right atrial pressure exceeds 10 mm Hg or the left atrial pressure exceeds about 20 mm Hg. A patient with both forward and congestive failure would be expected to have a cardiac output of less than 2 $L/min/m^2$ at rest and right and left atrial pressures greater than 10 or 20 mm Hg, respectively. Patients with arteriovenous fistulae or hyperthyroidism may have congestive heart failure and higher than normal cardiac output at rest. This type of heart failure is known as high-output failure. It is rarely necessary (or possible, in most practices) to measure cardiac output or left atrial pressure to diagnose heart failure. The physical examination, chest radiographs, and echocardiography generally

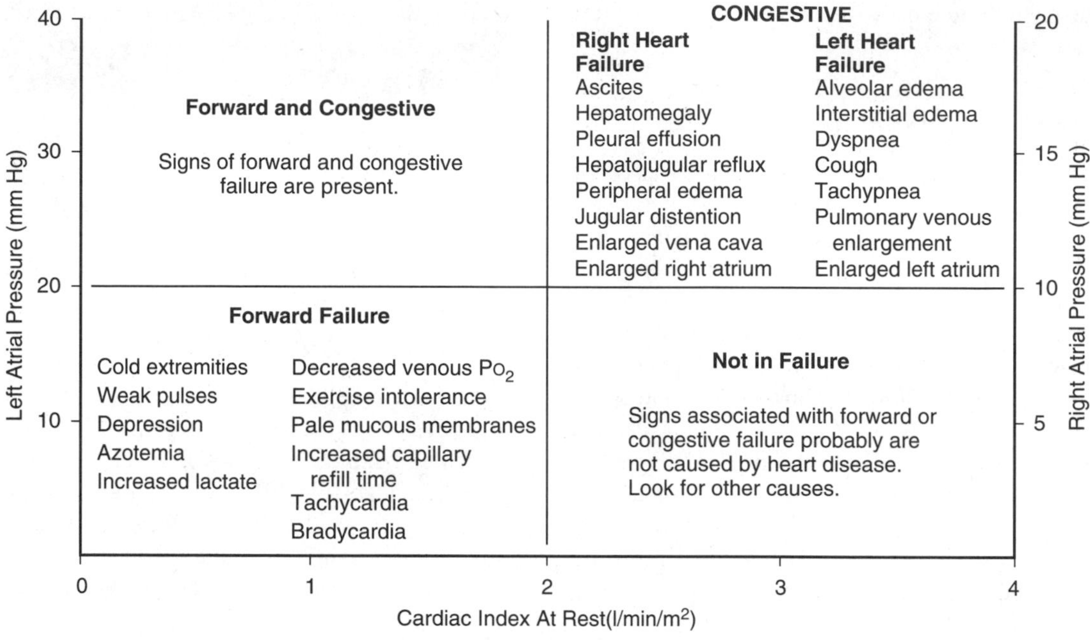

Figure 15-1

Relationship between hemodynamic data and clinical signs of heart failure.

provide enough information to make an accurate diagnosis of the type of heart failure and its cause. Figure 15-1 shows the relationship between signs of heart failure and hemodynamic measurements.

IDENTIFYING PATIENTS WHO MAY HAVE HEART FAILURE

CLIENT COMPLAINTS

In emergency practice, dyspnea, tachypnea, syncope, weakness, and collapse are the most common complaints associated with heart failure. Heart failure should be considered when a client seeks help for a pet with a cough (coughing is much more common in dogs with heart disease than in cats), weight loss, exercise intolerance, or abdominal distention.

PHYSICAL FINDINGS

Systolic murmurs with an intensity of 3 on a scale of 1 to 6, precordial thrills, diastolic murmurs, and diastolic gallop sounds generally are reliable signs of heart disease. The arterial pulse tends to be weak or normal in most types of heart disease, but animals with patent ductus arteriosus or aortic insufficiency may have a prominent pulse. Irregular pulses, pulse deficits, and changes in the quality of the heart sounds may be present in animals with cardiac arrhythmias. Animals with left heart failure show signs of dyspnea, tachypnea, exercise intolerance, cyanosis, and weakness. Animals with right heart failure show signs of venous distention, hepatomegaly, ascites, weakness, and weight loss. Patients with biventricular failure often develop pleural effusion in addition to signs of both right- and left-sided failure. Table 15-5 lists diseases that can cause heart failure. The diseases are listed in decreasing order of prevalence.

EMERGENCY TREATMENT OF CONGESTIVE HEART FAILURE

Pulmonary edema, pleural effusion, and severe ascites are the most common emergencies caused by congestive heart failure. Patients with pleural

TABLE 15-5 Common Causes of Heart Failure

Left heart failure in dogs
- Chronic degenerative valvular disease (mitral regurgitation)
- Dilated cardiomyopathy
- Patent ductus arteriosus
- Infective endocarditis
- Subaortic stenosis (usually with concomitant mitral dysplasia)

Right heart failure in dogs
- Pericardial disease
- Tricuspid regurgitation
- Pulmonic stenosis (usually with concomitant tricuspid dysplasia)
- Heartworm disease (heartworm disease may be the most common cause of right heart failure in areas with high infection rates)

Generalized (biventricular) heart failure in dogs
- Dilated cardiomyopathy
- Some dogs with severe left heart failure

Heart failure in cats
- Hypertrophic cardiomyopathy
- Restrictive cardiomyopathy
- Dilated cardiomyopathy
- Cardiomyopathy secondary to hyperthyroidism

effusion or ascites can be treated very effectively for the short term by simply removing fluid from the thorax or the abdomen. Care should be taken to avoid stress in patients with hypoxia or dyspnea caused by their effusions. These effusions will return unless proper medical treatment is started to reduce venous pressure. Pulmonary edema is more difficult to treat. Treatment consists of several different therapies that reduce pulmonary venous pressure while providing adequate oxygen delivery. Oxygen therapy maximizes the oxygen content of arterial blood, which provides some increase in oxygen delivery. Avoiding physical restraint, providing a calm, quiet environment, and using sedatives when needed minimizes oxygen consumption and reduces the work of the heart. Furosemide and venodilating drugs decrease pulmonary venous pressure by eliminating fluid from the body and dilating capacitance vessels (large veins). Arterial dilators reduce the regurgitant fraction in patients with mitral regurgitation and improve cardiac output by decreasing afterload. Positive inotropic drugs improve contractility and cardiac output in patients that have low-output failure in addition to congestive failure. When the simpler therapies already mentioned have failed, other options are available if the client has the desire and financial resources and if the necessary facilities exist. Positive-pressure ventilation can eliminate the work of breathing and improve oxygenation. Pulmonary artery catheterization can be used to measure cardiac output, pulmonary artery wedge pressure (PAWP), and central venous blood gases. Arterial catheterization can be used to measure blood pressure and arterial blood gases. This type of intensive monitoring can be used to identify the cause of treatment failure and to allow treatment to be targeted at the problem. Table 15-6 lists the goals of therapy for pulmonary edema and the therapies used to achieve them.

DIURETIC THERAPY

Water and salt retention is an important compensatory mechanism in heart failure. Diuretics are drugs that act on the kidneys to promote water and salt elimination. Furosemide is a potent diuretic that can be used to eliminate fluid from the body quickly. Furosemide's ability to decrease pulmonary venous pressure rapidly makes it one of the most effective emergency treatments for life-threatening pulmonary edema caused by congestive heart failure. Overzealous furosemide administration can cause dehydration, decreased cardiac output, azotemia, and electrolyte abnormalities.

OXYGEN THERAPY

Congestive heart failure often causes hypoxia and hypoventilation through hydrothorax and pulmonary edema. Oxygen therapy can improve oxygenation and reduce the work of breathing. It is extremely important to remember that oxygen therapy may cause only a small increase in the oxygen content of the blood. Oxygen therapy can lead to death if the method of administering oxygen increases patient stress or causes the patient to struggle. Many oxygen administration methods are

TABLE 15-6 Goals in Emergency Heart Failure Treatment

Goal	Therapy
Reduce oxygen consumption, minimize stress.	Avoid physical restraint, provide calm, quiet environment, use sedatives.
Increase oxygen content of blood.	Provide oxygen therapy.
Decrease venous pressure.	Administer furosemide, nitroglycerine paste.
Decrease regurgitant fraction, decrease afterload.	Administer arterial dilator.
Improve contractility and cardiac output.	Use positive inotropic drugs.
Eliminate the work of breathing, improve oxygenation.	Provide positive-pressure ventilation.
Improve the ability to identify problems and target therapy.	Perform hemodynamic monitoring, arterial and central venous blood gas monitoring.

available; if one method does not work, another can be tried. The success of therapy is measured by improved patient comfort and oxygenation, not by whether the patient has been forced to breathe increased concentrations of oxygen.

Almost every practice has the equipment needed to administer oxygen by face mask. A tight-fitting face mask with adequate oxygen flow can deliver 100% oxygen. Unfortunately, face masks are poorly accepted by most patients, and face masks cannot be used for long periods of time. Nasal insufflation can be used to deliver high concentrations of oxygen for long periods of time. Use the following technique to insert the catheter. Make a mark on a soft, flexible catheter to indicate the distance from the tip of the nose to the medial canthus of the eye. Instil a small amount of lidocaine solution in one nostril, apply some lubricant to the catheter, and insert it into the nostril, stopping when the mark is reached. Suture the catheter to the skin to keep it in place.

Use the following rule to determine the flow of oxygen. Every 50 ml/kg/min oxygen flow increases the inspired oxygen concentration by 7% above the normal value of 21%. For example, an oxygen flow of 1.5 L/min administered to a 10-kg patient should provide an inspired concentration of 42%. It is important to humidify the oxygen when using a nasal catheter. The gas in an oxygen cylinder contains almost no moisture and can cause severe drying of the mucous membranes in the upper respiratory tract. Oxygen cages are well tolerated by most patients, but they require high oxygen flows and do not allow hands-on monitoring of the patient. Oxygen cages should be designed to remove exhaled CO_2 and cool the cage.

VASODILATOR THERAPY

Vasodilating drugs are effective in treating both congestive and low-output heart failure. Venodilating drugs expand the capacity of the circulatory system by dilating veins, which reduces preload and venous pressure. Venodilation can reduce congestion but will not improve cardiac output. Arterial vasodilators decrease systemic vascular resistance, which reduces afterload, improves cardiac output, reduces the regurgitant fraction in animals with valvular disease, and decreases the work of the heart. The main disadvantage of arterial vasodilators is that they lower blood pressure. It is possible to select a vasodilator that acts on veins, arterioles, or a combination of the two. Drugs that block the enzyme that converts angiotensin I to angiotensin II (angiotensin-converting enzyme inhibitors) are the most commonly used vasodilators. They also benefit the patient by decreasing the sodium and water retention seen in heart failure by decreasing the plasma concentration of aldosterone. However, these drugs do not take effect quickly enough to be useful in emergency heart failure treatment.

POSITIVE INOTROPIC THERAPY

Positive inotropic drugs increase stroke volume by increasing contractility. With the exception of

TABLE 15-7 Drugs Used to Treat Heart Failure

Drug	Dosage
Drugs used to minimize stress	
Morphine	0.5 mg/kg SQ or IM for dogs
Oxymorphone	0.05 mg/kg SQ or IM for dogs and cats
Acepromazine	0.03 mg/kg SQ or IM for dogs and cats
Drugs used to decrease venous pressure or preload	
Furosemide	2-8 mg/kg IM, IV, or SQ for dogs A dosage of 4-8 mg/kg q 1-4 hr is used for fulminant pulmonary edema and 2-4 mg/kg q 8-12 hr for maintenance 2-4 mg/kg IM, IV, or SQ for cats
Nitroglycerin	4-15 mg topically for dogs 3-4 mg topically for cats
Drugs used to decrease afterload	
Hydralazine	0.5-3 mg/kg q 12 hr PO for dogs
Sodium nitroprusside	0.5-10 µg/kg/min IV for dogs
Drugs used to increase contractility	
Dobutamine	2-20 µg/kg/min IV for dogs
Dopamine	2-10 µg/kg/min IV for dogs
Amrinone	1-3 mg/kg IV followed by 10-100 µg/kg/min IV for dogs

drugs such as digoxin, positive inotropes are most useful for improving cardiac output or blood pressure for short periods of time. Sympathomimetic drugs such as dopamine and dobutamine lose their effectiveness over time because their use causes a decrease in the number of receptors. In addition, positive inotropes can cause tachycardia, cause arrhythmias, increase afterload, and increase the work of the heart.

SYMPATHOMIMETIC DRUGS

Sympathomimetic drugs mimic the effect of stimulating the sympathetic nervous system and work by stimulating adrenergic receptors on the cells of the heart and blood vessels. Dopamine and dobutamine are the sympathomimetic drugs used most often to treat heart failure. Dobutamine increases contractility without causing a significant increase in heart rate or vascular resistance. This combination of properties makes dobutamine a good choice for treating heart failure in patients with myocardial failure or mitral regurgitation. Dopamine is useful when poor contractility is associated with hypotension.

BIPYRIDINE DERIVATIVES

Amrinone and milrinone are positive inotropic drugs that work by inhibiting phophodiesterase. Both amrinone and milrinone cause vasodilation in addition to increased contractility, and both can be used when sympathomimetic drugs such as dopamine and dobutamine are no longer effective. These drugs are rarely used in veterinary medicine because they are expensive and most of their effects can be achieved with other drugs. Table 15-7 lists drugs used to treat heart failure.

MONITORING THERAPY FOR HEART FAILURE

Animals with dyspnea caused by heart failure appear anxious and often are unwilling to sit or lay down. Affected animals often assume a characteristic posture, with the feet spread apart, elbows abducted, and the head and neck extended. Tachypnea usually is present, with respiratory rates often greater than 60 breaths per minute. If therapy has been effective in treating pleural effusion or pulmonary edema, the patient's attitude should improve, the respiratory rate should decrease, mucous membrane color should improve if the patient was cyanotic, and the animal may be able to lie down or sleep. Improvement of pulmonary edema on chest radiographs usually takes longer than improvement of clinical signs.

Monitoring Vasodilator Therapy

Vasodilator therapy should improve cardiac output or pulmonary edema. Improved cardiac output can be monitored by looking for signs of increased perfusion, such as warming of the extremities, increased venous oxygen tension, and a decreased blood lactate. Blood pressure should be measured whenever arteriolar vasodilating drugs are used to maintain mean blood pressure around 70 mm Hg. Venodilating drugs reduce venous pressure and should therefore decrease CVP and PAWP.

Monitoring Positive Inotropic Therapy

Positive inotropic therapy should improve cardiac output. This is most commonly monitored by looking for signs of improved cardiac output. Decreases in blood lactate, increased venous oxygen tension, or measured cardiac output provide a more objective assessment of therapy. In addition to increasing contractility, positive inotropic agents can cause vasoconstriction, vasodilation, increased heart rate, or cardiac arrhythmias. Vasoconstriction generally causes an increase in CVP, PAWP, and arterial blood pressure (ABP). Vasodilation may cause a decrease in CVP, PAWP, or ABP depending on the increase in cardiac output. The electrocardiogram (ECG) is helpful in detecting cardiac arrhythmias or sinus tachycardia. Safe, effective use of sympathomimetic drugs requires monitoring of at least the ECG and blood pressure and assessing perfusion.

Monitoring Diuretic Therapy

Diuretic therapy should quickly produce an increase in urine production when furosemide is used. This elimination of fluid should result in a decreased respiratory rate and improved oxygenation and ventilation. Weighing the patient and palpating the urinary bladder to determine its size may be useful for establishing a baseline before diuretic therapy is started. The loss of volume can be estimated by measuring the volume of urine, measuring the increase in weight caused by urine soaked up in a disposable diaper, or noting patient's weight loss during treatment. Electrolyte and acid-base disturbances can be caused by diuretic therapy, so these values should be monitored. The loss of preload can cause a decrease in cardiac output. This can result in prerenal azotemia or signs of low-output failure.

CARDIAC ARRHYTHMIAS

Client Complaints

Cardiac arrhythmias should be considered whenever an animal experiences syncope, weakness, or collapse. Cardiac arrhythmias should not be considered a primary disease. Instead, cardiac arrhythmias occur as a result of some other disease that affects the heart. Table 15-8 lists several diseases that are common in emergency medicine and have a high incidence of cardiac arrhythmias.

Signs of Cardiac Arrhythmias

An ECG should be recorded to determine whether a cardiac arrhythmia is present whenever changes in the character of heart sounds, tachycardia,

Table 15-8 Emergencies in Which Cardiac Arrhythmias Are Common
Trauma
Splenic tumors
Gastric dilation volvulus
Canine dilated cardiomyopathy
Urethral obstruction in cats
Heat-induced illness
Feline cardiomyopathies

bradycardia, irregular heart rhythm, pulse deficits, or changes in arterial or jugular pulse are present.

Medical Treatment of Cardiac Arrhythmias

The efficacy of antiarrhythmic therapy has not been determined in most forms of heart disease found in dogs and cats. In humans the use of certain antiarrhythmic drugs was found to decrease survival in patients with certain forms of heart disease. Consider the following principles before deciding whether to use antiarrhythmic drugs to treat an arrhythmia.

- Treating the primary disease may eliminate the arrhythmia.
- Arrhythmias that cause hypotension or poor perfusion should be treated.
- Prolonged tachycardia can damage the heart even when blood pressure and cardiac output are adequate.
- The arrhythmia should be treated if it has the potential to progress to a more severe arrhythmia or cardiac arrest. Multiform ventricular premature contractions (VPCs), R on T phenomenon, more than 20 VPCs per minute, ventricular flutter, and ventricular tachycardia greater than 130 per minute generally are considered to have the potential to become more dangerous.
- When the decision is made to treat an arrhythmia, it is important to select an antiarrhythmic drug based on its ability to eliminate the arrhythmia balanced against the risk of proarrhythmic effects, hypotension, decreased contractility, altered atrioventricular conduction, and interactions with other drugs.

Ventricular Fibrillation Treatment

The use of a electrical defibrillator is the only effective method of treating ventricular fibrillation. Successful treatment of ventricular fibrillation depends on diagnosing and treating the patient as soon as possible after ventricular fibrillation occurs. Current recommendations for treating ventricular fibrillation in humans are to attempt to defibrillate as soon as a diagnosis of ventricular fibrillation is made using 200 J. If this is unsuccessful, two more attempts should be made using 200 to 360 J. The first three attempts should be made without interrupting to perform cardiopulmonary resuscitation (CPR). If the first three attempts are unsuccessful, three more attempts should be made after 1 minute of CPR. This pattern is continued until the patient is no longer in ventricular fibrillation. This method of treating ventricular fibrillation can be used in dogs if the electrical dosage is modified to take into account the smaller body size. The initial dosage, for electrodes placed externally on the chest wall, should be 2 to 3 J/kg, with subsequent attempts made at 2 to 5 J/kg. For electrodes placed directly on the heart, the initial dosage should be 0.2 J/kg, with subsequent attempts made at 0.2 to 0.5 J/kg. The use of excessive electrical dosages for defibrillation can result in death or damage to the heart.

Ventricular Tachycardia Treatment

Lidocaine, procainamide, and quinidine are the drugs used most often in the emergency treatment of ventricular arrhythmias in the dog. Lidocaine and β-blockers such as propranolol or esmolol are the drugs used most often to treat cats. Lidocaine generally is considered the drug of choice for treating ventricular tachycardia in the dog. Lidocaine has very little effect on myocardial function. Blood pressure and cardiac output usually are unaffected when lidocaine is used. Adverse reactions such as depression or twitching are treated by discontinuing the drug, and convulsions are treated by discontinuing the drug and giving diazepam. Rapid intravenous administration of quinidine, and to a lesser extent procainamide, can cause dangerous hypotension and decreased cardiac output. β-Blocking drugs can exacerbate heart failure and cause bradycardia and bronchospasm. Esmolol has an extremely short duration of action, and any adverse reaction caused by the drug should stop soon after the drug is

TABLE 15-9 Drugs Used to Treat Ventricular Arrhythmias

Lidocaine	2-4 mg/kg IV over 1-3 min followed by 40-100 μg/kg/min IV for dogs
	0.5 mg/kg IV slowly for cats
Procainamide	5-15 mg/kg IV q 6 hr for dogs
Quinidine	5-15 mg/kg IM q6-8 hr for dogs
Propranolol	0.01-0.1 mg/kg IV slowly titrated to effect in dogs
	0.04 mg/kg IV slowly for cats

TABLE 15-10 Drugs Used to Treat Supraventricular Arrhythmias

Propranolol	0.01-0.1 mg/kg IV slowly titrated to effect in dogs
	0.04 mg/kg IV slowly in cats
Esmolol	0.25-0.5 mg/kg IV, 50-200 μg/kg/min IV in dogs
Verapamil	0.05-0.15 mg/kg IV titrated to effect over 15-30 min in dogs
Diltiazem	0.05-0.25 mg/kg IV titrated to effect in dogs

discontinued. Ventricular tachycardia that causes cardiac arrest should be treated like ventricular fibrillation (Table 15-9).

Atrial Fibrillation Treatment

Reestablishing normal sinus rhythm in patients with long-standing atrial fibrillation, particularly atrial fibrillation coexisting with other forms of heart disease, usually is impossible. Most often therapy consists of using digoxin and a β-blocker to slow the ventricular rate and improve cardiac function. Animals that have recently developed atrial fibrillation and do not have significant heart disease are the best candidates for conversion to normal sinus rhythm. The use of quinidine is the most common form of antiarrhythmic therapy used, but direct current cardioversion has also been used successfully.

Supraventricular Tachycardia Treatment

β-Blocking drugs, such as esmolol and propranolol, or calcium channel–blocking drugs, such as verapamil and diltiazem, are commonly used to treat supraventricular tachyarrhythmias. Mechanical methods such as the precordial thump often are effective, and vagal maneuvers such as ocular pressure and carotid sinus massage sometimes are effective. A precordial thump is administered by striking the chest wall over the heart with the side of the fist. Precordial thumps can injure a patient or cause ventricular fibrillation if the thump occurs during the vulnerable period on the ECG (R on T phenomenon; Table 15-10).

Bradyarrhythmia Treatment

Sinus bradycardia, sinus arrest, and second-degree atrioventricular block often respond to treatment with anticholinergic drugs such as atropine or glycopyrrolate. Anticholinergic drugs usually are not effective in treating third-degree atrioventricular block, but sympathomimetic drugs such as isoproterenol or dopamine often can be used to increase the ventricular rate to an acceptable level. Drug therapy is ineffective in treating the bradycardia associated with sick sinus syndrome. Pacemaker implantation is the best long-term therapy for most patients with bradyarrhythmias (Table 15-11).

Hyperkalemia Treatment

Hyperkalemia can be treated by giving drugs that cause potassium to move from the vascular space to the intracellular space, such as bicarbonate or insulin, or by giving calcium, which antagonizes the effect of potassium on the heart. Definitive treatment for hyperkalemia should be started as soon as possible because the effect of calcium, bicarbonate, or insulin therapy is short lived. Glucose is given when insulin is used to treat hyperkalemia to prevent hypoglycemia (Table 15-12).

TABLE 15-11 Drugs Used to Treat Bradyarrhythmias

Atropine	0.01-0.04 mg/kg IV, IM, or SQ for dogs and cats
Glycopyrrolate	0.005-0.01 mg/kg IV, IM, or SQ for dogs and cats
Isoproterenol	0.01-0.1 μg/kg min IV for dogs
Dopamine	2.5-10 μg/kg/min IV for dogs

TABLE 15-12 Drugs Used to Treat Hyperkalemia

Calcium gluconate 10%	0.5-1 ml/kg given over 15 min for dogs and cats
Sodium bicarbonate	0.5-2 mEq/kg IV given over 20 min for dogs and cats
Regular insulin	0.1-0.25 U/kg IV immediately followed by 1-2 g/U glucose to prevent hypoglycemia for dogs and cats

MONITORING CARDIAC ARRHYTHMIA TREATMENT

Continuous ECG monitoring increases the safety and effectiveness of antiarrhythmic therapy. Arterial blood pressure and clinical signs of perfusion should be monitored to determine whether antiarrhythmic therapy has improved cardiac function. Changes in the P-R interval, QRS duration, and Q-T interval on the ECG may be important signs of toxicity for some antiarrhythmic drugs. Vomiting, twitching, convulsions, and syncope are a few physical signs that can be associated with toxicity from antiarrhythmic drugs.

PACEMAKER THERAPY

Anticholinergic or sympathomimetic drugs, such as atropine or isoproterenol, are not always effective in treating bradyarrhythmias. Temporary pacing, which can be accomplished without anesthesia, is a safe and effective method for treating bradyarrhythmias. The equipment needed to insert a temporary pacemaker consists of a pacing generator, a pacing lead, and a percutaneous introducer sheath or a catheter designed for inserting a pacing lead. The pacing lead generally is inserted into the right jugular vein and advanced into the cranial vena cava, through the right atrium and the tricuspid valve and into the right ventricular chamber near the apex using a fluoroscope to determine the location of the lead. If a fluoroscope is not available, the location of the lead can be determined using the ECG. Once the pacing lead is in place, the length of catheter inserted into the jugular vein and the rate, sensitivity, and settings of the pacing generator should be noted.

CAVAL SYNDROME

Caval syndrome is complication of heartworm disease that can occur in both dogs and cats. Caval syndrome occurs when large numbers of heartworms enter the right atrium and entwine themselves in the tricuspid valve apparatus, causing acute and severe tricuspid regurgitation. The heart is not the only organ affected. Hemolysis occurs when red blood cells shear as they are forced through the entangled worms. This results in hemoglobinuria. Analysis of the CBC and serum chemistry in dogs with caval syndrome may indicate liver and renal dysfunction and signs of disseminated intravascular coagulation.

CLIENT COMPLAINTS

Owners of dogs with caval syndrome typically notice anorexia, weakness, and depression. Some owners may complain that the animal has hemoglobinuria (dark brown urine), dyspnea, or cough. Many animals with caval syndrome present in a state of shock.

Physical Findings

Pale mucous membranes, prolonged capillary refill time, weak pulses, distended jugular veins, ascites, icterus, and dyspnea may be identified on physical examination. Chest auscultation may reveal a systolic murmur, split second heart sound, or gallop sound.

Surgical Treatment of Caval Syndrome

The presence of heartworms in the right atrium and vena cava is associated with high mortality. Patients with caval syndrome often present in shock and must be stabilized before heartworm removal is attempted. Fluid therapy usually is needed to improve poor perfusion, but care must be taken to avoid exacerbating preexisting right heart failure. The anesthetic protocol selected should minimize further depression of the cardiovascular system. In many animals the procedure can be performed with local anesthesia. For general anesthesia, the lowest possible concentration of inhalational anesthetic should be used; 100% oxygen and positive-pressure ventilation can be used to improve oxygenation and eliminate hypercapnea. The procedure usually is performed with the patient in lateral or dorsal recumbency. After the surgical site is prepared, an incision is made over the jugular vein. The jugular vein is then freed from the surrounding tissue. An incision is made in the jugular vein, and alligator forceps are inserted and passed into the heart. Worms are grasped gently and removed. This technique allows one or more worms to be removed at a time from the right atrium and vena cava. Two-dimensional echocardiography can be used to visualize the heartworms and direct the forceps.

Monitoring

Even with treatment, mortality is high in caval syndrome. CVP monitoring is useful for managing fluid therapy and assessing the prognosis. A CVP of 20 cm H_2O or higher is associated with a poor prognosis. Arterial blood pressure, mucous membrane color, capillary refill time, extremity temperature, and urine production should be monitored to evaluate perfusion.

CARDIAC TAMPONADE AND PERICARDIAL EFFUSION

Fluid can accumulate in the pericardial sac for many reasons. Neoplasia and pericarditis are the most common causes of pericardial effusion and generally produce signs of right heart failure caused by chronic pericardial effusion. Trauma, atrial tears, and some cases of right atrial hemangiosarcoma are the most common causes of acute cardiac tamponade. When fluid accumulates slowly in the heart, the pericardium stretches and the heart has time to compensate for the increased pressure on the heart. Effusions that develop slowly tend to produce large volumes of pericardial fluid and cause signs of right heart failure. When fluid accumulates quickly, there is no time for compensation to occur, and even a small volume of fluid in the pericardial sac can cause signs of shock. Echocardiographic examination of the heart is very sensitive in detecting even small amounts of pericardial fluid.

Client Complaints

Lethargy, dyspnea, anorexia, and collapse are the most common reasons for owners to seek help for dogs with acute signs of pericardial effusion. Abdominal distention, lethargy, anorexia, and cough are common client complaints for dogs with chronic signs of pericardial effusion. Sudden death, collapse, or a history of trauma may cause clients to seek help for an animal with cardiac tamponade.

Clinical Signs

Ascites, jugular venous distention, cachexia, tachycardia, and weak pulses are common findings. Auscultation may reveal muffled heart sounds, murmurs, or friction rubs. Signs of shock accompanied by signs of increased systemic venous pressure should raise suspicion of cardiac tamponade.

Treatment of Cardiac Tamponade and Pericardial Effusion

Pericardiocentesis rapidly relieves the signs caused by increased pressure in the pericardium. The patient should be prepared by shaving the hair on the right side of the chest over the region of the heart. After scrubbing the shaved area, local anesthetic is infiltrated into the tissues between the fourth and fifth intercostal spaces at the level of the costochondral junction. Ultrasound imaging can be used to determine the best location. A 16-gauge over-the-needle catheter is recommended for the typical patient, usually a large breed dog. Most clinicians cut several side holes in the catheter before insertion. The catheter is inserted through the chest wall and into the thoracic cavity. It may be possible to feel the catheter contact the pericardium as the catheter is advanced. Once the catheter has entered the pericardium, fluid flashes into the stylet, and the catheter can be advanced over the needle. The ECG should be monitored during the procedure to help determine whether the needle has contacted the myocardium. Contact with the myocardium is indicated by ventricular premature beats. A small sample of the fluid can be taken to see whether it will clot and to check the hematocrit. As the pericardial fluid is removed, the heart rate may decrease and the ECG may show increased amplitude.

Monitoring

Most animals improve rapidly after the fluid is removed from the pericardium. If the patient does not improve or worsens, there may be active bleeding in the case of cardiac tamponade or a complication of pericardiocentesis, such as laceration of a coronary artery, but these complications are rare. CVP monitoring may help with the initial diagnosis of cardiac tamponade or pericardial effusion. Blood pressure should be monitored if cardiac tamponade is suspected.

FELINE AORTIC THROMBOEMBOLISM

Feline aortic thromboembolism is a devastating complication of myocardial disease. Thrombi develop in the heart, usually in the left atrium, and then travel into the systemic arteries. These thromboemboli usually lodge in the distal aorta, where they often cause posterior paresis, paralysis, and pain. Mortality is very high in aortic thromboembolism, with 63% of the patients being euthanized or dying during the initial episode. Animals that survive sometimes lose skin, toes, or even a leg to ischemic necrosis.

Client Complaints

Most owners seek help for their cats because of acute paralysis and pain. Few owners are aware of preexisting heart disease.

Clinical Signs

In addition to paralysis and pain, the rear legs are cold and pale or cyanotic. The femoral pulses are nonexistent or very weak. There may be a heart murmur, gallop sound, or irregular heart rhythm. Some cats may show signs of dyspnea or tachypnea.

Treatment

Patients should be handled carefully because many have severe underlying heart disease. In one study, 66% of the animals had radiographic signs of congestive heart failure. Treating pleural effusion and pulmonary edema may be as urgent as treating the aortic embolus. Three forms of treatment are available: supportive, surgical, and thrombolytic. In supportive treatment the patient is treated for pain and given heparin to prevent clot growth. Some clinicians may use vasodilators to promote collateral circulation. Cats that survive the initial episode may recover gradually over a period of days to weeks. The clot can be removed by aortic arteriotomy (although the mortality is high) or by the use of an embolectomy catheter. Anesthesia for

Table 15-13 Goals of Therapy in Feline Aortic Thromboembolism

Stabilize preexisting heart disease.
Administer analgesics for pain.
Use vasodilators to improve collateral circulation (the effectiveness of this therapy is unproven).
Administer heparin to prevent clot growth.
Use tissue plasminogen activator, streptokinase, or surgery to eliminate the clot.
Administer warfarin, heparin, or aspirin to prevent future clot formation.

aortic embolectomy in a cat with severe heart disease is particularly challenging and should be performed in an environment where the patient can be monitored intensively and supported during the procedure. Thrombolytic therapy can be used to remove the embolus from the aorta without the need for anesthesia and surgery. Unfortunately, thrombolytic therapy is expensive, requires intensive patient monitoring and support, and is associated with a high mortality from complications of therapy. A 50% mortality rate with tissue plasminogen activator therapy. Surgery and thrombolytic therapy are most likely to be effective when they are started as early as possible in the course of the disease. The effectiveness of aspirin and warfarin to prevent the formation of new thromboemboli has not been determined, but it appears that in many cats thromboembolism reccurs despite therapy. Table 15-13 summarizes the goals of therapy for feline aortic thromboembolism.

CONCLUSION

The veterinary technician plays a very important role in diagnosing and treating cardiovascular emergencies. They are one of the most common types of problems seen in the small animal practice. Understanding the clinical signs of cardiac problems is just the beginning. Various drugs and other therapies are used to treat cardiovascular problems quickly and effectively. The animal in cardiac distress must be handled very carefully and with a good understanding of the many types of cardiovascular problems that commonly affect dogs and cats.

BIBLIOGRAPHY

Abbott JA: Traumatic myocarditis. In *Current veterinary therapy,* ed 12, Philadelphia, 1995, WB Saunders.

Atkins CE: Caval syndrome in the dog, *Semin Vet Med Surg (Small Anim)* 2(1):64, 1987.

Berg JR, Wingfield W: Pericardial effusion in the dog: a review of 42 cases, *J Am Anim Hosp Assoc* 31:492, 1995.

Berk WA, Shea MJ, Crevey BJ: Bradycardic responses to vagally medicated bedside maneuvers in healthy volunteers, *Am J Med* 90:725, 1991.

Bonagura JD, Lehmkuhl LB: Fluid and diuretic therapy in heart failure. In DiBartola SD (ed). *Fluid therapy in small animal practice,* Philadelphia, 1992, WB Saunders.

Bossaert LL: Fibrillation and defibrillation of the heart, *Br J Anaesth* 79:203, 1997.

Brockman DJ, Washabau RJ, Drobatz KJ: Canine gastric dilatation/volvulus syndrome in a veterinary critical care unit: 295 cases (1986-1992), *J Am Vet Med Assoc* 207(4):460, 1995.

Brown WA: Congenital heart disease. In August JR, ed: *Consultations in feline internal medicine,* Philadelphia, 1997, WB Saunders.

Buchanan JW: Causes and prevalence of cardiovascular disease. In *Current Veterinary Therapy,* ed 11, Philadelphia, 1992, WB Saunders.

Buttrick ML, Riedesel DH, Selcer BA, et al: Hypoxemia in the acutely traumatized canine patient, *Vet Emerg Crit Care* 2(2):73, 1992.

Calvert CA, Hall G, Jacobs GJ, et al: Clinical and pathologic findings in Doberman pinschers with occult cardiomyopathy that died suddenly or developed congestive heart failure: 54 cases (1984-1991), *J Am Vet Med Assoc* 210(4):505, 1997.

Cobb M, Mitchell AR: Plasma electrolyte concentrations in dogs receiving diuretic therapy for cardiac failure in small animals, *J Small Anim Pract* 33:526, 1992.

Davis H: *Role delineation survey,* 1997, Academy of Veterinary Emergency and Critical Care Technicians, San Antonio.

DeLellis LA, Kittleson MD: Current uses and hazards of vasodilator therapy in heart failure. In *Current Veterinary Therapy,* ed 11, Philadelphia, 1992, WB Saunders.

Drobatz KJ, Macintire DK: Heat induced illness in dogs: 42 cases (1976-1993), *J Am Vet Med Assoc* 209(11): 1894, 1996.

Ettinger SJ: In Ettinger SJ, Feldman EC, eds: *Textbook of veterinary internal medicine,* Philadelphia, 1995, WB Saunders.

Forrester JS, Diamond G, Chatterjee K, et al: Medical therapy of acute myocardial infarction by application of hemodynamic subsets (first of two parts), *N Engl J Med* 295(24):1356, 1976.

Fox PR: Current uses and hazards of diuretic therapy. In *Current Veterinary Therapy,* ed 11, Philadelphia, 1992, WB Saunders.

Hamlin RL: To treat or not to treat ventricular arrhythmias in the dog, *ACVIM Forum Proceedings,* 1991.

Hamlin RL: Therapy of supraventricular tachycardia and atrial fibrillation. In *Current Veterinary Therapy,* ed 11, Philadelphia, 1992, WB Saunders.

Harpster NK: Boxer cardiomyopathy. In Kirk RW, ed: *Current veterinary therapy,* ed 8, Philadelphia, 1983, WB Saunders.

Harpster NK: The pericardium. In Gourley IM, Vasseur PB, eds: *General small animal surgery,* Philadelphia, 1985, Williams & Wilkins.

Harpster N: Pulmonary edema. In *Current veterinary therapy,* ed 10, Philadelphia, 1989, WB Saunders.

Harpster NK: Warfarin therapy in the cat at risk of thromboembolis. In *Current Veterinary Therapy,* ed 12, Philadelphia, 1995, WB Saunders.

Hoskins JD, Hagstad HV, Hribernik TN, et al: Heartworm disease in dogs from Louisiana: pretreatment clinical and laboratory evaluation, *J Am Anim Hosp Assoc* 20:205, 1984.

Hunt GB, Malik R, Church DB: Ventricular tachycardia in the dog: a review of 28 consecutive cases, *Aust Vet Pract* 20(3):122, 1990.

International Small Animal Cardiac Health Council: *Recommendations for the diagnosis of heart disease and the treatment of heart failure in small animals,* 1994, International Small Animal Cardiac Health Council, 1994, p. 30-32.

Jacobs GJ: Adding cardiovascular drugs to the CHF treatment plan, *Vet Med* 84:499, 1989.

Jacobs GJ: Treating cardiomyopathy in dogs and cats, *Vet Med* 91(6):544, 1996.

Keene BW, Bonagura JD: Therapy of heart failure. In *Current Veterinary Therapy,* ed 12, Philadelphia, 1995, WB Saunders.

Keye ML, Rush JE, Helio SA, et al: Ventricular arrhythmias in dogs with splenic masses, *Vet Emerg Crit Care* 3(1):33, 1993.

Kienle RD, Thomas WP, Pion PD: The natural history of canine congenital subaortic stenosis, *J Vet Intern Med* 8(6):423, 1994.

Kittleson MD: Cardiovascular physiology and pathophysiology. In Slatter DH (ed). *Textbook of small animal surgery,* Philadelphia, 1985, WB Saunders.

Kittleson MD: Left ventricular function and failure, *Compend Contin Educ* 16(3):287, 1994.

Knapp DW, Aronohn MG, Harpster NK: Cardiac arrhythmias associated with mass lesions of the canine spleen, *J Am Anim Hosp Assoc* 29:122, 1993.

Knowlen GG, Oliver NB, Kittleson MD: Contractility: a review, *J Vet Intern Med* 1(4):188, 1985.

Laste NJ, Harpster NK: A retrospective study of 100 cases of feline distal aortic thromboembolism: 1977-1993, *J Am Anim Hosp Assoc* 31:492, 1995.

Marino DJ, Matthiesen DT, Fox PR, et al: Ventricular arrhythmias in dogs undergoing splenectomy: a prospective study, *Vet Surg* 23(2):101, 1994.

McCurnin DM, Sceli DE, Arp LH: Surgical treatment of aortic embolism in a cat, *Vet Med Small Anim Clin* 67(4):387-390, 1972.

Miller MS, Tilley LP: Treatment of cardiac arrhythmias and conduction disturbances. In: *Manual of canine and feline cardiology,* Philadelphia, 1995, WB Saunders.

Monnet E, Orton EC, Salman M, et al: Idiopathic dilated cardiomyopathy in dogs: survival and prognostic indicators, *J Vet Intern Med* 9(1):12, 1995.

Olivier NB, Kittleson MD, Knowlen GG: Cardiac preload physiology and clinical implications, *J Vet Intern Med* 1(2):81, 1985.

Opie LH: *Drugs for the heart.* Philadelphia, 1995, WB Saunders.

Pascoe PJ, Haskins SC, Ilkiw JE, et al: Cardiopulmonary effects of halothane in hypovolemic dogs, *Am J Vet Res* 55(1):121, 1994.

Rawlings CA, Calvert CA, Glaus TM, et al: Surgical removal of heartworms, *Semin Vet Med Surg (Small Anim)* 9(4):200, 1994.

Rush JE: Emergency therapy and monitoring of heart failure. In *Current Veterinary Therapy,* ed 11, Philadelphia, 1992, WB Saunders.

Schaer M: Hyperkalemia in cats with uretheral obstruction: electrocardiographic abnormalities and treatment, *Vet Clin North Am* 7(2):407, 1977.

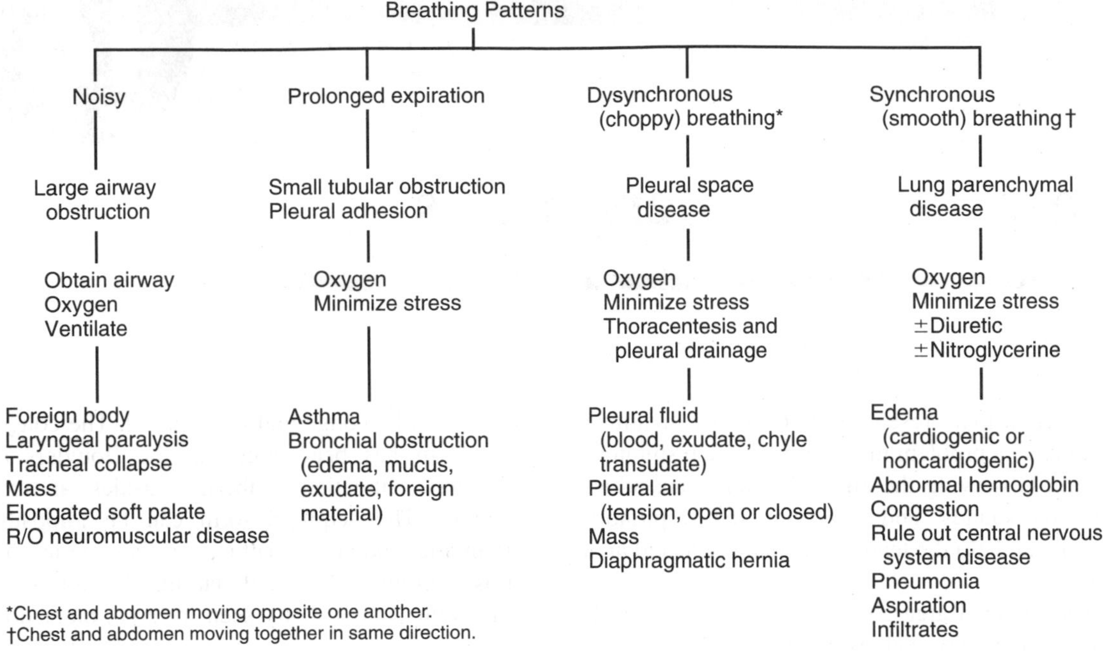

Figure 16-1

Breathing patterns. (Courtesy of Rebecca Kirby, DVM. Reprinted with permission from Murtaugh RJ: Acute respiratory distress, *Vet Clin North Am Small Anim Pract* 24(6):1043, 1994.)

tion. Corticosteroids are administered intravenously (dexamethasone 0.2 to 1.0 mg/kg twice daily) to reduce the inflammation and edema. Fluid therapy is used with caution. Some animals with upper airway obstruction can develop pulmonary edema.

Surgical treatment is recommended once the animal has been stabilized. It involves removing or repositioning the laryngeal cartilages. Intensive postoperative care is necessary because of the possible complications. These animals should be placed under 24-hour observation for 1 to 3 days. Antibiotics and corticosteroids are continued. Patients should be fed boluses of food and ice cubes to reduce the risk of aspiration for 12 to 24 hours post operatively. Owners must be instructed to keep the animal quiet and avoid excessive exercise for 6 to 8 weeks. Tranquilizers are recommended for the very active animal.

Foreign bodies partially blocking the upper airway in the form of sticks, balls, or other objects can be removed manually using forceps after sedation. The animal should be placed in a quiet environment and given flow-by oxygen. Trying to restrain the animal can cause additional stress and possibly dislodge the foreign body, allowing it to move further down into the airway. Once the foreign body is removed, the airway must be examined for possible trauma to any of the structures. The animal must be monitored for any other complications, which can include swelling or pulmonary edema.

TRACHEA

Tumors, tracheal stenosis and collapse, and intraluminal occlusion can cause tracheal obstructions. An acute onset of coughing and dyspnea is observed. High-frequency rales can be heard where the foreign body is lodged if it is only a partial obstruction. Collapse and respiratory arrest occur in animals with complete obstructions. These animals need a tracheostomy (Box 16-1).

The ideal presentation allows the time to preoxygenate the animal, sedate it, and then perform the technique. Many times an emergency tracheostomy (slash tracheostomy) is needed to save the animal's life.

Once the airway has been established and the animal has been stabilized, further diagnostic procedures can be performed.

Tracheal collapse is a common condition that often affects toy breeds and middle-aged to older dogs. It occurs when the tracheal ring does not maintain its rigidity. The trachea collapses dorsoventrally to form a flattened oval or slitlike lumen.

Presentation. Animals with a collapsed trachea usually have a history of coughing and signs of respiratory distress. Exercise intolerance is noted. Radiographs and endoscopy can confirm the condition.

Treatment. Medical therapy including bronchodialators, cough suppressants, and antiinflammatory drugs often is successful. Some animals with severe collapse need surgical intervention. Ring prosthetics made out of syringe cases, surgical stents, or a tracheal ring resection and anastomosis are a few of the techniques used to repair a collapsed trachea.

Postoperative care includes 24-hour observation, antibiotics, and corticosteroids. Cage rest with only light exercise is recommended.

Trauma to the trachea can result from dog fights, poor intubation or extubation techniques, and cords or chains placed around the animal's neck. Establishing a functional airway is the primary goal in all these situations. Once this has been accomplished, further stabilization techniques can be performed.

LOWER AIRWAY DISEASE

Feline Bronchial Disease

Bronchitis is a common cause of respiratory distress in cats. It has also been called feline asthma, which can be misleading. There are many forms of bronchial disease, and feline asthma is one of those forms. It most often affects young to middle-aged cats of any breed. The bronchitis can be caused by allergens, irritants, and infectious agents, but often the cause cannot be determined.

Presentation. Common clinical signs include respiratory distress characterized by prolonged expiration, coughing episodes, and wheezing. Vomiting and retching can occur after a severe coughing episode. Expiratory wheeze may be noted upon auscultation. No breath sounds may be noted in the more severe cases because of airway obstruction.

Diagnosis. Cardiac disease can cause very similar clinical signs and must be ruled out before treatment is administered. Bronchial disease is confirmed by evaluating a complete blood count, thoracic radiographs, and a tracheal or bronchoalveolar lavage. A fecal float should be evaluated to rule out a lung worm infestation.

Treatment. The cat in respiratory distress must be stabilized before any procedures can be performed. Oxygen therapy can begin immediately, using a stress-free technique. Short-acting glucorticoids (prednisolone sodium succinate 10 to 20 mg/kg intravenously) is highly recommended. This can be given intramuscularly if the intravenous injection is too stressful. Bronchodilators are used in conjunction with the steroids and antibiotics if indicated.

PARENCHYMAL OR GAS EXCHANGE DISEASE

Pneumonia

Pneumonia is an inflammation of the lungs with accompanying consolidation. Pneumonia can be caused by more than one agent. Viral, bacterial, fungal, and chemical causes are possible. Viral pneumonia usually is self-limiting, but some forms can be life-threatening.

Box 16-1 Establishing an Airway

The following procedures are performed when an endotracheal tube cannot be placed. These situations include head or facial trauma, spinal injuries, and upper airway obstructions.

Transtracheal Catheterization

A 14- or 16-gauge over-the-needle catheter or commercially available transtracheal catheter is placed through the tracheal rings. Commercially available transtracheal catheters are made with guarded tubing to prevent kinking once they are advanced into the trachea (see figure). This is a temporary solution until a more permanent airway can be established.

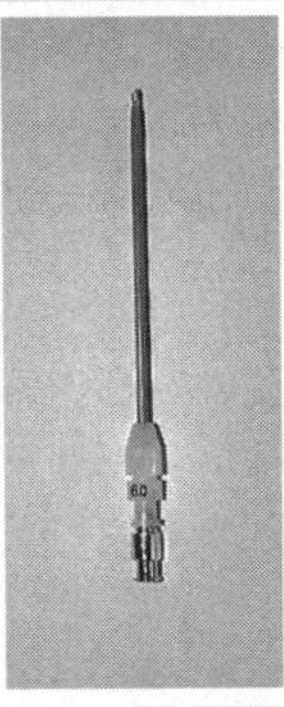

Procedure

1. When possible and appropriate, the anterior neck of the animal should be surgically prepped.
2. Identify the cricothyroid membrane between the cricoid and thyroid cartilages.
3. Stabilize the trachea with thumb and index finger.
4. Insert the catheter between the rings in the midcervical region, directing it caudally. A loss of resistance is felt once the trachea is punctured.
5. Aspirate air to ensure proper position.
6. Administer O_2 at 50 ml/kg/min.
7. Administer O_2 at 100 ml/kg/min if airway obstruction is present. Watch for chest expansion, then press on chest and abdomen in attempt to dislodge foreign body.
8. Tracheotomy is necessary if cyanosis does not resolve.
9. Maintain control of catheter position at all times. High oxygen pressures can dislodge catheter from the airway.

Possible Complications

Barotrauma
Pneumomediastinum
Bleeding
Catheter dislodgement
Subcutaneous emphysema
Hematoma
Tracheoesophageal fistula

Tracheotomy

An incision is made through the skin and muscles of the neck overlying the trachea. A tube 1 to 1.5 sizes smaller than what would be used for orotracheal intubation is placed through the incision. Commercially made

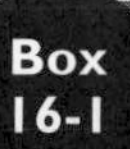

Box 16-1 Establishing an Airway—cont'd

Tracheotomy—cont'd

tracheotomy tubes are available. Tracheostomy tubes can be made out of endotracheal tubes by using the following method (see figure).

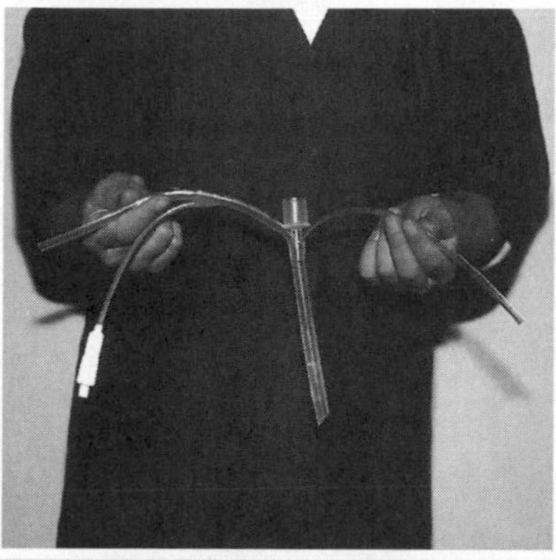

1. Remove 15-mm adapter from endotracheal tube.
2. Estimate how long the tube should be. Mark the length on the tube.
3. Cut tube in two places, starting proximally, down to the center of the tube. Avoid cutting the airline. Stop at the mark.
4. Replace the 15-mm adapter at the junction of the cut.
5. Shorten the split ends and place two holes at either end to be used for stabilizing.

Procedure

1. Administer general anesthesia or sedation with a local block around site of incision.
2. Surgically prepare the area.
3. Position animal in dorsal recumbency with neck extended back. Place a rolled towel under the neck to cause dorsal flexion of the cervical region. The animal's head can be stabilized by using tape over the jaw.
4. Make a ventral midline incision from approximately the first to the eighth tracheal ring.
5. Part the two sternohyoid muscles on the midline. Continue blunt dissection down to the tracheal rings.
6. Elevate the trachea using hemostats or fingers.
7. Make a transverse incision between the fourth and fifth ring.
8. Place stay sutures through the skin and tracheal cartilage adjacent to the transverse incision on either side of the opening.
9. Insert tube into opening and tie into place.

Slash tracheostomy is necessary for an animal in respiratory arrest with a complete upper airway obstruction or severe head trauma. This procedure is performed without a surgical prep. Scissors or a blade rather than blunt dissection is used to expose the trachea.

Complications

Obstruction from excessive secretions
Nosocomial pneumonia
Laryngeal stenosis
Tube dislodgement
Subcutaneous emphysema

Presentation. An animal with viral pneumonia presents with a fever, severe cough, rapid respiration, and possibly bloody mucus. Chest sounds consist of rhonchi, rales, and diminished breath sounds. Vomiting and lethargy also can be present. Blood gases reveal a low Po_2 caused by impairment of diffusion by pulmonary exudate and a low Pco_2 caused by hyperventilation. Some of the common causes of viral pneumonias are *Chlamydia* (psittacosis or ornithosis), and adenovirus. *Streptococcus pneumoniae, Staphylococcus pyogenes,* and *Klebsiella pneumoniae* commonly cause bacterial pneumonias. Other common causal agents are *Mycoplasma pneumoniae* and *Rickettsia burnetii.*

Pneumonias cause inflammation of the parenchyma of the lung, primarily the bronchi. Exudate forms and flows into the alveoli, plugging the alveoli and small airways. This process renders them airless, resulting in consolidation.

One of the most common forms of pneumococcal pneumonia is *Streptococcus pneumoniae.* Staphylococcal pneumonia often results as a secondary infection and usually is bronchial rather than lobar. Lung abscess and empyema are complications of staphylococcal pneumonia and are very destructive to tissue. *Rickettsia burnetii* is a type of pneumonia common to goats, sheep, and cattle. This form of pneumonia can be zoonotic to humans. Chemical pneumonias can be caused by using inhalants containing substances such as ammonia, nitrogen dioxide, cadmium, and fat or oil aerosol or from aspiration of stomach content.

Diagnostic Testing. Microbiological testing is used to determine the particular type of pneumonia that is present. A tracheal wash can be performed to collect the necessary specimen. Radiographic examination also is a valuable tool for evaluating the effects of specific types of pneumonia. Radiographs will reveal collapsed lobes or atelectasis, pleural effusion, and other effects of various pneumonias. Blood work and electrocardiography are helpful in determining the physiologic effects of this type of pneumonia. Polymorphonuclear leucocytosis is common in bacterial pneumonia. Blood gas analysis should be done to evaluate respiration; low to high $Paco_2$ may be present depending on the severity and duration of the disease. $Paco_2$ is reduced; pH could be normal to low, indicating respiratory acidosis.

Acidosis can result from CO_2 retention and ventilation-perfusion mismatch. $Paco_2$ measurement is very important because it indicates whether ventilatory assistance is needed. The electrocardiograph (ECG) will indicate any previous cardiac abnormalities or pending cardiac arrhythmias.

Treatment. Specific treatment depends on laboratory and radiographic diagnostic tests and physical assessment because there are so many types of pneumonia. The primary treatment for early-onset pneumonia is antibiotic therapy. Which antibiotic is appropriate depends on the type of pneumonia. In more advanced stages of pneumonia, standard treatment for respiratory emergencies is needed. This could consist of basic oxygen support or ventilation support and control. For minor respiratory distress such as tachypnea, flow-by oxygen is started with 100% oxygen. The results of arterial blood gas analysis indicate the severity of the respiratory distress. A $Paco_2$ greater than 60% and a pH greater than 7.60 indicate uncompensated respiratory acidosis. This also indicates that ventilatory support is needed.

Tracheal bronchial hygiene and fluid administration are important in these animals. Cardiac monitoring is also imperative, especially in the more debilitated patient. Septic shock can occur in more advanced cases of pneumonia. The patient should be monitored for fluid input and output, blood pressure, cardiac function, and acid-base status. In more advanced cases of pneumonia, tracheostomy may be necessary for adequate tracheal bronchial hygiene. Specific antibiotics can be selected based on laboratory cultures and titers.

PULMONARY CONTUSION

One of the most common types of pulmonary parenchymal injury in household pets is pulmonary contusion caused by chest trauma. The problem results from blood inside the alveolar and interstitial space. This blood interferes with the adequate exchange of oxygen and CO_2 at the alveolar capillary membrane.

Presentation. Depending on the degree of contusion, symptoms can vary from mild pain and dyspnea to total inability to move air in and out of the lung. Other complications of pulmonary contusion could be laceration, broken ribs, pneumothorax, hemothorax, pneumomediastinum, diaphragmatic hernia, and shock caused by fluid loss.

Treatment. Because so many conditions present with pulmonary contusions, each condition must be evaluated individually, with emphasis on respiration, circulation, and fluid volume. As with all trauma conditions, careful examination is imperative.

The patient is monitored on a 24-hour basis. Blood pressure, ECG, and arterial blood gas are critical aspects of adequate patient care. Wounds must be dressed and evaluated regularly, and splints and supports must be checked at regular intervals.

Pulmonary Edema

Pulmonary edema is defined as an abnormal accumulation of fluid in the extravascular tissues and lungs. This problem can be caused by increased pulmonary capillary pressure, leaking of the alveolar capillary membrane caused by trauma, or low plasma protein levels. Increased capillary permeability is the cause of edema. The most common cause of pulmonary edema is left heart failure. Trauma, sepsis, oxygen toxicity, hypoalbuminemia, airway obstruction, chemical inhalation, and pancreatitis are only a few of the conditions that can lead to pulmonary edema.

Presentation. The patient may present with blood tinged frothy mucus. This may not be observed in the earlier stages. Restlessness, labored respiration, crackling breath sounds on auscultation, and rapid, irregular heart rate also can be noted. Radiography shows pulmonary venous congestion and air space edema. Vascular markings are very clear in upper lung fields, and pleural effusion can be present. The heart shadow usually indicates an enlarged heart, particularly the left ventricle. Arterial blood gas would indicate a low Po_2, with a low to high $Paco_2$ depending on the severity of the edema and the stage of the condition. pH usually is low, indicating respiratory acidosis. There could also be a mixed acidosis, respiratory and metabolic. One of the classic symptoms of pulmonary edema is engorgement of the neck veins.

The cause of the edema must be determined before proper treatment can begin. Fluid overload, hyperalbuminemia, upper airway obstructions, and increased membrane permeability caused by shock are possible causes of pulmonary edema.

Treatment. The patient with pulmonary edema needs oxygenation to help alleviate the dyspnea. Assisted ventilation with positive end-expiratory pressure (PEEP) may be necessary for severe cases.

Airway care is especially challenging. Frequent airway suctioning may be needed to remove the fluid that usually accumulates with this disease. Suctioning must be performed carefully and for short duration. Suctioning for long periods further reduces interalveolar pressure, increasing the permeability of the alveolar capillary membrane.

Two forces in normal physiology work to maintain positive pressures in the alveolar capillary network. Plasma oncotic pressure usually is higher than transcapillary pressure; this higher pressure is what keeps fluid from entering the airspace of the alveoli through leakage from the capillaries. Fluid regulation usually can be managed with diuretics. Furosemide (lasix) is a common diuretic recommended at 2 to 4 mg/kg intravenously. When using diuretics, one must be careful to avoid hypovolemia. Bronchodilators may also be helpful for reducing the work of breathing. Corticosteroids have been indicated for shock.

Airway care and monitoring physiologic parameters for O_2 saturation, blood pressure, and cardiac status with ECG are necessary. Ventilator use also may be indicated. Specific anesthesia and sedation monitoring is of particular importance because many anesthetics and sedatives can increase the

thoracic drainage system or pump. Active air flow is determined by observing the bubbles in the water seal drainage system. As the pneumothorax begins to heal, the bubbles become less frequent.

A light chest wrap is used for additional support. An Elizabethan collar is used to prevent the animal from pulling the tube out.

Supplemental oxygen can be given via face tent or in an oxygen cage if hypoxia is present. Pulse oximetry can be used to determine oxygen saturation.

PLEURAL EFFUSION

The lining of the thoracic cavity and the outer surface of the lung is called the pleural lining. The lining covering the outer portion of the lung is called the visceral pleura, and the lining covering the diaphragm and the mediastinum is called the parietal lining. These two linings usually are separated by a thin layer of fluid. This eliminates friction between the two surfaces. A collection of excess fluid between the visceral and parietal pleura is known as pleural effusion. Normally the fluid in the pleural space flows from the interstitial tissue on the parietal side to the interstitial tissue of the lung by an absorptive force. An imbalance in this force impedes the flow of water, electrolyte, and protein. Some causes of pleural effusion are cancer, heartworm, congestive heart failure, chylothorax, hemothorax, hypoalbuminemia, infections, trauma, and idiopathic conditions.

Presentation. Clinical signs can include dyspnea, restlessness, cough, and lethargy. Respiration is labored with abdominal contraction. Lung auscultation indicates increased bronchial sounds. Cardiac sounds may be decreased. The degree of symptoms depends solely on the amount of fluid present and the rate of fluid formation.

Radiographic examination is the best way to diagnose pleural effusion. It is possible to determine whether the effusion is unilateral or bilateral and the extent of the effusion. The type of fluid can be determined by obtaining a sample. This is accomplished by performing a pleural tap. The tap also can be performed to relieve the pressure caused by the fluid accumulation. A chest tube may be necessary, with a continual closed-suction system attached.

The fluid is evaluated for contents such as blood, pus, or empyema. It is analyzed for cell count and differential as well as biochemical content and cytology.

Treatment is based on what is found in the fluid analysis. Blood, chyle (milky-looking aspirate), and protein can indicate conditions such as pyothorax, hemothorax, or chylothorax. It is important to determine the cause so appropriate treatment can be administered. Pleural biopsy may be necessary if cancer is suspected.

Continual monitoring and assessment of the animal's status is essential during stabilization and treatment. Pulse oximetry is monitored to determine oxygen saturation. Oxygen therapy and maintenance of a thoracic drainage tube also may be necessary.

DIAPHRAGMATIC HERNIA

Diaphragmatic hernia occurs when the contents of the abdomen herniate into the thoracic cavity. It is usually caused by blunt trauma to the chest or abdomen. A congenital form has been noted but rarely presents as an emergency.

Animals with a diaphragmatic hernia present with varying degrees of dyspnea, abdominal breathing, cyanosis, and shock. (The degree of respiratory distress depends on the degree of trauma and displacement of the organs.) Many other forms of trauma to the chest and abdominal wall also can be noted.

Radiographs and ultrasound can be used to diagnose the diaphragmatic hernia. Radiographic diagnosis can be challenging if pleural effusion or pulmonary contusions are present. The abdomen may feel empty on physical examination. Heart and lung sounds may be diminished on auscultation.

Treatment. Diaphragmatic hernia usually is secondary to trauma. The animal must be stabilized before hernia repair can be considered. An emergency surgery must be performed if the stomach is entrapped or a loop of bowel strangulated. Surgical intervention ultimately is needed to correct the problem.

The animal must be monitored closely for signs of deterioration and respiratory distress. Elevating the animal's front end may move the abdominal contents out of the thoracic cavity toward the abdominal cavity. This alleviates some of the pressure in the thoracic cavity.

Flail Chest

Flail chest occurs after severe trauma to the thoracic wall. A rib segment is broken off and becomes a free-floating segment. Pain and dyspnea are observed.

The animal must be maintained on oxygen and analgesics. Cage rest is necessary. Surgical intervention may be necessary to stabilize the flail segment.

Any animal that arrives to the emergency center in respiratory distress must be handled with care. A stressful environment may cause the patient to go into respiratory arrest. All tools needed to handle this type of emergency must be readily available.

CONCLUSION

The method of respiratory support veterinary professionals provide is very different from the patient's natural respiration. Lung ventilation is performed by creating a negative pressure in the chest, allowing air to flow into the lungs. Respiration takes place as an exchange between carbon dioxide and oxygen at the tissue level. When applying mechanical devices to the lung, we create an abnormal situation that can have side effects and complicate the course of treatment. Pulmonary barotrauma, impeded venous return, renal shutdown, tracheal malaise, and pneumothorax are some of the potential complications.

Anesthesia in itself can cause other complications, such as suppressed respiratory function and central nervous system depression. By being aware of these complications and the factors that create them, we can take steps to minimize or eliminate them. Knowledge of the equipment and drugs used in emergency care is essential to successful patient care.

BIBLIOGRAPHY

Braund KG, Shores A, Cochrane S, et al: Laryngeal paralysis polyneuropathy complex in young dalmations, *Am J Vet Res* 55:534, 1994.

Buback JL, Booth HW, Hobson HP: Surgical treatment of trachea collapse in dogs: 90 cases (1983-1993), *J Am Vet Med Assoc* 208:308, 1996.

Burbridge HM: A review of laryngeal paralysis in dogs, *Br Vet J* 151:71-82, 1995.

Cole RB: *Essentials of respiratory disease,* ed 2, Philadelphia, 1975, JB Lippincott.

Farzan S: *A concise handbook of respiratory disease,* Reston, Va, 1978, Reston Publishing Co.

Fingland RB: Treatment of tracheal collapse. In Bojrab JM, Ellison GW, Slocum B, eds: *Current techniques in small animal surgery,* Baltimore, 1998, Williams & Wilkins.

Hedlund CS: Tracheostomies in the management of canine and feline upper respiratory disease, *Vet Clin North Am Small Anim Pract* 24:873, 1994.

Moise NS, Wiedenkeller D, Yeager AE, et al: Clinical, radiographic and bronchial cytologic features of cats with bronchial disease: 65 cases (1980-1986), *J Am Vet Med Assoc* 194:1467, 1989.

Murtaugh RJ: Acute respiratory distress, *Vet Clin North Am Small Anim Pract* 24(6):1041, 1994.

Spearman CB, Sheldon RL, Egan DF: *Egan's fundamentals of respiratory therapy,* ed 4, St Louis, 1982, Mosby.

Stephen I, Bistner BS, Ford RB: *Handbook of veterinary procedures and emergency treatment,* Philadelphia, 1995, WB Saunders.

Chapter

Gastrointestinal Emergencies

Gastrointestinal emergencies are a common problem in veterinary medicine. They are often easy to diagnose because nausea (in the form of drooling or retching), vomiting, and diarrhea are very apparent. Some of the signs, such as restlessness, shivering, abnormal posture, and crying, are more subtle. Patients usually have some degree of pain on abdominal palpation, but this is quite variable. Animals usually do not show signs of pain if they are severely depressed, and some are more stoic than others.

This chapter addresses the common emergency conditions affecting the gastrointestinal system, including clinical signs and treatment options. Gastrointestinal emergencies to be discussed include problems affecting the esophagus, stomach, small intestine, large intestine, and pancreas. Close attention to history and accurate questioning of the owner are vital to early diagnosis, choice of appropriate diagnostic tests and treatment, and prevention of unnecessary expenses.

The technician's responsibilities for the patient with gastrointestinal emergencies include taking the history, performing physical examinations and laboratory analyses, taking radiographs of the abdomen and chest, assisting with ultrasound examination, readying the operating room (OR) and endoscopy equipment, monitoring anesthesia, assisting in the OR, and providing postoperative care. The technician often is the one who sees the patient the most and therefore detects patient discomfort more acutely and provides the most insight about how the patient is progressing.

Equipment List

- Stomach tubes
- Nasogastric feeding tubes
- 14- to 18-gauge over-the-needle catheters for gastrocentesis
- Complete surgical packs
- Warmed sterile saline for lavage during surgery

VOMITING

Vomiting is an active expulsion of gastrointestinal contents. It is preceded by signs of nausea such as restlessness, salivation, and repeated swallowing attempts followed by forceful contractions of the abdomen and diaphragm and the expulsion of food or fluid. The act of vomiting ultimately is initiated in the medullary vomiting center, which receives input from the chemoreceptor trigger zone (CRTZ), higher central nervous system (CNS) centers, vestibular system, and peripheral sensory receptors. Knowing which of these mechanisms is responsible enables practitioners to treat the vomiting patient appropriately. For instance, if a dog is vomiting because persistent gastric distention is stimulating the peripheral sensory receptors, it would be far better to place a nasogastric (NG) tube for stomach decompression than to treat the patient with a phenothiazine derivative.

Vomiting must be differentiated from regurgitation. Regurgitation implies an esophageal disorder, and close attention must be paid to the possibility of underlying aspiration pneumonia. Regurgitation is not preceded by signs of nausea, and there is no active expulsion of food or fluid. It often occurs very soon after drinking or eating. Food, if present in the vomitus, is undigested.

Projectile vomiting is most commonly associated with a pyloric outflow obstruction or a complete proximal intestinal obstruction. This can be either mechanical, as in the case of a foreign body, or functional, as in the case of pyloric or duodenal thickening or a mass (benign or malignant) compressing the pylorus. Vomiting of white fluid suggests a disorder of gastric or esophageal origin, and yellow suggests gastric vomiting with some bile coming from the duodenum. Green indicates bile and duodenal vomitus or a significant amount of bile that has refluxed into the stomach and immediately been vomited. Both yellow and green fluid can be associated with pancreatitis. Brown fluid suggests reflux of fecal material from further down the small intestine. It usually has a fecal odor as well. Frank blood in the vomitus (hematemesis) implies esophageal, gastric, or duodenal bleeding from erosions or ulceration, whereas "coffee grounds," or black flecks, indicate gastric or duodenal vomitus with the presence of digested blood (where hydrochloric acid has denatured the hemoglobin). Often blood may not be visible grossly, but chemistry strips can be used to confirm that blood is present.

Vomiting should be characterized as precisely as possible in all patients (Box 17-1). The frequency and amount of vomitus being produced are important to note because fluid therapy is dictated largely by ongoing losses. In addition, it is important to note the timing of the episodes as related to food or water ingestion. The presence of blood or foreign material is noted also because this may determine therapy.

Box 17-1 Vomiting Assessment

- Is it regurgitation (no nausea or active expulsion of GI contents)?
- Is it vomiting (nausea and abdominal contractions or active expulsion of GI contents)?
- Is it projectile?
- Is it nonproductive?
- What color is it (white, yellow, green, brown, red)?
- Is blood present (red, black, or chemistry strip evidence)?
- How frequently is it occurring?
- How much volume is being vomited?
- What is the consistency (fluid, foam)?
- When does it occur (after drinking, after eating, after medication)?

GI, Gastrointestinal.

DIARRHEA

As with vomiting, characterizing diarrhea is important in determining the underlying cause (Box 17-2). It is important to note whether the diarrhea is frequent, whether straining accompanies the passage of feces, and whether frank blood (hematochezia) or black digested blood (melena) is present. High frequency usually is associated with large intestinal diarrhea, as is straining. The presence of frank blood usually indicates colitis; however, patients with hypermotility disorders may have blood in the stool that is coming from the distal jejunum or ileum. The color of the stool, the presence of odor, and the presence of undigested food or foreign material should be noted because these are important clues about the health of the gastrointestinal tract. The odor of certain types of bacteria and blood being digested is very characteristic.

Box 17-2 Diarrhea Assessment

- How frequently does the diarrhea occur?
- How much volume is produced?
- What is the consistency (watery, soft, undigested food, foreign material)?
- Is blood present (red, black)?
- Does the animal have tenesmus?
- Is there an odor?

FIRST AID MEASURES

Owners often call veterinary hospitals indicating that a pet has evidence of a gastrointestinal disorder. They may report vomiting or retching, diarrhea, or ingestion of foreign material. Some descriptions are very obvious emergencies, such as nonproductive vomiting and abdominal distention in a 2-year-old dog; however, some problems are not so easy to diagnose. In almost all situations the patient should be seen because many patients who seem to have a minor problem based on the owner's description may actually have a very serious or even life-threatening problem.

If the owner declines to bring in the pet on an emergency basis, he or she should remove food for at least 24 hours and water for at least 4 hours. When water is reintroduced, ice cubes or several teaspoons to tablespoons of water (depending on the size of the patient) or electrolyte solution should be offered every 1 to 2 hours. The owner should be advised to have the pet examined immediately if vomiting recurs. If the pet does well with water for 12 hours, several teaspoons to tablespoons of a bland diet can be offered every 3 to 4 hours. If the pet vomits again, examination is highly recommended. If the emergency call comes in at night, it may be appropriate to have the owner withhold all water and food and have the pet examined first thing in the morning.

If the pet has ingested foreign material or a potential toxin, it may be appropriate to have the owner induce vomiting at home and then either bring the pet in for examination and treatment or monitor the pet at home. Vomiting should never be induced if the patient has an altered level of consciousness or is having breathing difficulties. It also is contraindicated with the ingestion of a caustic toxin, a petroleum-based product, or a foreign body that may get stuck or cause trauma to the stomach, esophagus, or oral cavity as it is being expelled.

DIAGNOSIS

Patients presenting with gastrointestinal emergencies may be stable or critical or any grade in between. In critically ill patients, rapid assessment is followed by immediate resuscitative measures, and there may be no time initially to take a full history or to perform a complete physical examination. A more complete history can be taken and a complete physical examination can be performed in stable patients before treatment.

Patients with an acute abdomen secondary to gastrointestinal emergencies may be unstable from a respiratory and cardiovascular standpoint; therefore, on presentation a primary survey examination (evaluation of level of consciousness, airway, breathing, and circulation) should be completed within 30 to 60 seconds, and abnormalities should be treated as indicated. For instance, a patient that presents obtunded with shallow respiration should be intubated and positive-pressure ventilation should be instituted. (This will help respiration and protect the airway against aspiration.) Depending on the severity of the patient's condition, resuscitation may be needed before a complete physical examination is performed. A very brief history is obtained at this time, if possible; however, resuscitation should not be delayed in the critically ill patient while a complete history is obtained. Instead, permission to start treatment should be obtained from the owner immediately. Once the primary survey is completed and resuscitation instituted, if necessary, a secondary survey or complete physical examination is performed. Vital signs are taken at this time. Rectal thermometers may induce a vagally mediated arrest in the severely bradycardic or hypotensive patient and should be avoided in these patients. Rectal temperatures also should be avoided in patients with rectal trauma or rectal bleeding. Instead, axillary or auricular temperatures should be taken. Rectal temperatures in patients with a dilated rectum may be very inaccurate because of the presence of air; the tip of the thermometer must be in contact with rectal mucosa. If there is concern about the accuracy of the rectal temperature, axillary, auricular, or colonic temperatures (using a long thermometer probe) can be taken. Toe web temperatures can be taken and compared with rectal temperatures. If the patient is perfusing normally, the ΔT should be less than 7° F.

The jugular vein should be clipped and evaluated for distention, filling time (less than 4 seconds), and relaxation time (less than 2 seconds) because this will provide a crude estimate of central venous pressure (CVP). Patients with surgical conditions of the abdomen may have concurrent pneumothorax, secondary aspiration pneumonia, or metastatic disease, and close attention should be paid to the ventilatory pattern, the presence of cough, and bilateral auscultation of the thorax. Blood pressure (BP) should be monitored as part of the initial examination because fluid resuscitation depends to a large extent on the patient's BP. A Doppler ultrasonic blood flow detector or an oscillometric device can be used; the Doppler is preferred because it allows the clinician to evaluate perfusion or flow as well as BP. In addition, many arrhythmias can be detected with a Doppler. If the patient has any auscultable evidence of an arrhythmia or is unstable from a cardiovascular standpoint, a lead II electrocardiogram should be assessed. Patients with myocardial hypoxia or ischemia secondary to circulatory shock often have ventricular premature contractions (VPCs) or ventricular tachycardia. These arrhythmias also are common in patients with splenic disease (i.e., gastric dilation and volvulus with concurrent splenic torsion).

The abdomen should be palpated, auscultated, and percussed with the goal of localizing pain and detecting fluid waves, gas-filled organs, or solid masses. A rectal examination should be performed and the presence of blood noted. The ventral abdomen should be clipped because petechiation or ecchymoses may indicate thrombocytopenia, a coagulopathy, or disseminated intravascular coagulation (DIC). If there is any doubt about the possibility of trauma, the abdomen (and the flank and thoracic regions) should be clipped of all hair and a visual examination done. Petechia, ecchymoses, abrasions, puncture wounds, and deformity or protrusion should be noted. Periumbilical hemorrhage can be seen with a hemoabdomen, and periumbilical masses can be seen with pancreatic carcinoma. Distended superficial abdominal veins are consistent with increased intraabdominal pressure, which can be associated with decreased preload and decreased cardiac output. The technician should always be alert for subtle signs of abdominal discomfort or changes in the skin that may reflect problems.

Diagnostic tests are needed to determine the extent of the disease and confirm the diagnosis. Resuscitation of the critically ill patient should not be delayed while tests are being performed unless those tests are needed to guide resuscitation. Laboratory work, including packed cell volume (PCV), total solids (TS), azostick, and glucose should be part of a stat data base. Many patients with sepsis are hypoglycemic and need an intravenous bolus of 25% dextrose (1 to 2 ml/kg body weight) followed by dextrose supplementation in the fluids. Ideally a complete blood cell count with microscopic evaluation of a blood smear for the differential, electrolytes, blood gas (venous or arterial), activated clotting time (ACT) or prothrombin time (PT), activated partial thromboplastin time (aPTT), blood chemistries, fecal (direct smear, flotation, and possibly zinc sulfate test), parvovirus test, and urinalysis should be performed. The choice of tests may vary based on the presenting complaint. Survey abdominal radiographs are always indicated. Chest radiographs should be evaluated preoperatively in every injured patient and in any patient in whom aspiration pneumonia or metastases are a potential concern. Contrast studies including barium series may be needed. Barium should not be used if there is concern about gastrointestinal perforation or aspiration. Water-soluble contrast material should be used instead. Abdominal ultrasound can be useful for diagnosis of some gastrointestinal emergencies, but because ultrasound waves do not pass through air, ultrasound is of limited use in diagnosing most gastrointestinal emergencies. Abdominocentesis or diagnostic peritoneal lavage may be indicated. Fluid should be evaluated for PCV, protein level, white blood cell count, and chemistries (as indicated) and evaluated microscopically. Elevations in amylase or lipase indicate pancreatic or small bowel injury or inflammation. Vegetable fibers, degenerative white blood cells, and those with intracellular bacteria indicate gastrointestinal content contamination and septic peritonitis.

MEDICAL TREATMENT

Some gastrointestinal emergencies can be managed medically, and some warrant emergency surgery (within minutes to hours of presentation); therefore, it is important to determine rapidly whether surgery is indicated. Acute abdominal conditions that warrant emergency surgery include trauma-related disease (penetrating wound to gastrointestinal tract), gastrointestinal obstruction (foreign body, neoplasia), gastrointestinal accident (gastric or intestinal torsion or volvulus, intussusception), peritonitis, and vascular accident (Box 17-3).

Oxygen should be provided to any patient showing signs of shock by flow-by using high flow rates (3 to 15 L/min), nasal oxygen cannula, or oxygen hood. One or two large-bore peripheral catheters (14 to 16 gauge in medium and large dogs, 18 to 20 gauge in small dogs and cats) should be placed. A central line should be placed if CVP monitoring is indicated. A central venous catheter also is indicated in all "crashing" patients, and a cutdown should be performed if the animal is extremely hypovolemic so that a large catheter (8- to 14-French feeding tube) can be inserted. CVP monitoring is indicated in any patient who presents with signs of moderate to severe shock, any patient in whom large volumes of fluids are being used for resuscitation, and any patient in whom fluid overload is a concern.

Fluids of the appropriate type are the most important therapy for patients with gastrointestinal emergencies. Fluid deficits should be replaced using replacement crystalloid solutions (e.g., lactated Ringer's solution, Normosol-R, Plasmalyte-A) over the first 8-12 hours in the stable patient; however, in the unstable patient it may be necessary to replace this deficit in 2-6 hours. In the critically ill, collapsed patient, perfusion abnormalities should be corrected as quickly as possible, with fluids given until BP is greater than 90 mm Hg systolic, heart rate approaches normal for the breed, digital pulses are palpable, and the patient's mentation has im-

Box 17-3 Treating the Patient with Vomiting or Diarrhea

Monitor vital signs q 4-8 hr (temperature, respiratory rate and effort, heart rate, pulse rate, BP, electrocardiogram, CVP, mucous membranes, capillary refill time).

NPO until vomiting is under control.

Crystalloid fluid support
- Correct dehydration over 2-6 hr if critical, 8-12 hr if stable.
- Replace ongoing losses.
- Help restore euvolemia (CVP 5-8 cm H_2O, urine production 1-2 ml/kg/hr).
- Correct electrolyte and acid-base imbalances.

Colloid fluid support
- Normalize intravascular volume and organ perfusion (BP > 110 mm Hg, CVP 5-8 cm H_2O, urine output 1-2 ml/kg/hr).
- Fresh frozen plasma if albumin < 2.0 g/dl.
- Red cells or hemoglobin if PCV < 25%.

Nasogastric tube decompression.

± Antiemetics.

± Antiulcer medications (H_2 blockers, ulcer-coating agents).

± Antibiotics.

Nutritional support.

Monitor PCV/total solids, glucose, blood urea nitrogen, electrolytes, venous and arterial blood gas q 8-24 hr.

In critical patients monitor coagulation parameters, albumin q 12-24 hr.

BP, Blood pressure; *CVP,* central venous pressure; *NPO,* nothing by mouth; *PCV,* packed cell volume.

proved. Usually 30 to 90 ml/kg of crystalloids and 10 to 20 ml/kg of a synthetic colloid are needed. Alternatively, if pressures are almost nonexistent, 7% hypertonic saline (1 ml/kg) with dextran 70 or hetastarch (3 ml/kg) can be given to effect. Because approximately 70% of crystalloids have left the intravascular space within 1 hour, in most cases intravenous colloids are needed because the volumes needed to resuscitate these animals with crystalloids alone may lead to tissue edema (peripheral, gut, and pulmonary).

After resuscitation or in the patient that does not need fluid resuscitation, fluid rates and types of fluid administered depend on the patient's status. Crystalloids should be provided at maintenance rates, and the rate should be increased to replace ongoing losses. Electrolytes (sodium, potassium, chloride, ionized calcium, magnesium) should be monitored at least daily. Fluid type and supplements should be adjusted as indicated. Potassium often is supplemented at 20 to 40 mEq/L based on the patient's level. Magnesium should be supplemented in the face of hypomagnesemia or hypokalemia that is nonresponsive to potassium supplementation. Glucose levels should be monitored at least daily in stable patients and dextrose should be supplemented as indicated. Patients with hypoglycemia may need more frequent monitoring.

Synthetic colloids are indicated during the postresuscitation period if the albumin is less than 2.0 g/dl, if the colloid osmotic pressure is low, or if it is suspected that the patient has ongoing protein losses. Constant-rate infusions of up to 20 ml/kg/day may be needed. If the albumin is less than 2.0 g/dl, plasma also is indicated. If it is suspected or confirmed that the patient has DIC, then heparin at 50 to 75 U/kg subcutaneously every 8 hours may be indicated. The heparin can be added to the plasma to help activate the antithrombin; however, the heparin should not be given more frequently than every 8 hours. Packed red blood cells or whole blood should be administered to keep the packed cell volume at approximately 30%. If red cell products are not available, a hemoglobin substitute can be used (oxyglobin, Biopure, Cambridge, MA).

Broad-spectrum antibiotics covering aerobic and anaerobic bacteria are indicated if infection is a concern. Antibiotics to counteract anaerobic infections are especially important in patients with diarrhea that is suspected to have infectious causes. Antibiotics should be used with great caution if infection is not suspected. Inappropriate antibiotic use can lead to bacterial overgrowth and severe diarrhea. In addition, they can lead to bacterial resistance and severe nosocomial infection problems. Like all other medications, they should be administered intravenously in the vomiting patient. Antiemetics are indicated if there is intractable vomiting. Pain control often includes opioid infusions or epidural morphine. Very small dosages of acepromazine may be useful if the patient is very anxious. Acepromazine should be used with extreme caution in hypotensive patients because of its α-adrenergic blocking effects.

Antiemetics

Antiemetics are classified based on the mechanism of action; therefore, it is important to know the cause (or suspected cause) of the vomiting. NG tubes are underused antiemetic devices. Many patients vomit because of gastric distention or gastric motility disorders. Poor gastric emptying may lead to fermentation of food and subsequent nausea. NG tubes can be used to remove fluid (and sometimes liquefied food), thus decreasing vomiting. They also remove air very well if positioned dorsally in the stomach. Ill patients often have gastric distention caused by aerophagia. This air often does not move well through the gastrointestinal tract and may cause delayed gastric emptying.

There are several classes of antiemetic medication. Phenothiazines (acepromazine, chlorpromazine, perchlorperazine) act at the higher CNS centers as well as at the CRTZ. They also have weak anticholinergic action. Trimethobenzamide acts at the CRTZ. Metoclopramide acts by enhancing gastric emptying and increasing lower esophageal sphincter tone and acting centrally at the CRTZ. Anticholinergics act by decreasing gastrointestinal secretions and motility; however, these agents are almost never indicated because they can lead to ileus. Butorphanol is a fairly effective antiemetic that counteracts the nausea caused by certain medications (especially chemotherapeutic agents) and may help decrease vomiting caused by pain. Parenteral antiemetics should be used in most vomiting patients because oral medications can cause vomiting and gastrointestinal absorption is unreliable.

SURGICAL TREATMENT

Surgical treatment is indicated in many gastrointestinal emergencies. The sun should never rise or set on an esophageal or gastrointestinal obstruction. Valuable time can be saved if the veterinary technician has the OR ready so that an emergency celiotomy can be done within minutes. At least three people—a surgeon, assistant surgeon, and anesthetist—are needed to treat these patients. Balanced anesthesia with close BP monitoring (ideally with a Doppler ultrasonic flow detector) and ventilation is essential. In the unstable patient, efforts should be made to use anesthetic agents that are least damaging to the cardiovascular system, and the anesthetist should try to keep the animal at the lightest possible level of anesthesia to minimize cardiovascular depression. Effective use of analgesia with intravenous or intrathecal opioids minimizes the general anesthetic needed, makes the patient more comfortable, and reduces patient morbidity both preoperatively and postoperatively. Many of these patients do not ventilate well under anesthesia and may need hand ventilation or mechanical ventilation. Anesthetic ventilators that have become available recently are very easy to operate and allow the technician to attend to other important anesthetic tasks.

The entire abdomen, including the inguinal regions and flanks, should be clipped and surgically prepared. The caudal third of the thorax also should be clipped and surgically prepared. This provides adequate exposure in anticipation of a full exploratory celiotomy, including the exposure of the inguinal canals for additional venous access and extension into the chest via a parasternal approach if needed. A full exploratory celiotomy consists of a ventral midline incision from the xiphoid to near to the pubis, and this should be anticipated in every patient with a gastrointestinal surgical emergency.

Every effort should be made to prevent hypothermia because this promotes vasoconstriction and poor tissue perfusion, decreases immune function, and prolongs coagulation times. This is especially important in intestinal surgery, where the intestines often must be placed outside the abdomen. Supplemental heat can be provided by various means; the patient always should be protected to ensure that burns do not occur. Patients should be placed on warmed surgical tables or on warm water circulating blankets. Warm air circulating blankets also can be used. As much of the patient's body as possible should be wrapped in blankets, bubble wrap, or plastic to help retain heat. Warming devices can be placed around the head and neck. Intravenous fluids should be warmed before administration and kept warm during administration (by keeping them in a commercial warming unit or running the administration tubing through a warm water circuit or warm water bath). When the abdomen is open, the exposed contents should be covered with laparotomy pads or towels as much as possible to prevent evaporative heat and water loss.

The abdomen should be lavaged adequately with warm sterile saline before closure. Usually, 1 to 3 L is needed. Lavage helps to flush out any contamination, reduce adhesions, and rewarm the patient. The temperature of the irrigation fluid should be 100° to 105° F.

Ideally, an NG tube is placed at the time of surgery, before the abdomen is closed, so that the surgeon can verify its placement. The NG tube allows postoperative decompression and early enteral nutritional support. An esophagostomy, gastrostomy, duodenostomy, or jejunostomy tube may be needed for postoperative nutritional support. If it is anticipated that the patient will not be eating normally for at least 3 days postoperatively, then a feeding tube should be placed.

Before extubation the oropharynx should be evaluated for signs of regurgitation. If vomitus is noted, the oropharynx should be suctioned and strong consideration should be given to lavage and suction of the esophagus. This is often indicated in patients with gastric dilation and volvulus, in whom passive regurgitation is common. Lavage and suction of the esophagus help prevent silent aspiration and pneumonia. Failure to remove gastric contents from the esophagus and pharynx can lead to inflammation, erosion, and possibly ulceration of these areas.

POSTOPERATIVE CARE

Postoperatively, all vital signs should be monitored closely, including level of consciousness, respiratory rate and effort, heart rate, pulse rate, pulse strength, BP, temperature, mucous membrane color, and capillary refill time. CVP should be monitored in critically ill or injured patients. Electrocardiographic monitoring should be performed in all patients with arrhythmias or those at risk for arrhythmias. Generally, vital signs are taken every 30 to 60 minutes in the immediate postoperative period until the patient is sternal. If the condition is critical, vital signs should be monitored more frequently or even continuously. Recumbent patients should be turned every 2 to 4 hours. If there is any concern about silent regurgitation and aspiration, the head and neck should be kept slightly elevated (30 degrees).

Ideally, high levels of supplemental oxygen should be provided in the immediate postoperative period to all patients because recent research has shown that this improves healing in patients who have undergone intestinal surgery. This may not be feasible or necessary in most veterinary patients; however, supplemental oxygen definitely is recommended in critically ill or injured patients after surgery.

Intravenous fluids should be continued until the patient is drinking normally. The type of crystalloid to be administered, the use of colloids, and the rate of administration vary depending on the patient's status and underlying disease process. Synthetic colloids should be used in all hypovolemic patients and in patients with a low colloid osmotic pressure or albumin less than 2.0 g/dl. If the patient is anemic, red blood cells or a red blood cell substitute (Oxyglobin, Biopure, Cambridge, Massachusetts) may be indicated. Fresh frozen plasma should be provided to the patient with albumin less than 2.0 g/dl, prolonged coagulation times, or risk for DIC. Antibiotics may be needed. Liberal use of parenteral analgesics is indicated to keep the patient comfortable.

Postoperative laboratory work in the critically ill or injured patient should consist of a minimum of a PCV, TS, and glucose. Ideally, venous blood gas, electrolytes, blood urea nitrogen, and albumin should be checked. Intravenous fluids (type, rate, and supplements) should be adjusted based on results. These tests should be repeated every 8 to 24 hours. Complete blood cell counts and coagulation parameters should be monitored every 24 to 48 hours depending on the patient's status.

Psychological support for both the pet and the owner, physical therapy (range-of-motion exercises), frequent turning, skin and hair care (often including a closed urinary catheter system to keep the patient dry), and respiratory therapy (stimulation to take deep breaths frequently) are essential.

Nasogastric Tubes

NG tubes are used for both stomach decompression and enteral nutrition. Decompression is indicated in all patients in whom significant volumes of air or fluid are accumulating. Gastric distention is one of the major triggers for vomiting; therefore, if gastric distention can be prevented the frequency of vomiting can be reduced. NG tubes should be placed in all patients who are aerophagic, have a tendency to bloat, are vomiting frequently, have gastric motility disorders or megaesophagus, or are at risk for silent regurgitation and aspiration. In addition, NG tubes should be placed postoperatively in all patients. Animals undergoing an exploratory celiotomy will not have normal gastric motility for at least 24 hours. If air and excess fluid are suctioned, vomiting can be prevented and gastric motility returned to normal more rapidly. Suctioning is indicated every hour initially until it is determined that large volumes of air and fluid are not accumulating. (Fluid volumes of up to 1 ml/kg/hr may be normal.) Continuous suction devices can be used if prolonged frequent suctioning is indicated. Once air is no longer being suctioned and volumes of fluid being suctioned decrease to less than 1 ml/kg/hr, the frequency of suctioning should be reduced to every 4 to 6 hours. If large volumes of fluid are being aspirated, electrolytes must be monitored closely.

Nutritional Support

Enteral nutrition should be started as soon as possible. Initially, microenteral nutrition is used. Microenteral nutrition is composed of electrolytes and dextrose (2.5% to 5%) given in small volumes. The fluid is infused via the NG tube starting at rates of 0.1 to 0.25 ml/kg/hr as a bolus or constant-rate infusion. This rate is slowly increased up to 1 ml/kg/hr over 24 to 48 hours depending on the patient. Once this is tolerated, a liquid diet can be provided via the NG tube or gruel of canned food (small amounts) is offered orally. In medically managed patients microenteral nutrition can be started within the first 12 to 24 hours after admission. Microenteral nutrition is started within 6 hours postoperatively or as soon as the patient is sternal, normothermic, and normotensive. It has been shown that glucose solutions delivered to the gastric mucosa help prevent gastric ulceration and may help improve splanchnic blood flow, thereby decreasing the chance for bacterial translocation. Clinically the use of microenteral feeding appears to be associated with a quicker return to normal enteral nutrition. This may be because microenteral nutrition helps preserve gastrointestinal function.

Blue food coloring should be added to the liquid if there are any concerns about aspiration. This helps determine whether any fluid suctioned from the oropharynx or trachea (in the case of intubated patients) contains the nutritional supplement. Based on the color of fluids aspirated from the stomach, clinical assessment of gastric emptying can be made.

When patients cannot tolerate enteral nutrition, parenteral nutrition is indicated. Partial parenteral nutrition containing 3% amino acids and glycerol (ProcalAmine, B. Braun Medical Inc., Irvine, California) is available commercially. Alternatively partial parenteral nutrition solutions of 3% amino acids (3% Fre Amine III, McGaw Inc., Irvine, California) and 3% dextrose can be administered. These solutions are hyperosmolar and ideally are administered via central venous catheters; however, they can be administered effectively via peripheral intravenous catheters. These solutions act primarily as protein-sparing solutions and do not provide total nutritional support. Therefore they should be used only for short-term nutritional support. Total parenteral nutrition is indicated in any patient that is not expected to be able to tolerate enteral nutrition for at least 5 to 7 days.

Duodenostomy or Jejunostomy Feeding Tubes

Duodenostomy or jejunostomy tubes are placed in anticipation that the upper gastrointestinal tract, including the stomach and pancreas, will need a rest, with no food being presented to the stomach for at least several days. Liquid diets that are polymeric (which must be digested) or monomeric (which are not digested) are given as constant-rate infusions through these tubes. They allow early and progressive feeding in such conditions as pancreatitis and complicated gastric surgery. Generally 1 to 2 ml/kg/hr is administered throughout the day and tapered off at night. The exit site of these tubes is cleaned every day and antibiotic ointment is placed around the exit site to help prevent infection.

The Importance of Record Keeping

Continued 24-hour care is ideal in all gastrointestinal emergencies. The watch word is *diligent care* from the time of arrival through the course of hospitalization. All monitoring and treatments must be recorded. A flowchart should be used to record this information in a chronological order. This is vital because it is often difficult to remember what happened hours after the event. To decrease morbidity from things such as inadequate fluid support, inadequate use of antiemetics, and insufficient nutritional support, accurate, thorough recordkeeping is essential.

SPECIFIC GASTROINTESTINAL EMERGENCIES

FOREIGN BODIES

Foreign bodies are one of the most common causes of vomiting in the young dog or cat; however, animals of any age can ingest foreign material. Fortunately, many foreign bodies pass or are vomited without serious consequence, but these materials often cause a partial or complete obstruction of the gastrointestinal tract, and endoscopic or surgical intervention is needed to remove the material.

Esophageal Foreign Bodies. Esophageal foreign bodies sometimes are treated differently from gastrointestinal foreign bodies and are dealt with separately.

History and Clinical Signs. History is very important in diagnosing an esophageal foreign body. The animal may present with signs of drooling, excessive swallowing, dysphagia, and apparent vomiting (which on closer questioning is determined to be regurgitation). Animals with an upper or midesophageal foreign body may present with signs of respiratory distress because the foreign material may be compressing the trachea. Harsh lung sounds may indicate aspiration pneumonia.

Diagnosis. Some foreign bodies are palpable. Radiographs and esophagoscopy can then be used to locate the material if it is not readily visible. Barium should not be used if a perforation is suspected, low osmolarity nonionic contrast material should be used.

Treatment. Dehydration and perfusion should be corrected before anesthesia and antibiotics are started. Suctioning any esophageal fluid or contrast material will aid in observing and removing the material and preventing aspiration pneumonia. General anesthesia should be used, and a cuffed endotracheal tube must be in place. Foreign material often lodges at the base of the heart, and significant bradycardia may be present. Anticholinergics often are used to help decrease salivation and prevent severe bradycardia.

Removal often can be done by the oral route using a rigid or flexible endoscope. A rigid endoscope and a "mechanic's helper" or mare uterine biopsy forceps are most useful. It is important to use generous amounts of lubrication (water-soluble jelly and water). The lubrication can be placed at the location of the foreign body using a stiff polyethylene catheter with its tip placed at the junction of the foreign body and the esophageal mucosa. By gentle manipulation after lubrication, the foreign body is brought close to the end of the rigid endoscope and all three (foreign body, grasper, and endoscope) are pulled out together.

If the foreign body is still stuck or if it can be manipulated into the stomach, then surgery is necessary. A gastrotomy may be used to remove very distal esophageal foreign bodies; however, the surgeon must be prepared to do an esophagotomy. The technician should anticipate that the lumen of the esophagus will not be sterile, and as the lumen is entered suction will be needed to aspirate contents to avoid contamination. A separate area on the operating table should be designated for placing all instruments used to remove the foreign body and close the mucosal layer. Clean instruments are used to close the outer muscularis serosal layer of the esophagus (after irrigation) and the cervical area or thorax to help minimize contamination.

Postoperatively, a gastrostomy feeding tube may be placed to bypass the esophagus while allowing enteral nutritional support. Some clinicians may prefer to use a small flexible esophagostomy tube (with its tip distal to the surgery site). The authors are not aware of any contraindications for the use of esophagostomy tubes for postoperative feeding after esophageal surgery.

Gastrointestinal Foreign Bodies

History and Clinical Signs. History from an owner is the most useful factor in early diagnosis of a foreign body. Early signs of a gastrointestinal foreign body include nausea, vomiting, and inappetance. Vomiting usually persists until the material has passed, been vomited, or is removed. The character of the vomiting may indicate the location of the problem and the degree of obstruction. Abdominal pain may or may not be present depending on the duration of the problem and degree of obstruction.

Diagnosis. The gastrointestinal foreign body may be directly palpable on physical examination. Abdominal pain is a warning sign, and splinting may indicate the presence of a surgical disorder. Vomiting at the time of or at the conclusion of palpation of the abdomen is a significant indicator that the animal has a surgical abdomen. Survey radiographs may reveal radioopaque foreign bodies, and an abnormally gas-distended loop of bowel may indicate an obstruction. A barium series may be needed to locate the material. Water-soluble contrast material rather than barium should be used if there is any concern about bowel perforation. A loss of detail on radiographs suggests the possibility of peritonitis, and an immediate diagnostic peritoneal lavage to detect white blood cells, plant material, and bacteria is indicated. Laboratory work should include electrolytes, a complete blood cell count, and blood chemistries. If there is a concern that the patient may have peritonitis or be developing systemic inflammatory response syndrome (SIRS), then coagulation parameters including a platelet estimate and an ACT or PT and aPTT should be obtained because this patient is at risk for DIC. If the patient is critically ill, an antithrombin (AT) level should be assessed if available.

Treatment. The patient with a foreign body may present in a stable condition, in hyperdynamic shock, or in decompensatory (hypodynamic) shock. Fluid therapy should be guided by the patient's status. Those that are stable can be rehydrated more slowly. Those in shock need rapid volume replacement with crystalloids and colloids. Many patients with intestinal foreign bodies cannot be stabilized completely until surgery.

Surgical removal is indicated in the vast majority of these patients and in all patients with significant clinical signs or a radiographic pattern of distended bowel loops. In some patients rehydration "relubricates" the bowel and allows the material to pass, but this is uncommon. In the critically ill or unstable patient, prompt surgery may be needed because pressure necrosis can lead to bowel perforation. It is best to operate early, even if there is only a slight chance of a foreign body. A foreign body that is very radioopaque and appears round in some radiographic views and thin in others may be a penny. Unfortunately, most pennies contain zinc, which can cause a hemolytic anemia. Therefore, if there is any suspicion that the animal may have ingested pennies, they should be removed immediately by endoscopy or gastrotomy. Safety pins, straight pins, and other identifiable gastric or intestinal foreign bodies should be removed if clinical signs are apparent. The only time a watch-and-wait attitude should be taken is if there are no clinical signs. In these cases, serial radiographs should be taken to monitor the progress of the object. These objects generally pass out of the gastrointestinal tract without any problems. However, if the object has a string attached to it, exploratory surgery should be performed. If there is any doubt about the nature of the foreign body or whether it will pass, surgery should be performed.

During gastrointestinal surgery, the entire tract should be explored. The technician should anticipate the same concerns as with esophageal surgery regarding contamination. Broad-spectrum antibiotics should be given before the lumen of the gastrointestinal tract is incised.

Gastric Dilation and Volvulus

Etiology and Pathophysiology. The cause of gastric dilation and volvulus (GDV) is not clearly understood. Twisting causes a one-way valve effect at the gastroesophageal junction, allowing swallowed air to enter the stomach but not leave. Gas accumulation also may result from carbon dioxide–producing bacteria and from carbon dioxide diffusion associated with trapped blood in the gastric mucosa, submucosa, and muscle wall. Gastric acid and bicarbonate from the pancreas and saliva also can lead to carbon dioxide production.

GDV has been associated with more than 100 clinical entities. It is typically seen in large, deep-chested dogs but can occur in any size dog and typically an underlying cause is never discovered. It has been observed in patients who ingest foreign material, in those with chronic debilitating diseases, altered gastric emptying, neuromuscular diseases, or respiratory difficulty, and in hospitalized animals that are very nervous. As in humans, it is most common in older patients.

The key effect with distention and rotation (which can also occur to some extent with distention alone) is partial to complete blockage of the portal vein. The degree of venous obstruction of the portal vein is variable. Microcirculatory sludging, activation of the coagulation system, neutrophil and platelet activation, adhesion, liberation of cytokines, endothelial swelling and cleft opening, and profound regional ischemia may progress rapidly. Nearly all splanchnic organs are affected by the distention and rotation of the stomach. The liver, pancreas, small intestine, and stomach all become ischemic.

The physiologic effects of GDV lead to hypovolemic shock. A large amount of the patient's functional blood volume is trapped in the veins of the splanchnic circulation. Because of vena caval obstruction, which is caused by the distention, blood is trapped in the systemic veins in the caudal portion of the body. A cardiogenic form of shock also results from cytokine liberation, myocardial depressant factor, and myocardial necrosis. Septic or endotoxic shock also occurs and may play a very significant role in the posttreatment period. Without aggressive treatment, almost all patients with GDV die. With aggressive treatment, which involves surgery within an hour, more than 90% of patients may survive. With delayed treatment, mortality rates can be as high as 80%.

History and Clinical Signs. Patients commonly present with a history of attempting to vomit or nonproductive retching. Abdominal distention may or may not be noted by the owner. The onset usually is acute and often associated with eating a fairly large meal. It also may be associated with dietary indiscretion such as ingestion of unleavened bread, garbage, or poorly digestible treats. There may be a history of gastrointestinal disease or previous episodes of bloating.

On presentation, dogs usually show some degree of circulatory shock. Pressure on the diaphragm caused by a progressively dilating stomach may compromise lung expansion and lead to ventilatory compromise. Salivation, nausea, and nonproductive retching may or may not be present.

Diagnosis. The patient usually is restless and attempting to retch nonproductively and may have abdominal distention. Because GDV occurs mainly in deep-chested dogs, the abdominal distention may not be evident until late in the disease because the stomach is contained under the rib cage. The gas-distended stomach may be detectable on percussion of the cranial abdomen. Because the dog may be in hyperdynamic shock or in a stage of decompensatory shock, findings vary from tachycardia, tachypnea, bounding pulses, and injected mucous membranes to collapse, respiratory distress, and weak, thready pulses.

A right lateral radiograph should be taken. On occasion, the volvulus is not evident on the right lateral view, so if there is a high index of suspicion, a left lateral radiograph should taken. A characteristic shelf sign with compartmentalization supports a diagnosis of a gastric volvulus.

Treatment. Immediate treatment should consist of oxygen, if the dog is showing any signs of shock, and volume replacement with crystalloids and synthetic colloids. The electrocardiogram (ECG) should be monitored because these dogs are prone to ventricular arrhythmias. The stomach should be decompressed only after volume replacement has been started because of the potential for worsening the hypovolemic shock. Rapid-onset corticosteroids (dexamethasone sodium phosphate at 4 to 8 mg/kg intravenously or methylprednisolone sodium succinate at 15 to 30 mg/kg intravenously) usually are given and broad-spectrum antibiotics started. Coagulation parameters should be monitored closely because these patients are at risk for DIC. BP should be monitored closely.

Gastrocentesis to decompress the stomach is performed using 14- to 18-gauge needles or catheters after percussion to identify the best insertion location. This usually is followed by immediate surgery (ideal) or nasogastric or orogastric tube placement and lavage for those in normal anatomic position (based on a right lateral radiograph) with stable vital signs. In the latter patient, surgery still should be performed within the next 1 to 2 hours. Owners refusing surgery are given the option of anesthetizing the dog and placing a large-bore orogastric tube and lavaging the stomach until the effluent is clear. If the effluent is bloody or very dark, then it is recommended that surgery be performed immediately because this indicates the likelihood of gastric necrosis. Until the stomach is placed back into normal anatomic position, the patient continues to be at high risk. The stomach will continue to have an embarrassed blood supply that cannot be assessed.

Immediate surgery is indicated for several reasons. It can be difficult to confirm that the stomach is in its correct anatomic position without surgery. In addition, it is almost impossible to determine whether gastric necrosis or active hemorrhage is present (usually from tearing of the short gastric vessels) or whether the spleen is thombosed (secondary to partial or complete torsion) without performing surgery. Gastric lavage can be performed before or during surgery; however, a stomach tube can be passed into a twisted stomach. It is also possible to pass a stomach tube through the wall of an ischemic stomach, and excessive force should not be used.

INTESTINAL ACCIDENTS

Other intestinal disorders necessitating rapid surgical intervention include intestinal intussusception and mesenteric volvulus.

History and Clinical Signs. If seen early in the disease process, these patients may present only with signs of not acting normally, with possible restlessness and nausea. Late in the disease they may present with a history of vomiting, diarrhea (which may or may not be hemorrhagic), abdominal distention, and abdominal pain.

Diagnosis. Palpation may reveal an intussusception; however, in the case of a sliding intussusception that may reduce itself intermittently, diagnosis can be challenging. In these animals, abdominal palpation generally is painful, and significant splinting may be present. Gut sounds may or may not be present. Survey radiographs may reveal gas-distended loops of bowel, but in some cases a barium series may be needed. Surgical exploration must be done as soon as possible. In the case of a mesenteric volvulus, endotoxic shock commonly leads to death, and surgery is indicated immediately upon presentation. Prognosis with mesenteric volvulus is grave.

Treatment. These patients must be resuscitated with oxygen, crystalloids, and colloids. Close monitoring is needed because these patients may have a complicated preoperative, operative, and postoperative course. Surgery is performed as soon as possible. Most often, resection is necessary. If more than one intussusception has occurred, enteroplication is needed in many cases to prevent recurrence. Enteroplication is a procedure by which the small intestine is folded back and forth and sutured together from the duodenum to the colon.

HEMORRHAGIC GASTROENTERITIS

History and Clinical Signs. Hemorrhagic gastroenteritis (HGE) is indicated by the presence of blood (frank or digested) in the vomitus or diarrhea. A characteristic foul odor to the stool is identified, most often with rectal examination. Onset may be peracute or more chronic. In peracute cases, profound septic shock often is present.

Diagnosis. Because of the multiple causes of blood in the vomitus or stool, many tests may be needed for diagnosis. In an emergency, the most important laboratory tests include those that assess the degree of anemia or hemoconcentration, a complete blood cell count, fecal parvovirus test, coagulation parameters, and radiographs to rule out the presence of a foreign body. Abdominal radiographs usually reveal a small to moderate amount of gas throughout the small and large intestine, but a characteristic obstructive pattern is not observed. A barium series, endoscopy, and possibly exploratory surgery may be needed to diagnose and treat the patient. Parvovirus enteritis may appear as a "surgical abdomen," but fortunately the antigen test usually is positive, obviating surgery. Gram staining of the material obtained from a rectal examination generally shows many large gram-positive rods, and anaerobic culture reveals many *Clostridium* species. *Escherichia coli* often is cultured from the stool of these patients, but without serotyping it may be difficult to determine whether they are pathogenic. If the cultures are hemolytic on blood agar, the organism is presumed to be pathogenic.

Treatment. Intravenous fluids should be given according to the parameters noted on presentation, the degree of perfusion abnormality, and the underlying disease. In the patient with idiopathic HGE, rapid boluses of crystalloids may be needed to restore a normal hematocrit and normal rheology. In the poorly perfused patient with parvovirus, colloids may be needed as part of the initial resuscitation. Because of third-spacing of fluids into the gut, in the patient with HGE it is very easy to underestimate the volume of fluids needed. Close attention must be paid to maintaining normal heart rates, normal BP, and normal CVP. (Monitoring the strength of metatarsal pulses can be used as a crude estimate of BP if indirect or direct BP monitoring is not available. Clipping the area over the jugular vein and monitoring the degree of jugular filling when the vein is held off and the degree of runoff provides a crude estimate of CVP and right heart function if a central venous line and CVP monitoring are not available.) Intravenous broad-spectrum antibiotics should be used to cover the range of pathogens that could be contributing to endotoxin and exotoxin effects in the seriously ill patient. Sucralfate and H_2 blockers also are indicated in many cases. Because many patients with HGE may be at risk for hypoalbuminemia and SIRS, close monitoring for complications associated with SIRS (e.g., DIC, acute respiratory distress syndrome, left heart failure) is strongly recommended. Plasma may be needed early in the disease course to replace albumin, AT, and clotting factors.

In the case of severe gastric ulceration and bleeding, lavage of the stomach with ice water may be necessary. Some cases of gastrointestinal ulceration may warrant surgical intervention, especially if perforation is suspected.

Rectal Emergencies

History and Clinical Signs. Rectal emergencies usually are caused by trauma, neoplasia, or severe perianal fistulas. Passing blood through the rectum or active bleeding is the most common complaint. With more chronic disease, these patients present with a history of tenesmus, diarrhea, or passing ribbonlike stools. Active bleeding from the rectum or perirectal tissue or tenesmus usually is present on examination.

Diagnosis. Traumatic wounds or actively hemorrhaging perianal fistulas often are diagnosed based on visual inspection. Rectal examination or proctoscopy is used to diagnose other conditions. Basic laboratory tests should be performed and coagulation parameters analyzed.

Treatment. Active external hemorrhage should be controlled with external pressure. Because of the pain and discomfort, intravenous sedation often is needed before treatment with external pressure can begin. It may be necessary to follow direct pressure with cauterization under sedation, general anesthesia, or epidural anesthesia. In some instances the bleeding warrants formal eversion of the rectal wall, location of the bleeding site, and ligation of the vessels. Complete ablation may be needed to control tumors that are bleeding significantly. Fluid resuscitation should be provided as indicated. Antibiotics should be provided to control anaerobic and aerobic coliform bacterial infection.

Pancreatitis

History and Clinical Signs. These patients may present with signs similar to those of other gastrointestinal emergencies. Anorexia and intermittent vomiting may be the only signs in cats. Dogs typically have a history of dietary indiscretion followed by nausea, vomiting, and anorexia. Diarrhea may be present late in the disease. Abdominal pain is present, and in mild cases it can be localized to the right upper quadrant of the abdomen. If seen early in the disease process, these patients may present only with signs of not acting normally, with possible restlessness and nausea. Late in the disease they may present with a history of vomiting, diarrhea (which may or may not be hemorrhagic), abdominal distention, and abdominal pain.

Diagnosis. Ultrasound can be very useful in diagnosing pancreatitis in dogs, but false negatives are common in cats. Abdominal fluid evaluation via abdominocentesis or diagnostic peritoneal lavage (DPL), is the test of choice to determine the need for an exploratory celiotomy.

Treatment. The pancreas releases vasoactive substances that lead to varying degrees of shock, vasculitis, and coagulopathies. Fluid therapy is the cornerstone of treatment for pancreatitis. Crystalloids, synthetic colloids, and plasma often are indicated. Abdominal lavage clinically appears to help these patients, probably by diluting enzymes and other factors from the inflamed pancreas. Patients with pancreatitis often are in pain, and opioids should be used as frequently as needed to control the pain. Peritoneal lavage often helps decrease the pain associated with pancreatitis. The surgical management of pancreatitis is controversial. If the patient has signs of peritonitis, a pancreatic abscess, or phlegmon, is not clinically improving after several days of medical management, or is deteriorating, surgery is indicated. A jejunostomy feeding tube should be placed for nutritional support in all patients who undergo surgery for pancreatitis. Medical treatment of pancreatitis is controversial. In the past it was recommended not to feed patients with pancreatitis for 5 to 7 days. Recent studies in humans have shown that oral feeding can be provided as long as there is no clinical exacerbation of the pancreatitis. The authors recommend trickle feeding with small amounts of a liquid low-fat diet.

Peritonitis

History and Clinical Signs. Patients that have an acute rupture or perforation of a hollow viscus (usually secondary to trauma) may present with signs of not acting normally, with possible restlessness and nausea. Late in the disease they may present with a history of vomiting, diarrhea (which may or may not be hemorrhagic), abdominal pain, and possibly abdominal distention. These patients present in varying degrees of shock depending on the length of time they have been sick and the cause of the peritonitis.

Diagnosis. Peritonitis may be diagnosed with abdominocentesis. Abdominal ultrasound can be useful in helping to determine the cause. Diagnostic peritoneal lavage is the test of choice to confirm peritonitis if other tests have been equivocal. Because patients with peritonitis may have many systemic abnormalities, complete laboratory work is recommended. Abnormalities should be corrected as indicated.

Treatment. These patients need fluid resuscitation, antibiotics, and analgesics. A complete exploratory surgery is indicated as soon as possible after diagnosis and initial resuscitation. After complete exploration through an incision that extends from the xiphoid process to the pubis, all sources of the sepsis are removed or repaired depending on visual assessment of viability. Omental wrapping is performed after complete irrigation of repaired stomach, small intestine, or colon. Serosal patching may be indicated for bowel surgery. In this technique, the wall of an intact section of jejunum including the serosa generally is used to cover (like a patch) the defect of the repaired areas of another hollow viscus. A jejunostomy feeding tube is placed to deliver nutritional support beginning immediately after anesthetic recovery.

The abdominal cavity is left open to allow drainage and admit air. The use of open abdominal drainage in the management of the septic abdomen has improved survival significantly for the following reasons:

- Allowing the abdomen to remain open ventrally prevents the retention of septic exudate at the visceral-parietal peritoneal interfaces (common with simple tube drainage); more effective drainage is provided by this method.
- Keeping a large wound open into the abdomen allows air to be actively or passively insufflated into the peritoneal cavity, which raises the redox potential (Po_2 of 100 mm Hg inside the abdomen with open abdominal drainage versus Po_2 of 20 to 40 mm Hg within the peritoneal cavity when the abdomen is closed).

The common organisms associated with bacterial peritonitis are mostly microaerophilic or completely anaerobic (e.g., *Escherichia coli* and *Clostridium perfringens,* respectively). Allowing air to continue to bathe the peritoneal surfaces suppresses the growth of these organisms and the accumulation of toxic byproducts (exotoxins). Peritoneal macrophage function also is enhanced by the increased redox potential accompanying the open drainage technique, which also helps suppress aerobic and enteric microaerophilic bacteria proliferation.

Beginning Open Drainage. After thorough, copious irrigation with a balanced electrolyte solution until the effluent is clear, the abdomen is dried as much as possible with suction and laparotomy pads. The caudal aspect of the incision is closed to avoid the difficulties of applying dressing between the rear limbs. To protect the patient from evisceration, a loose, simple, continuous suture using monofilament suture material is placed into the external rectus sheath of the rest of the abdominal incision. A gap of 2 to 3 cm is left in the average-sized dog.

Several sterile absorbent pads (cotton, polyester) or towels are laid over the ventral abdominal incision line and a circumferential dressing is applied using a circular cotton, stretchable gauze bandage to hold the pads in place. An absorbent, disposable "diaper" or "blue pad" with a plastic outlining is then wrapped around the dressing to prevent strikethrough of the abdominal pads from urine and contamination from the environment. The dressing–blue pad combination is secured with adhesive tape or elastic woven stretch tape. While the peritoneal cavity is open the patient must be observed carefully to ensure that the dressing stays in place. In male dogs, closed, chronic catheterization of the urinary bladder usually is performed as long as the abdomen is open to prevent urine strikethrough.

Postoperative Abdominal Dressing Management. The abdominal dressing generally is changed two or three times per day or when it becomes saturated with abdominal fluid and exudate. The patient is kept in sternal recumbency or standing as much as possible to encourage drainage into the dressing, aided by gravity. The abdominal dressing under the blue pad is examined every 6 to 8 hours for strikethrough. When this occurs, the dressing is changed. The animal is placed in dorsal recumbency after the intravenous administration of a light sedative (oxymorphone, diazepam, ketamine), if necessary. The outer dressing is removed and the absorbent pads replaced using sterile technique. If the small intestine or omentum adheres to the pads being removed, these tissues are gently teased off the pads, with the operator wearing sterile gloves and using saline in a small sterile syringe. After the old pads are removed, the wound is inspected for evidence of necrosis. If it is observed, it must be removed surgically. This is not common, fortunately.

New inner pads are placed and the "trapdoor" or circumferential dressing is replaced and the sedation reversed if desired. The amount of fluid lost through the drainage can be estimated by weighing the dressings removed and comparing this weight to that of a similar amount of dry dressings. The difference in weight of the dressings represents the amount of fluid drained, with 1 g equal to 1 ml fluid. The amount of protein lost also can be estimated by measuring the concentration of total protein in the fluid and multiplying this number by the estimated amount of fluid drained. Fluid can be examined microscopically to follow the cellular changes in the abdominal cavity.

Open Abdominal Drainage Medical Management. Patients with open abdominal drainage are prone to the loss of large volumes of fluids, electrolytes, and protein. Enteral replacement of these losses is preferred over parenteral replacement; however, intravenous fluid support usually is needed in these patients. Plasma administration usually is needed to replace peritoneal albumin losses.

Daily physical activity and movement should be encouraged for several reasons. Activity facilitates peritoneal drainage. Physical movement also encourages deep breathing. These patients are prone to develop pneumonia, and deep breathing and chest physiotherapy (percussion, postural drainage, and nebulization) are indicated to prevent or treat it.

Antibiotic therapy is best guided by culture and sensitivity results. Before the results are available, it should be assumed that a mixed infection is present. Gram staining of the exudate can help confirm this.

Concluding Open Drainage. The abdomen should be closed when there is no further strikethrough of the abdominal dressing for approximately 18 to 24 hours, which usually occurs after 3 to 4 days. At that time the patient is taken back to the operating room and, under general anesthesia, the dressings are removed, culture taken, and the loose, continuous sutures in the abdominal wall pulled tight and tied. The subcutaneous tissues are then irrigated thoroughly. The skin and subcutaneous tissues are closed.

Second-Look Laparotomy and Deep Local Drain Use. If the drainage from the abdomen does not begin to decrease within 4 days, becomes worse in character (more prevalent, fecal-like, biliary-like), a second-look laparotomy is recommended. A second-look laparotomy also may be elected if the initial repair or tissue viability was believed to be tenuous. A second laparotomy also is done in cases with deep intraabdominal abscesses or septic disease processes that may lead to deep abscess formation (e.g., suppurative necrotizing pancreatitis). In most of these cases, placing deep abdominal drains is also recommended. This is because in these closed areas, omentum, mesentery, and other nearby organs help form a pocket that cannot be drained well with open abdominal drainage alone. Deep localized abdominal drainage using silicone rubber multiple-fenestrated gravity and suction drains keeps the area evacuated. These drains have been used in suppurative pancreatitis, suppurative cholecystitis-cholangiohepatitis, and areas of previously evacuated intraabdominal abscesses.

POISONINGS

History and Clinical Signs. History from an owner is essential in the accurate diagnosis and treatment of most toxicities because clinical signs can vary widely. If the toxin is suspected or identified, it is essential to get accurate and detailed information on the chemical or chemicals involved so that a poison control center can be contacted for information on expected effects, treatment, and prognosis.

Diagnosis. Identifying a specific toxin takes a high index of suspicion. The clinician should work closely with poison control centers—both local human centers and the National Animal Poison Control Center at the University of Illinois. Local emergency clinics may also have information. Blood, urine, and gavage samples may be needed for assay to identify suspected toxins, and samples should be taken on admission whenever possible. If the animal has vomited at home, the owner should be instructed to save the contents in a plastic bag and bring it in with the animal.

Treatment. Vomiting should be induced as soon as possible in the patient ingesting a suspected or unknown toxin unless vomiting is known to be specifically contraindicated. Hydrogen peroxide and salt can be given by the owner at home and generally are very effective in inducing vomiting. The dosage of hydrogen peroxide is 1 to 2 teaspoons of 3% peroxide per 10 kg body weight. This can be repeated three times at 5-minute intervals. Salt, which is a much less preferred emetic, can be given at a dosage of one eighth of a teaspoon per 10 kg body weight. The sooner the toxin is out of the system, the less likely are toxic effects; even making the animal vomit in the car on the way to the clinic is a good idea. Apomorphine also can be used to induce vomiting. A 6-mg tablet is now more pure and therefore much more potent than before. The tablet should be mixed with 6 ml saline, and 1 ml of the suspension should be given intravenously per 10 kg body weight.

If significant and early emesis does not occur, gastric lavage should be performed. Most often this is performed under general anesthesia with a cuffed endotracheal tube in place to guard the airway. Activated charcoal should be administered via a gavage or nasogastric tube. Air should be aspirated from the stomach before the dog is awakened and the esophagus should be lavaged with saline or water and suctioned to prevent silent aspiration on recovery.

Further treatment in most cases is symptomatic unless a specific antidote is known. Fluid diuresis is indicated in many cases. Seizure activity, ventilation and oxygenation, BP and perfusion, cardiac rhythms and rates, renal function, and coagulation are just some of the parameters that should be controlled and maintained as normal as possible. Treatments such as dialysis may be needed if ethylene glycol has been ingested.

CONCLUSION

Animals with gastrointestinal distress can deteriorate very quickly, especially when vomiting and or diarrhea is present. Almost all calls from owners involving an animal with some form of gastrointestinal distress should be considered emergencies. It is very difficult to evaluate this type of problem, and what may be described as mild discomfort may be life threatening.

Surgery for gastrointestinal emergencies is very challenging. The facility must be equipped with a highly skilled team to stabilize and monitor these patients throughout treatment.

BIBLIOGRAPHY

Crowe DT, Devey J: Clinical experience with the use of a modified surgical technique for placement of a jejunostomy feeding tube in 47 patients, *J Vet Emerg Crit Care* 7:7, 1997.

Devey JJ, Crowe DT: Microenteral nutrition. In Bonagura JD, ed: *Current veterinary therapy,* ed 13, Philadelphia, 2000, WB Saunders.

Greif R, Akca O, Horn EP, et al: Supplemental perioperative oxygen to reduce the incidence of surgical-wound infections. Outcomes Research Group, *N Engl J Med* 342(3):161, 2000.

King LG, Donaldson MT: Acute vomiting, *Vet Clin North Am (Small Anim Pract)* 24:1189, 1994.

Windsor ACJ, Kanwar S, Li AGK, et al: Compared with parenteral nutrition, enteral feeding attenuates the acute phase response and improves disease severity in acute pancreatitis, *Gut* 42:431, 1998.

Chapter 18

Metabolic and Endocrine Emergencies

Metabolic and endocrine emergencies are some of the most demanding and critical conditions treated in the intensive care unit; with careful patient monitoring, however, they can be some of the most rewarding cases. This chapter discusses diabetic ketoacidosis, hypoadrenocorticism, hypercalcemia, hypocalcemia, and hypoglycemia.

Equipment List

Basic supplies needed for stabilization
A selection of catheters suitable for the jugular vessels
Multilumen intravenous catheters
Regular insulin
Insulin syringes
50% Dextrose
Potassium phosphate
Sodium bicarbonate
Dexamethasone sodium phosphate
Desoxycorticosterone pivalate
Prednisone and prednisolone
Fludrocortisone acetate
Calcium gluconate 10% solution
Calcium chloride 10% solution
Furosemide
Calcitonin
Electrocardiograph monitor
Infusion pumps
Blood chemistry analyzers
Blood glucose monitor

DIABETIC KETOACIDOSIS

Diabetic ketoacidosis (DKA) is a complicated form of diabetes mellitus that can be fatal in dogs and cats. Patients with insulin-dependent diabetes mellitus have an absolute or relative insulin deficiency. As a result, the body's cells (except the brain and heart) are unable to take up glucose via insulin-dependent insulin receptors located in the cell membrane. Insulin deficiency initiates lipolysis (the breakdown of stored body fat into fatty acids) and promotes the conversion of the released fatty acids into glucose precursors in the liver via β-oxidation. Additionally, the body experiences increased secretion of the stress hormones, glucagon, cortisol, catecholamines, and growth hormone. These hormones are gluconeogenic and promote β-oxidation. The by-products of β-oxidation are ketoacids (acetoacetate, β-hydroxybutyrate, acetone), which cause acidosis.

Presentation

Diabetes mellitus in dogs can occur from 4 to 14 years of age, with most patients presenting in the range of 7 to 9 years. Females are affected nearly twice as frequently as males. Diabetes seems to be common in poodles, miniature schnauzers, beagles, and dachshunds and has a genetic basis in keeshonds and golden retrievers. There may be a genetic basis in cairn terriers and miniature pinschers. Diabetes mellitus can be diagnosed at any age in the cat; however, most are 6 years or older. No breed predisposition has been identified, but neutered males are predominantly affected.

Most patients show typical signs of diabetes mellitus (Box 18-1). Polyuria, polydipsia, weight loss, and muscle wasting are most common. Dermatologic signs include unkempt hair coat and flaky, dry skin. Some patients, usually cats, develop a diabetic neuropathy, typically in the form of a plantigrade stance in the pelvic limbs. Careful evaluation for concurrent illness is essential, especially for pancreatitis, which can cause a painful cranial or right cranial abdomen. As the acidosis worsens, patients present with anorexia, vomiting, dehydration, weakness, lethargy or depression, hypotension, coma, panting, or Kussmaul breathing. The breath has a distinctive acetone odor. See Table 18-1 for a list of common clinicopathologic abnormalities.

TREATMENT

The major focus of the treatment of DKA is to replace sufficient amounts of insulin to stablize the patient's metabolic condition. Electrolyte, mineral, and acid-base status must be corrected concurrently. If an underlying cause of the diabetes or concomitant infection (urogenital, skin, respiratory, abscess) is identified, this must also be treated.

Initial insulin therapy should be regular insulin delivered intravenously or intramuscularly. The greatest control can be achieved with a constant-rate infusion of intravenous regular insulin at 0.05 to 0.5 u/kg/hr for dogs and 0.05 to 0.2 u/kg/hr for cats. A constant-rate infusion pump is needed for this technique. Changing the rate of the infusion changes the speed at which the blood glucose decreases in the patient. Regular insulin can be placed in lactated Ringer's solution or 0.9% sodium chloride solution for initial therapy. Insulin adheres to plastic, and 30 to 50 ml of the insulin solution should be allowed to flow through the line to saturate the tubing before the infusion starts. Insulin is damaged by ultraviolet light, and fresh infusions should be made very 24 hours. Insulin infusions are administered at slower rates than non–insulin-containing solutions used for rehydration. A double-lumen central line or a second intravenous catheter in another vein is needed.

Insulin also can be administered intramuscularly. The initial dose of 0.2 u/kg is followed by subsequent doses of 0.1 u/kg. The half-life of regular insulin is approximately 2 hours, and redosing is needed every 3 to 6 hours, but it is important to consider the response to the previous insulin dose before determining when the next dose is given (i.e., if the serum glucose concentration is decreasing at an appropriate rate, it may be inadvisable to redose the insulin, even if the patient is still hyperglycemic).

With both intravenous and intramuscular dosing, the goal is to have the serum glucose concentration decline 50 to 100 mg/dl/hr. If the glucose declines more rapidly, there may be significant complications. The brain produces neurogenic osmoles (small molecules that attract water) in an effort to maintain adequate hydration in the face of a hyperosmolar environment. It takes time for these neurogenic osmoles to be depleted in the brain. Rapid changes in serum glucose concentrations cause marked reductions in the osmolality of the blood. The brain then becomes hyperosmolar and

Box 18-1 The Most Common Clinical Signs Associated with Diabetes and Ketoacidosis

Polyuria
Polydipsia
Weight loss
Muscle wasting
Vomiting
Anorexia
Dehydration
Lethargy or depression
Weakness
Panting or Kussmaul breathing
Ketotic breath
Plantigrade stance (cats, usually)
Dry flaky skin
Polyphagia (nonketotic)

TABLE 18-1 Common Initial Clinicopathologic Values Associated with Diabetic Ketoacidosis

Complete Blood Cell Count	Serum Chemistry Profile	Urinalysis	Blood Gases
Usually normal	Hyperglycemia	Glucosuria	Decreased P_{CO_2}
Leukocytosis (if infection present)	Increased liver enzyme activities	Ketonuria	Decreased total bicarbonate
Polycythemia (if dehydrated)	Azotemia	Proteinuria	Acidemia
Anemia of chronic disease	Hypercholesterolemia	Bacteriuria	Decreased base excess
	Hyperlipidemia	Pyuria	
	Hypertriglyceridemia	Hematuria	
	Hyperlipasemia (if pancreatitis present)	Submaximal urine concentration	
	Hyperamylasemia (if pancreatitis present)		
	Hyponatremia		
	Hypokalemia		
	Hypochloremia		
	Decreased total CO_2		
	Increased serum osmolality		

attracts water. This can cause cerebral edema, seizures, coma, and death. If signs coincide with a rapid drop in the blood glucose concentration, add dextrose to the fluids to produce a 5% to 10% solution to maintain the blood glucose in the range of 250 to 300 mg/dl. Treat the cerebral edema with mannitol. This is a very rare complication.

Once the patient has been stablized, longer-acting insulin can be used. In dogs, the initial dosage is 0.5 u/kg once or twice daily based on the glucose curve. An initial dosage of 1 to 3 u/cat once or twice daily depending on the glucose curve is recommended. Most dogs and cats ultimately need lifelong twice-daily insulin injections. See Table 18-2 for a comparison of insulin types and administrations. All insulin types (including regular insulin) should be refrigerated to maintain a constant temperature. Regular insulin does not settle, so there is no need to resuspend it. All the other types of insulin settle out, and gentle resuspension is needed. All insulins should be protected from sunlight and ultraviolet light because it degrades the insulin. It is recommended that bottles of insulin be discarded 3 months after initial use, regardless of the amount left in the bottle. Most insulin comes in the concentration of 100 u/ml (U-100). Insulin syringes designed for U-100 insulin should be used because they measure 1 u/0.01 ml more accurately than a 1-cc (tuberculin) syringe.

All patients need intravenous fluid therapy for rehydration. Rehydration helps to improve cardiac output and tissue perfusion, provides fluid diuresis to remove ketoacids and other retained organic acids, and helps to correct acid-base and electrolyte imbalances. The use of isotonic crystalloid fluids (lactated Ringer's solution, 0.9% sodium chloride) is preferred. The fluid rate should be calculated to provide maintenance fluid volume plus dehydration deficit volume (percentage dehydration multiplied by the body weight in kilograms) delivered over a 24- to 48-hour period. In some severely dehydrated and critically ill patients, the dehydration deficit must be delivered more rapidly, over a 6- to 12-hour period. Monitor lung sounds, respiration rate, and respiratory effort closely to ensure that the patient does not become overhydrated.

TABLE 18-2 Insulin Types, Time to Maximal Effect and Duration of Action for Cats and Dogs

Type	Route of Administration	Time Until Onset of Action	Time Until Maximal Effect		Duration of Action	
			Cats	Dogs	Cats	Dogs
Regular	IV	Immediate	0.5-2 hr	0.5-2 hr	1-4 hr	1-4 hr
	IM	10-30 min	1-4 hr	1-4 hr	3-8 hr	3-8 hr
	SQ	10-30 min	1-5 hr	1-5 hr	4-10 hr	4-10 hr
Lente	SQ	15-60 min	2-8 hr	2-10 hr	6-14 hr	8-24 hr
NPH	SQ	0.5-3 hr	2-8 hr	2-10 hr	4-12 hr	6-24 hr
Ultralente	SQ	2-8 hr	4-16 hr	4-16 hr	8-24 hr	8-28 hr
PZI	SQ	1-4 hr	3-12 hr	4-14 hr	6-24 hr	6-28 hr

Adapted from Nelson RW: Diabetes mellitus. In: Ettinger SJ, Feldman EC, eds: *Textbook of veterinary internal medicine,* Philadelphia, 1995, WB Saunders, p. 1526.

Most patients with DKA need potassium supplementation. Diabetes mellitus and especially ketoacidosis cause total potassium depletion through a shift of potassium out of the cells into the serum to replenish renal losses and to help offset acid-base imbalances. Treatment of DKA further decreases potassium concentrations through dilution from the fluid therapy, insulin-mediated uptake of potassium by the cells, correction of acidemia, and continued renal losses. Measure serum concentrations of potassium before treatment and follow the recommendations in Table 18-3. If in-house serum chemistries are not available, supplement potassium at a rate of 0.055 to 0.11 mEq KCl/kg/hr while waiting for pretreatment serum biochemical analysis. Potassium supplementation should be avoided in patients with oliguria or anuria, hyperkalemia, hypocalcemia, or hyperphosphatemia.

TABLE 18-3 Potassium Supplementation Recommendations for Diabetic Patients

Serum Potassium (mEq/L)	Amount to Supplement	
	mEq K^+/L*	mEq K^+/kg/hr
>3.5	20	0.055
3.0-3.5	30	0.083
2.5-3.0	40	0.110
2.0-2.5	60	0.165
<2.0	80	0.220

*Amount supplemented to 1 L fluids if delivered at a maintenance rate of 66 ml/kg/day.

Shifts in body phosphorus occur in a similar fashion as potassium. Treatment of DKA also decreases phosphorus by mechanisms similar to those by which it decreases potassium. Phosphate bonds are the main energy storage vehicle for the cells (especially red blood cells, skeletal muscle, and brain), and phosphorus is important for 2.3-diphosphoglycerol's role in oxygen dissociation in the red blood cell. Most dogs and cats have normal serum phosphorus and phosphate concentrations, and phosphate should be supplemented with 0.01 to 0.03 mmol phosphate/kg/hr (potassium phosphate has 3.3 mmol phosphate/ml) for 6 to 24 hours in the intravenous fluids. The calcium in lactated Ringer's precipitates out some of the phosphate, so 0.9% sodium chloride is a better choice in patients that are severely hypophosphatemic. Dogs and cats with a phosphorus concentration of 1.5 mg/dl or less need 0.03 to 0.12 mmol phosphate/kg/hr. Close monitoring is needed for these patients. Phosphate supplementation should be avoided in patients with oliguria or anuria, hyperphosphatemia, hypocalcemia, or hyperkalemia.

Intravenous bicarbonate therapy is controversial. Most patients with DKA improve with insulin and fluid therapy alone. If the plasma bicarbonate concentration is 11 mEq/L or less, or total venous CO_2 is 12 mEq/L or less (total $CO_2 - 1$ = plasma bicarbonate concentration), bicarbonate therapy can be considered, especially if the venous blood pH is 7.0 or less. Bicarbonate should be used only if venous blood gases can be monitored. The amount of bicarbonate (in mEq) needed to correct the acidosis to a plasma bicarbonate of 12 mEq/L over a 6-hour period is

$$\text{Bicarbonate (mEq)} = BW_{kg} \times 0.4 \times [12 - \text{Patient's bicarbonate (mEq/L)}] \times 0.5$$

where BW_{kg} is the body weight in kilograms. Bolusing bicarbonate is not advised. The acid-base status must be rechecked 6 hours after the bicarbonate infusion starts. Additional bicarbonate therapy can be used until the bicarbonate concentration is 12 mEq/L or greater.

Patients that are not eating and have hypoglycemia (less than 70 mg/dl) from their insulin therapy may need dextrose supplementation to their intravenous fluid therapy. If a constant-rate infusion of regular insulin is being used, stop the insulin infusion and recheck the blood glucose in 30 to 60 minutes. If the blood glucose continues to decline or the concentration is below 60 mg/dl, then initiate dextrose therapy. Remember that dextrose is converted into glucose, which enters the cells with potassium and phosphorus via insulin-mediated glucose receptors. Dextrose therapy is not needed unless there is hypoglycemia or the blood glucose concentration drops too rapidly. If the patient is experiencing signs of insulin shock and has neurologic signs of hypoglycemia, administer a bolus of 50% dextrose at a dosage of 1 ml/kg intravenously and then add enough dextrose to the infusion to create a 5% to 10% dextrose intavenous drip, which can be maintained as needed.

Antibiotics should be used as needed based on signs of infection. Urogenital tract infections are most common. Sampling the urine for culture before antibiotic therapy is advised.

MONITORING

Most of the monitoring evaluates the response to treatment and early identification of common complications. Patients should be weighed twice daily to monitor rehydration and to make sure they do not gain too much weight (more than the estimated dehydration, 1 L = 1 kg). Monitoring the respiration rate and effort and the lung sounds also helps prevent volume overload. The urine output should be evaluated carefully. Initially, urine output is lower than volume input because of dehydration, but once the patient is rehydrated, urine output should closely match intake and input.

Electrolytes should be measured every 4 to 8 hours. Because they change for similar reasons, changes in the potassium concentration can be correlated with the phosphorus concentration if phosphorus cannot be measured as frequently as potassium. Decreases in the potassium or phosphorus concentrations should be addressed promptly. The acid-base status also must be monitored closely. In patients with severe disturbances, venous blood gases should be monitored every 6 hours until stable, then once daily.

Urine color should be monitored continuously and a packed cell volume should be measured once or twice daily. Take note of the serum color. Severe hypophosphatemia causes the red blood cell membranes to destablize and results in acute hemolysis, which manifests as hemoglobinuria, hemolyzed serum, and a rapidly decreasing packed cell volume. The urine also should be checked daily for ketones. The separated serum can be checked with a urine dipstick in a similar fashion to detect ketonemia. Ketones may persist in the urine for 1 to 5 days after the ketotic state resolves. Because urinary tract infections are very common in patients with diabetes mellitus, sign of bacterial infection (e.g., foul odor, cloudiness, hematuria, strangury) should be noted daily.

Blood glucose should be monitored every 2 hours. In some severely affected patients, every 1 hour measurements are needed initially to ensure that the blood glucose is not decreasing too rapidly. The ideal rate of decline in the blood glucose is 50 to 100 mg/dl/hr. If blood glucose drops below 60 mg/dl, neuroglycopenic signs may occur, such as weakness, depression, lethargy, coma, bradycardia, or seizures. If the patient is eating, feed it. If not, intravenous dextrose therapy can be used. As previously mentioned, if the blood glucose drops too quickly, cerebral edema may occur, so careful attention to mental status is necessary.

With careful monitoring and anticipation of complications, these patients can do quite well. It is important to remember that no two patients with DKA are the same, and nothing is routine about this disease.

HYPOADRENOCORTICISM (ACUTE ADDISONIAN CRISIS)

Hypoadrenocorticism (Addison's disease) is a deficiency in the production of mineralocorticoids (aldosterone) or glucocorticoids (cortisol) in the adrenal glands. Destruction of the adrenal gland by immune-mediated causes is the likely cause of most cases of primary hyoadrenocorticism. Iatrogenic primary hypoadrenocorticism occurs if the adrenal cortex is destroyed by mitotane. Secondary hypoadrenocorticism, which is decreased production of adrenocorticotropic hormone (ACTH) by the pituitary gland, causes glucocorticoid deficiency only. Iatrogenic secondary hypoadrenocorticism occurs when there is a sudden withdrawal of exogenous high-dose or long-term glucocorticoid therapy.

Mineralocorticoids (aldosterone) are important in regulating body electrolyte status. Aldosterone promotes sodium and chloride reabsorption in exchange for potassium and hydrogen ions in the connecting segment and the collecting tubules of the renal nephron. Free water travels with the sodium. A lack of aldosterone results in sodium, chloride, and free water loss in the urine, with retention of potassium, hydrogen ions, and calcium. The resultant severe electrolyte imbalances and dehydration cause the shock and cardiotoxic events in an Addisonian crisis.

Glucocorticoids (cortisol) are important for many body systems. Gastrointestinal integrity is the major consequence of cortisol deficiency. Poor vascular perfusion of the intestinal mucosa, decreased mucus production, and gastrointestinal ulceration have clinical manifestations. Glucocorticoids also are important gluconeogenic hormones and are one of the four primary stress hormones.

PRESENTATION

Hypoadrenocorticism is an uncommon disease of dogs and an extremely rare disease in cats. Both species are treated similarly. The disease generally is seen in young dogs (mean 4 to 4.5 years, range 2 months to 12 years) and middle-aged cats. In dogs, 70% to 85% of the affected dogs are female. There appears to be no breed predilections in cats; however, in dogs, Great Danes, Portuguese water dogs, rottweilers, West Highland white terriers, and Wheaton terriers are at increased risk. The disease is inherited in standard poodles and Leonbergers.

Clinical signs and symptoms vary. They range from mild signs to severe or fatal signs with acute crisis. The history may reveal a waxing and waning course. The most common signs in the dog are anorexia, vomiting, lethargy or depression, and weakness. Some patients also have weight loss, diarrhea, melena, shaking or shivering, polyuria, and polydipsia. In cats, lethargy, anorexia, vomiting, weight loss, polyuria, and polydipsia are the most common clinical signs (Table 18-4).

Dogs often are depressed and dehydrated. Pale, tacky oral mucous membranes with slow capillary refill time are common. In severely affected patients, shock, collapse, coma, and seizures can occur. Weak pulses and bradycardia can result from hyperkalemia. An electrocardiogram in patients with hyperkalemia may reveal tall, spiked T waves with a narrow base. The QRS complexes become wider and the P-R interval increases. The P waves become smaller and wider and, in severe hyperkalemia, disappear altogether (atrial standstill). Severely hyperkalemic patients may have QRS-T fusion, resulting in a wide-complex idioventricular arrhythmia followed by ventricular fibrillation and asystole (Figure 18-1). A similar clinical presentation has been reported in the cat. Because many of these are nonspecific signs, it is important to rule out severe gastrointestinal disease, renal disease, and whipworm infestation. See

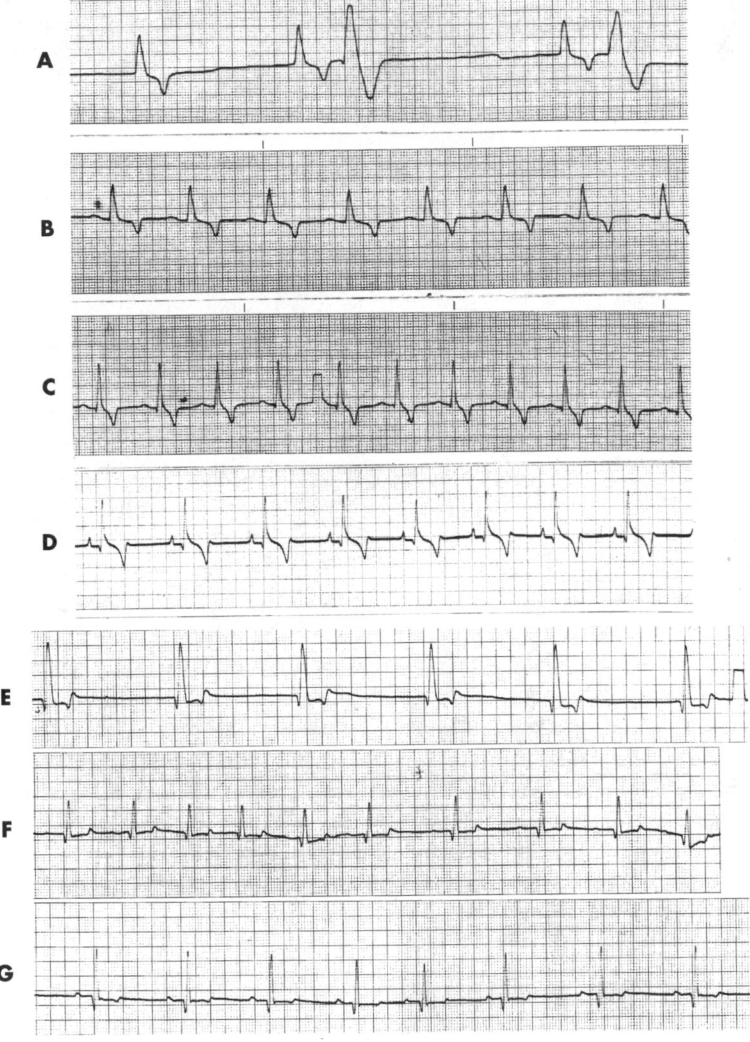

Figure 18-1

The electrocardiographic appearance of 2 dogs (Dog 1: **A, B, C, D;** and Dog 2: **E, F, G**) with hyperkalemia due to Addison's disease. In tracings **A** and **E** the effects of severe hyperkalemia (8.6 mEq/L and 9.4 mEq/L) are manifested as a lack of visible P waves, short and wide QRS complexes, and a slow heart rate. Note that the T waves are not of excessive amplitude. Tracing **A** also demonstrates ventricular escape beats, which are the wide and bizarre-looking QRS complexes following the more normal-appearing QRS complexes. This may be due to hyperkalemia, hypoxia, or both. Tracings **B** and **F** were obtained after treating each dog for 1 hour with IV 0.9% saline solution as the only treatment. This lowered the serum potassium concentration to 7.6 and 7.9 mEq/L, respectively. Note that the P waves have begun to return, the heart rate has increased, and the ventricular escape beats have disappeared. Also note the prolonged P-R interval (first-degree heart block); improved, but still widened QRS complexes; and a shortened Q-T segment. Tracings **C** and **G** were collected when the serum potassium concentrations were 6.2 and 5.9 mEq/L, respectively. The P-R interval and P, QRS, and T waves are of a shorter duration, and the R waves are taller. Tracing **D** demonstrates a more spiked T wave. This serum potassium concentration was 5.6 mEq/L. (From Feldman EC: In Ettinger SJ (Ed): *Textbook of veterinary medicine,* 2nd ed, Philadelphia, 1983, WB Saunders, p. 1664.)

Table 18-5 for a review of common clinicopathologic abnormalities.

TREATMENT

Patients with acute crisis or a significant number of clinical signs need hospitalization and treatment. Those with subtle or mild signs can be treated at home. The primary goals are to replace depleted volume rapidly, correct electrolyte status, and provide hormone replacement therapy.

Correcting hypovolemia and addressing electrolyte imbalances are the most important primary goals. The fluid of choice is 0.9% sodium chloride administered at a maintenance volume plus dehydration deficit volume (percentage dehydration times body weght in kilograms) over a 24-hour period. Rapid rehydration of the dehydration deficit over 4 to 12 hours may be necessary in some severely affected patients (Table 18-5).

Initially, parenteral glucocorticoid administration is advised. Once the patient is stable, mineralocorticoid support can be used. The glucocorticoid of choice is dexamethasone sodium phosphate. It is inexpensive and readily available. It is a water-soluble, rapid-onset steroid and it does not cross-react with the cortisol assay needed for the ACTH stimulation test. (See Table 18-6 for glucocorticoid dosage recommendations.) Once patients are more stable, those with primary hypoadrenocorticism can have mineralocorticoids added to their treatment. Desoxycorticosterone

TABLE 18-4 Clinical Signs Associated with Hypoadrenocorticism and Addisonian Crisis

Most Common (50%-100% of Patients)	Common (25%-50%)	Rare (<25%)
Lethargy and depression	Dehydration	Weak pulses
Anorexia	Diarrhea	Bradycardia (<60 bpm)
Vomiting weakness	Waxing and waning course	Melena
Weight loss	Collapse	Painful abdomen
	Hypothermia	Hair loss
	Previous response to therapy	
	Slow capillary refill time	
	Shaking	
	Polyuria	
	Polydipsia	

Adapted from Kintzer PP, Peterson ME: Hypoadrenocorticism in dogs. In Bonagura JD, (Ed): *Kirk's veterinary therapy XII.* Philadelphia, 1995, WB Saunders, p. 425.

TABLE 18-5 Clinicopathologic Findings in Patients with Hypoadrenocorticism

Most Common (50%-100% of Patients)	Common (25%-50%)	Rare (<25%)
Sodium : potassium ratio <27	Hypochloremia	Hyperbilirubinemia
Hyperkalemia	Decreased total CO_2	Eosinophilia
Azotemia	Hypercalcemia	Hypoglycemia
Hyponatremia	Increased liver enzyme activities (alanine aminotransferase and aspartate aminotransferase)	Lymphocytosis
Submaximal urine concentration	Anemia	

Adapted from Kintzer PP, Peterson ME: Hypoadrenocorticism in dogs. In Bonagura JD, (Ed): *Kirk's veterinary therapy XII.* Philadelphia, 1995, WB Saunders, p. 425.

Table 18-6 Commonly Used Steroid Replacement Medications and Dosages

Drug	Dosage, Route, and Frequency
Glucocorticoids	
Prednisolone sodium succinate	11-25 mg/kg IV q 2-6 hr
Dexamethasone sodium phosphate	1-3 mg/kg IV q 12 hr
Hydrocortisone sodium hemisuccinate	1-2 mg/kg IV q 8 hr
Hydrocortisone phosphate	1-2 mg/kg IV q 8 hr
Dexamethasone	2-4 mg/kg IV q 12-24 hr
Mineralocorticoids	
Desoxycorticosterone pivalate	1.1-2.2 mg/kg IM or SQ q 21-30 days
Fludrocortisone acetate	Dogs: 0.02 mg/kg PO q 24 hr or divided q 12 hr Cats: 0.1-0.2 mg/cat PO q 24 hr
Hydrocortisone acetate	1-2 mg/kg PO q 12 hr

pivalate (DOCP) is the most economical way to replace mineralocorticoids. DOCP is dosed at 1.1 to 2.2 mg/kg intramuscularly every 21 to 30 days. It has no glucocorticoid activity, so supplementation with prednisone or prednisolone at a dosage of 0.1 to 0.2 mg/kg/day probably will be necessary. Alternatively, fludrocortisone acetate is dosed at 0.01 to 0.02 mg/kg/day orally divided twice daily. Because fludrocortisone has some glucocorticoid activity, only about 50% of dogs need oral prednisone or prednisolone supplementation. The mineralocorticoid dosage should be based on clinical signs and electrolyte concentrations. The glucocorticoid dosage should be based primarily on the presence of gastrointestinal signs.

The hyperkalemia in some patients may warrant more than just fluid therapy. In patients with severe bradycardia or serious electrocardiographic abnormalities, serum potassium must be lowered more rapidly. Intravenous dextrose (1000 mg/kg diluted 1:1 with sterile water slow intravenous infusion) with regular insulin (0.5 u/kg intravenously) promotes cellular uptake of potassium and phosphorus. Supplementing the fluids with 0.01 to 0.03 mmol phosphate/kg/hr (potassium phosphate = 3.3 mmol phosphate/ml) helps prevent hypophosphatemia. In life-threatening cases of hyperkalemia, administer 10% calcium gluconate at a dosage of 0.5 to 1.0 ml/kg slow intravenous infusion over 15 to 30 minutes. Calcium provides important cardioprotective effects. Monitor the electrocardiograph (ECG) closely while administering the calcium. Bradycardia and Q-T interval shortening are indications to stop.

Monitoring

Careful monitoring of the heart rate and ECG is very important because fatal arrhythmias can occur. During initial therapy, the heart rate and rhythm must be recorded every 1 to 2 hours while a continuous ECG is monitored. Electrolytes should be measured every 4 to 6 hours initially. Once stable, they can be checked every 12 to 24 hours. Blood work to reevaluate for azotemia, hypercalcemia, and hypophosphatemia should be performed daily or every other day.

As with any dehydrated patient, weighing the patient twice daily and monitoring skin turgor are important. Measuring urine output is a good way to determine when patients are rehydrated or whether renal insufficiency exists.

Fludrocortisone therapy monitoring includes measuring the serum electrolyte, calcium, blood urea nitrogen (BUN), and creatinine concentrations every 2 to 4 weeks until the patient is stable. Once the patient is stable, monitoring every 3 to 6 months is sufficient. After the first DOCP injection, the serum electrolyte, calcium, BUN, and creatinine concentrations should be measured 3 weeks and 4 weeks after the injection. This will establish the duration of action of the DOCP. Most patients need injections every 21 to 30 days. Changes in the dosage are based on blood work abnormalities. If signs of gastrointestinal upset (nausea, anorexia, vomiting) occur, supplement with prednisone or prednisolone.

HYPERCALCEMIA

DEFINITION AND CAUSES

Hypercalcemia is the state of increased serum total calcium concentrations. If hypoalbuminemia exists, the calcium concentrations should be corrected in dogs using the following formulas:

$$\text{Corrected Ca} = \text{Ca (mg/dl)} - \text{Albumin (g/dl)} + 3.5$$

or

$$\text{Corrected Ca} = \text{Ca (mg/dl)} - [0.4 \times \text{Total protein (g/dl)}] + 3.3$$

These formulas do not apply to cats, although hypoalbuminemia also affects their serum calcium. Lipemia and hemolysis cause artifactual hypercalcemia. Also, young animals with physiologic bone growth have benign hypercalcemia.

The most common cause of persistent hypercalcemia is hypercalcemia of malignancy. Lymphoma is by far the most common malignancy causing hypercalcemia. Other neoplasms, such as anal sac adenocarcinoma, multiple myeloma, myeloproliferative disease, and solid tissue tumors have also been reported to cause hypercalcemia. Any neoplastic disorder could cause hypercalcemia. Other important rule-outs include renal insufficiency (most patients have normal serum calcium concentrations), primary hyperparathyroidism, and hypoadrenocorticism. Less common causes are granulomatous diseases such as fungal infections (blastomycosis), osteolytic bone lesions (primary or metastatic neoplasia, septic osteomyelitis), calciferol-containing rodenticide intoxication (hypervitaminosis D), oral calcium supplements, oral phosphate binders, thiazide diuretics, and plant intoxications (*Cestrum diurnum, Solanum malacoxylon, Triestum flavescens*). There is also an ill-defined syndrome of idiopathic hypercalcemia in the cat that warrants further in-depth evaluation. See Box 18-2 for a list of the most common causes of hypercalcemia.

Box 18-2 Causes of Hypercalcemia in Dogs and Cats

- Hypercalcemia of malignancy
  - Lymphoma (most common)
  - Anal sac adenocarcinoma
  - Multiple myeloma
  - Myeloproliferative disease
  - Solid tissue tumors
- Primary hyperparathyroidism
- Primary renal insufficiency
- Hypoadrenocorticism
- Chronic granulomatous diseases
- Fungal disease (blastomycosis)
- Osteolytic bone lesions
- Calciferol-containing rodenticides
- Hypervitaminosis D
- Plant intoxications
  - *Cestrum diurnum*
  - *Solanum malacoxylon*
  - *Triestum flavescens*
- Oral calcium supplements
- Oral phosphate binders
- Thiazide diuretics
- Idiopathic causes
- Hyperalbuminemia
- Laboratory error

Adapted from Chew DJ, et al: Disorders of calcium: hyperkalemia and hypocalcemia. In: DiBartola SP, ed: *Fluid therapy in small animal practice.* Philadelphia, 1992, WB Saunders Co, pp. 169 and 157.

PRESENTATION

Because there are many causes of hypercalcemia, there is no specific signalment at the time of presentation. Refer to the literature to review the signalments for the most common causes. See Table 18-7 for a list of clinical signs associated with hypercalcemia.

Hypercalcemia affects primarily four body systems: renal, gastrointestinal, neuromuscular, and cardiovascular. The most common renal signs are polyuria, polydipsia, and signs of renal failure. Calcium inhibits vasopressin receptors in the kidney and prevents free water reabsorption, creating nephrogenic diabetes insipidus. Very severe hypercalcemia (more than 15 mg/dl) can lead to tubular necrosis and renal failure and minerali-

TABLE 18-7 Clinical Signs Associated with Hypercalcemia

Common	Uncommon
Polyuria	Seizures
Polydipsia	Stupor
Anorexia	Coma
Vomiting	Constipation
Depression or lethargy	Electrocardiography abnormalities
Dehydration	Prolonged P-R interval
Weakness	Shortened Q-T segment
	Ventricular fibrillation
	Death

zation. Vomiting, anorexia, lethargy, and depression are common signs of renal failure. On physical examination, small kidneys suggest that the kidney disease has been chronic and may be the cause of the hypercalcemia. In some patients, signs of urolithiasis are present, and uroliths can be palpated in the urinary bladder or urethra.

Hypercalcemia reduces excitability of smooth, skeletal, and cardiac muscle and causes gastrointestinal dysfunction. Anorexia, vomiting, and constipation are most common. Firm stool can be felt in the colon. Alterations in skeletal muscle function cause generalized weakness (common) and muscle twitching (uncommon). Cardiac conduction abnormalities such as prolonged P-R interval, shortened Q-T segment, and ventricular fibrillation may be present but tend to be uncommon.

The most common direct effect of hypercalcemia on the central nervous system is lethargy. Rarely does this progress to seizures, stupor, or coma.

Careful palpation of the lymph nodes and abdomen is important. Lymphadenomegaly or organomegaly may support lymphoma or other neoplasia. A complete rectal examination to palpate for lymph nodes or pelvic canal tumors is essential. A waxing and waning history may suggest hypoadrenocorticism. Palpating the neck may reveal a parathyroid tumor.

Because hypercalcemia has many causes, additional laboratory values may help define the cause. Hyperphosphatemia without azotemia suggests a nonparathyroid cause. Hypophosphatemia or low normal phosphorus is most common with primary hyperparathyroidism or malignancy. Combinations of hyperphosphatemia with azotemia are difficult to assess because renal failure is both a cause and a result of hypercalcemia. Renal failure rarely causes calcium concentration to exceed 15 mg/dl. Serum ionized calcium is high with primary hyperparathyroidism or hypercalcemia of malignancy. Low or low normal ionized calcium is seen in patients with renal failure. Intact parathormone concentrations are high in primary hyperparathyroidism and renal failure and low normal or low in hypercalcemia of malignancy. Other electrolyte abnormalities such as hyponatremia with hyperkalemia are associated with hypoadrenocorticism.

Ancillary diagnostic tests such as radiography and ultrasonography can be used to evaluate for kidney size and architecture, bone lesions, urolithiasis, hepatic and splenic architecture, and lymphadenopathy. Fine needle aspirates, biopsies, and bone marrow analysis may be needed. An ACTH stimulation test can be used to rule out hypoadrenocorticism.

TREATMENT

Treatment focuses primarily on removing the underlying cause and on volume expansion. It is important not to allow treatment to inhibit the clinician's ability to identify the underlying cause. The cause in many cases may be readily identified but not immediately treatable. Therefore, supportive care is needed.

Volume expansion with intravenous 0.9% sodium chloride at a rate of 100 to 180 ml/kg/day is recommended. Fluids containing calcium such as lactated Ringer's solution should be avoided. Any dehydration deficit should be added into the fluid rate. In conditions of dehydration, the kidneys reabsorb sodium and calcium more effectively. Rehydration and volume expansion allow naturesis and calciuresis to occur. To prevent iatrogenic hypokalemia, potassium supplementation is necessary. Volume expansion is sufficient in most patients to resolve the hypercalcemia; however, some patients need additional supportive care.

Calciuretic diuretics can be used after rehydration and volume expansion have been completed. Furosemide, a loop diuretic, is the diuretic of choice. Thiazide diuretics should not be used. In the acute management of severe hypercalcemia, fuorsemide can be dosed at 5 mg/kg intravenously once, followed by a constant-rate infusion of 5 mg/kg/hr. Alternatively, a dosage of 2 to 4 mg/kg intravenously, intramuscularly, or orally given twice or three times daily can be used. Remember to maintain adequate hydration while using diuretic therapy.

Glucocorticoids increase renal calcium excretion, decrease gut calcium absorption, and decrease bone resorption. They are also cytotoxic to hematopoietic neoplasms such as lymphoma. It is very important to collect all diagnostic samples before glucocorticoid usage if lymphoid neoplasia is suspected. If hypoadrenocorticism is suspected, dexamethasone is the preferred glucocorticoid because it will not interfere with the cortisol assay. Glucocorticoids also help antagonize the effects of vitamin D intoxication. In the short term, steroids may reduce inflammation and hypercalcemia associated with granulomatous disease, but high-dose or intermediate- or long-term use may cause a progression of disease, especially fungal disease. Prednisone or prednisolone can be used at a dosage of 1 to 2 mg/kg orally, subcutaneously, or intramuscularly twice daily. Dexamethasone can be used at a dosage of 0.1 to 0.2 mg/kg intravenously, intramuscularly, subcutaneously, or orally twice daily.

Sodium bicarbonate therapy is controversial. Most clinicians reserve it to manage acute crises in the presence of metabolic acidosis. Ionized calcium concentrations decrease as serum pH rises because the calcium binds to serum proteins and bicarbonate ions. A dosage of 1 to 4 mEq/kg as a slow intravenous bolus has been recommended. It may take up to 24 hours to see results. Multiple dosing may be needed, but generally constant-rate infusions are not necessary. Refrain from using bicarbonate if calcium and acid-base status cannot be measured. Bicarbonate seems to work best in combination with other treatments.

Bone resorption inhibitors such as calcitonin, diphosphonates, and mithramycin are much less commonly used. Calcitonin (5 u/kg intravenously initially, then 4 to 8 u/kg subcutaneously every 6 to 24 hours) is a hormone that antagonizes parathormone. It is used as an antidote for calciferol-containing rodenticides. It can also be used as a temporary treatment for primary hyperparathyroidism. It is expensive, has a short duration of action, and can cause anorexia and vomiting. Diphosphonates (biphosphonates) are metal-complexing compounds that also inhibit calcitriol (active vitamin D) production by inhibiting 1-α-hydroxylase. Etidronate has limited use in veterinary medicine, but oral doses of 2.5 mg/kg orally twice daily for the dog and 5 mg/kg orally twice daily for the cat have been reported. It also is available as an intravenous solution. No intravenous dosage has been reported, but it is believed to be lower than the oral dosage. Pamidronate is a new diphosphonate. The intravenous dose is 1.3 to 2.0 mg/kg delivered in an IV solution with 0.9% saline over a 2-hour period. The dose is repeated 3 days later and can be used every 3 to 4 days to control the hypercalcemia. Mithramycin is a very expensive antineoplastic agent that is also a potent inhibitor of bone resorption. This medication has been used infrequently in veterinary medicine for treating hypercalcemia. A single dose of 25 μg/kg has been recommended, but once- or twice-weekly dosing may be needed to treat hypercalcemia effectively. Significant nephrotoxicity, hepatotoxicity, and myelosuppression can occur.

Monitoring

Weighing the patient twice daily, evaluating skin turgor, and monitoring urine output should be used to monitor hydration status. Ionized or serum calcium should be measured every 12 to 24 hours during initial therapy. Urinalysis (look for renal casts) and reevaluation of BUN and creatinine must be performed to monitor kidney function. Electrolytes must be followed to identify imbalances caused by fluid therapy. If ECG abnormalities are present, an ECG must be reevaluated every 12 to 24 hours. Phosphorus concentrations must be monitored because persistent hyperphosphatemia with hypercalcemia can result in tissue mineralization, especially if the product of the calcium times phosphorus concentrations is greater than 60.

HYPOCALCEMIA

Hypocalcemia is the state of decreased serum total calcium concentrations. If hypoalbuminemia exists, the calcium concentrations should be corrected in dogs using the following formulas:

$$\text{Corrected Ca} = \text{Ca (mg/dl)} - \text{Albumin (g/dl)} + 3.5$$

or

$$\text{Corrected Ca} = \text{Ca (mg/dl)} - [0.4 \times \text{Total protein (g/dl)}] + 3.3$$

These formulas do not apply to cats, although hypoalbuminemia also affects their serum calcium. Hypoalbuminemia is the most common cause of hypocalcemia in dogs and cats. It does not cause clinical signs because ionized calcium (physiologically active calcium) concentrations remain normal. See Box 18-3 for a list of causes of hypocalcemia in dogs and cats.

Box 18-3 Causes of Hypercalcemia in Dogs and Cats

Hypoalbuminemia
Primary renal insufficiency (including ethylene glycol intoxication)
Puerperal tetany (eclampsia)
Pancreatitis
Primary hypoparathyroidism
Severe intestinal malabsorptive disease
Phosphate enema administration
Secondary renal hyperparathyroidism
Iatrogenic causes
Postoperative thyroid or parathyroid surgery
Sodium bicarbonate oversupplementation
Intravenous phosphate oversupplementation
Dietary imbalance
Alkalemia
Laboratory error
Sample handling (collected in calcium-chelating anticoagulant)

Adapted from Chew DJ, et al: Disorders of calcium: hyperkalemia and hypocalcemia. In: DiBartola SP, ed: *Fluid therapy in small animal practice*. Philadelphia, 1992, WB Saunders Co, pp. 169 and 157.

Other common causes include chronic and acute renal failure, puerperal tetany (eclampsia), and acute pancreatitis. In renal failure, mass law interactions of calcium with hyperphosphatemia result in hypocalcemia. Additionally, decreased 1-α-hydroxylase activity and subsequent calcitriol (active vitamin D) production in the kidney significantly contribute to hypocalcemia. Puerperal tetany usually occurs within the first 21 days of lactation, generally in small-breed bitches. Eclampsia causes large amounts of calcium to be diverted into milk production. Acute pancreatitis causes hypocalcemia by mineralization of traumatized tissues and precipitation of calcium salts in saponified fat.

Hypoparathyroidism is an uncommon to rare disease of dogs and cats. It can be a spontaneous primary disease or an iatrogenic result of thyroid surgery (especially cats). It can also be a result of rapid reversal of chronic hypercalcemia or removal of a functional parathyroid tumor. In all cases, the lack of parathormone results in reduced gut absorption of calcium, decreased renal reabsorption of calcium, and unopposed osteoblastic activity (bone production).

Other causes include intestinal malabsorption, which is seen in patients with severe, diffuse gastrointestinal disease such as lymphangiectasia, inflammatory bowel disease, and infiltrative neoplasia (lymphoma, mast cell tumor). Ethylene glycol intoxication causes precipitation of calcium salts, usually in the urinary tract and soft tissues. Severely traumatized or necrotic tissue can take up calcium and cause mild hypocalcemia. Phosphate enemas (Fleet enemas) cause severe hyperphosphatemia and subsequent mass law effects with serum calcium. Phosphate enemas affect small dogs and cats more severely. Oversupplementation with sodium bicarbonate or intravenous phosphate infusions can cause iatrogenic hypocalcemia. Dietary vitamin D deficiencies are uncommon, as is chronic consumption of low calcium, high-phosphorus diets (all meat). Any condition that creates alkalosis will cause a shift from protein-bound (measured total serum calcium) to ionized calcium.

Laboratory error should be ruled out if the patient's sign do not correlate with the laboratory data. Sampling technique should be reviewed. Citrate, oxalate, and EDTA all chelate calcium and spuriously reduce serum calcium concentrations.

Presentation

Because there are many causes of hypocalcemia, there is no specific signalment at the time of presentation. Refer to the texts and literature to review the signalments for the most common causes. A careful history is extremely important in evaluating these patients (recent parturition, enemas given, toxin exposure, trauma, recent thyroid or parathyroid surgery, or historical cues of renal failure).

Hypocalcemia affects primarily the neuromuscular, cardiovascular, gastrointestinal, and respiratory systems. Neuromuscular excitability is increased by hypocalcemia. Clinical signs generally do not occur unless the calcium concentration is below 6.5 mg/dl in dogs. Acute hypocalcemia is associated with more severe clinical signs, whereas chronic hypocalcemia results in adaptation by the body, and patients may show few signs even with calcium concentrations less than 5.0 mg/dl. The most common neuromuscular signs are weakness, facial rubbing, muscle fasciculations or twitching, tetany, ataxia, and seizures. A fever may be recorded in patients that have excessive muscle activity. Common cardiovascular changes are bradycardia and ECG changes. These changes include prolongation of the S-T segment and Q-T segment and wide T waves or T-wave alternans (Figure 18-2). Anorexia and vomiting are common gastrointestinal signs and are the most common clinical signs seen in cats. Panting or respiratory arrest also can be seen. Other less common signs are polyuria and polydipsia. This may result from nephrocalcinosis secondary to conditions that cause hypercalciuria (hypoparathyroidism). A painful abdomen may be a sign of pancreatitis. (See Box 18-4 for common clinical signs associated with hypocalcemia.)

Treatment

Patients with clinical signs of hypocalcemia should be hospitalized and treated. Hypocalcemia caused

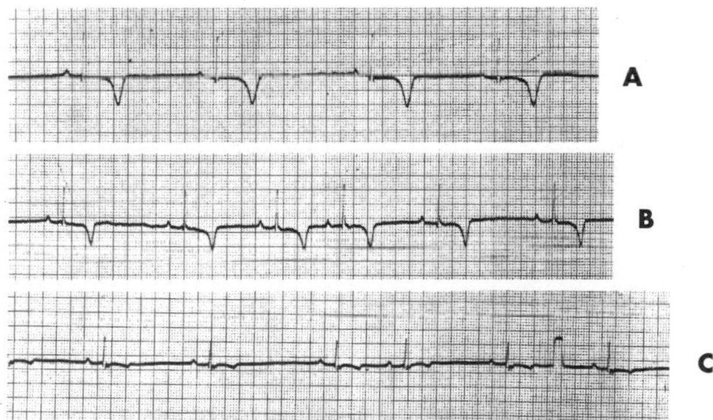

Figure 18-2

The electrocardiographic appearance of a dog with hypocalcemia secondary to primary hypoparathyroidism during various stages of treatment. Tracing **A** demonstrates prolonged S-T and Q-T segments, and prolonged (wide) and deep T waves. The serum calcium concentration was 4.0 mg/dl, and the electrolyte concentrations were within reference ranges. Tracing **B** shows improvements in S-T, Q-T, and T wave duration and amplitude as the serum calcium concentration has been increased to 6.2 mg/dl. Tracing **C** is from when the calcium concentration was returned to the reference range (9.7 mg/dl). The S-T, Q-T and T waves are normal. The three tracings also suggest diminishing R wave amplitude and increased heart rate as the serum calcium concentration rises to normal. (From Feldman EC, Nelson RW: *Canine and feline endocrinology and reproduction,* ed 2, Philadelphia, 1996, WB Saunders, p. 504.)

Box 18-4 The Most Common Clinical Signs Associated with Hypocalcemia

Muscle tremor or fasciculation
Facial rubbing
Weakness
Panting
Restlessness
Excitation
Disorientation
Hypersensitivity to stimuli
Stiff gait or ataxia
Prolapsed nictitans (cats)
Seizures
Posterior lenticular cataracts (hypoparathyroidism)
Fever
Electrocardiographic changes
- Bradycardia or tachycardia
- Prolonged S-T segment
- Prolonged Q-T segment
- Wide T waves
- T-wave alterans

Anorexia (especially cats)
Vomiting (especially cats)
Polyuria and polydipsia
Respiratory arrest

Adapted from Chew DJ, et al: Disorders of calcium: hyperkalemia and hypocalcemia. In: DiBartola SP, ed: *Fluid therapy in small animal practice*. Philadelphia, 1992, WB Saunders Co, pp. 169 and 157.

solely by hypoalbuminemia does not warrant treatment; the cause of the albumin deficit must be identified and treated. Treatment focuses on parenteral calcium salt therapy. Patients with severe hypocalcemia usually have primary or iatrogenic hypoparathyroidism or puerperal tetany (eclampsia) or have been given phosphate-containing enemas. Any cause could create signs severe enough to warrant treatment, however.

The two most commonly used parenteral calcium products are calcium gluconate 10% solution and calcium chloride 10% solution. Calcium chloride is three times more potent than calcium gluconate, but calcium gluconate is preferred because it causes much less vessel irritation and is not caustic if it extravasates. See Table 18-8 for dosing information. It is important to monitor the ECG while the calcium is being administered. Bradycardia and Q-T segment shortening are indications to temporarily stop the infusion. Acute treatment is by slow intravenous bolus infusion. After serious neurologic signs, tetany, and excessive muscle activity are stabilized, a constant-rate infusion of calcium can be given to prevent relapses, which can occur anywhere from 1 to 24 hours after a bolus infusion. If a bitch has puerperal tetany, any puppies should be removed. Long-term therapy may include oral calcium and vitamin D supplements (Table 18-8).

Laboratory testing (complete blood cell count, serum biochemistry profile, and urinalysis) is needed to evaluate these patients. Azotemia and submaximal urine concentration are hallmarks of renal failure and ethylene glycol intoxication. Although both increase anion gaps, ethylene glycol intoxication usually produces an anion gap of 40 mEq/L or greater. Increased amylase and lipase activities and an inflammatory leukogram are seen in patients with pancreatitis. These patients may also have a secondary hepatitis, as evidenced by increased liver enzyme activities and total bilirubin concentration. Hyperphosphatemia can be seen in patients with renal failure, ethylene glycol intoxication, and primary hypoparathyroidism and in those that have been given a phosphate-containing enema. The presence of increased total CO_2 concentrations supports alkalosis. Blood gases should be evaluated in these patients. Ancillary testing including ethylene glycol testing of the serum, radiography to help evaluate bone density and renal size and shape, ultrasonography of the abdomen to evaluate the kidneys, and intact parathormone concentrations can be helpful.

Monitoring

During initial management in severely affected patients, calcium concentrations should be measured every 4 to 6 hours, if possible. It is also important to monitor the ECG continuously. Bradycardia, Q-T interval shortening, vomiting, and cardiac arrest are signs to stop calcium administration. Neuromuscular signs may persist

TABLE 18-8 Commonly Used Calcium and Vitamin D Supplements and Dosages

Drug	Dosage, Route, and Frequency
Parenteral calcium	
Calcium gluconate 10% solution (9.3 mg Ca/ml)	Initial: 0.5-1.5 ml/kg slow IV Maintenance: 5-15 mg/kg/hr IV infusion or 1-2 ml/kg diluted 1 : 1 with saline SQ TID
Calcium chloride 10% solution (27.2 mg Ca/ml)	5-15 mg/kg/hr IV infusion
Oral calcium supplements	
Calcium carbonate	25-50 mg/kg/day
Calcium gluconate	25-50 mg/kg/day
Calcium lactate	25-50 mg/kg/day
Calcium chloride	25-50 mg/kg/day
Vitamin D supplements	
Dihydrotachysterol	Initial: 0.02-0.03 mg/kg/day PO Maintenance: 0.01-0.02 mg/kg PO q 24-48 hr
Calcitriol	2.5-10 ng/kg/day PO
Ergocalciferol	Initial: 4000-6000 U/kg/day PO Maintenance: 1000-2000 U/kg PO q 1-7 days

for 30 to 60 minutes after adequate correction of serum calcium concentrations. Repeat seizures and excessive muscle activity may cause hyperthermia severe enough to warrant tepid baths. If the patient has kidney disease or ethylene glycol intoxication, urine production and hydration status (body weight, skin turgor, packed cell volume) must be monitored closely. Fluid therapy is needed for patients with acute renal failure or ethylene glycol intoxication. Venous blood gases must be monitored every 12 to 24 hours initially in patients with alkalosis. Long-term monitoring of the stable patient includes monthly calcium concentration evaluation for the first 6 months, then every 3 to 4 months.

HYPOGLYCEMIA

Hypoglycemia is the state of decreased serum glucose concentration. Causes usually are divided into those that accelerate glucose removal and those that cause a failure of glucose production or secretion. It is always important to rule out improper sample handling and processing before pursuing a diagnostic evaluation of these patients. Red cells that are allowed to sit in the tube for more than 1 hour before separation show artifactual hypoglycemia. See Box 18-5 for a list of causes of hypoglycemia in dogs and cats.

Many disorders promote more rapid glucose removal from the plasma. Insulinomas are a rare tumor of the pancreatic B cells that have uncontrolled insulin secretion. This is the most common tumor associated with hypoglycemia in the dog. Other tumors (e.g., hepatoma, hepatocellular carcinoma, lymphoma, leiomyosarcoma, plasmacytoid tumors, oral melanoma, hemangiosarcoma, salivary gland adenocarcinoma) produce insulin-like proteins that are biologically active; however, it is likely that other factors are involved with paraneoplastic hypoglycemia. Some patients have such a large tumor burden that it consumes a disproportionately large amount of glucose to sustain its aberrant metabolic needs. Accidental iatrogenic overdosage of exogenous insulin is an important consideration in all diabetic patients. Increased red blood cell mass (polycythemia) causes hypoglycemia by using glucose to support the metabolic needs of the red blood cells. Patients with Fanconi syndrome or primary renal glucosuria lose glucose in their urine. Rarely do bitches in late-term ges-

Box 18-5 Causes of Hypoglycemia in Dogs and Cats

Delayed separation of serum from the red cells
Insulinoma
Extrapancreatic neoplasia
Neonatal hypoglycemia
Toy breed dog hypoglycemia
Hunting dog hypoglycemia
Intoxication
- Ethanol
- Salicylates
- Propranolol
- Ethylene glycol
- Oral hypoglycemic agents
- Iatrogenic insulin overdosage

Sepsis or endotoxemia
End-stage hepatic disease
Glycogen storage disease
Severe polycythemia
Late-term gestation
Prolonged seizure activity
Starvation or malabsorptive disease
Severe primary glucosuria or Fanconi syndrome
Hypoadrenocorticism

tation experience hypoglycemia because of high demand by the fetuses. Severe prolonged seizures cause increased consumption of glucose by the overactive skeletal muscle (seizures usually cause an increase in serum glucose because they increase cortisol and epinephrine secretion). Intoxications with ethanol, salicylates, propranolol, and oral hypoglycemic agents also are reported causes.

The most common diseases associated with a failure to produce or secrete glucose are neonatal hypoglycemia and toy breed hypoglycemia. With neonatal hypoglycemia, young puppies and kittens have low hepatic glycogen stores and a reduced ability to perform gluconeogenesis. Therefore, short periods of fasting can cause hypoglycemia. Starvation or malabsorptive gastrointestinal disease associated with preexisting systemic illness can deplete the liver of glycogen stores. After prolonged periods of physical exertion and little or no food consumption, hypoglycemia may occur, as in hunting dog hypoglycemia. An uncommon cause is end-stage hepatic insufficiency. Glucose homeostasis is one of the last functions to be lost with advanced liver disease.

Some diseases are a combination of mechanisms. Sepsis and endotoxemic shock promote increased glucose use by the body by altering metabolism and increasing insulin release. They also deplete hepatic glycogen stores making less glucose available for release. Patients with hypoadrenocorticism (Addison's disease) have an absence of counterregulatory cortisol, which facilitates increased insulin action (increased consumption) and decreased gluconeogenesis (decreased glucose secretion). This results in mild to moderate hypoglycemia.

Presentation

There is no specific signalment for patients with hypoglycemia; however, age, breed, and breeding status (i.e., young puppies and kittens, toy breed dogs, hunting breed dogs, pregnant bitches) are important in evaluating these cases. Hypoglycemia affects primarily the nervous and the musculoskeletal systems.

Nervous tissue relies on glucose as its primary energy source, and hypoglycemia causes central nervous system depression. Typical signs include lethargy, depression, ataxia, paraparesis, and, in some cases, seizures. Abnormal behaviors such as fly-biting, stargazing, and staring at walls also can be seen (Box 18-6). Hypoglycemia also stimulates appetite, and polyphagia may be a presenting sign. The skeletal muscle also needs large amounts of energy to maintain normal function. Patients with hypoglycemia display muscle weakness, collapse, muscle fasciculations, and exercise intolerance.

Many patients have few or no clinical signs. Some animals adapt to their presistent hypoglycemia and may have few clinical signs, even with blood glucose concentrations as low as 50 mg/dl. Those with paraneoplastic or a large neoplastic burden usually have obvious physical examination abnormalities. Additional laboratory evaluation may show a leukocytosis and abnormalities associated with specific organs that may be affected (e.g., liver, kidneys). Animals with plasmacytoid tumors can have hyperglobulinemia and proteinuria. Additional testing such as urine Bence-Jones

Box 18-6 The Most Common Clinical Signs Associated with Hypoglycemia

Depression or lethargy
Ataxia
Paraparesis
Seizures
Abnormal behavior
- Fly-biting
- Stargazing
- Staring at walls

Polyphagia
Muscle weakness
Collapse
Muscle fasciculation
Exercise intolerance

protein, bone marrow analysis, and radiographs of the skeleton are needed to verify the diagnosis. Animals with an insulinoma have an inappropriately high plasma insulin concentration in the face of hypoglycemia in two thirds to three quarters of patients. A fasted (8 to 12 hours) insulin : glucose ratio should be evaluated. An amended insulin to glucose ratio (AIGR) can be determined using the following formula:

$$\text{AIGR} = [\text{Plasma insulin } (\mu\text{U/ml}) \times 100] \,/\, [\text{Plasma glucose (mg/dl)} - 30]$$

If the plasma glucose is less than or equal to 30 mg/dl, then the denominator for the equation should be 1. Amended ratios above 30 indicate insulin-secreting tumors. Ratios between 19 and 30 are difficult to interpret, and testing must be repeated. If the ratio is below 19, an insulinoma is unlikely. False-positive results can occur if the patient's blood glucose is below 40 mg/dl.

Patients with end-stage liver disease or portovascular anomaly often have other clinical signs. Dogs and cats with portovascular anomaly often have stunted growth, are thin, and have polyuria and polydipsia. Usually they are juvenile to middle-aged. Gastrointestinal signs, icterus, and ascites are more common with end-stage liver disease or severe hepatic dysfunction. Laboratory findings that may be observed include anemia, microcytosis (especially portovascular anomaly), decreased BUN, hypoalbuminemia, and increased serum liver enzyme activities. The fasted and 2-hour postprandial bile acid concentrations are elevated. Urinalysis may reveal urate crystals (especially portovascular anomaly), bilirubinuria, and low urine concentrations.

Animals with sepsis are very ill. These cats and dogs are shocky and febrile and have injected mucous membranes when they are in the hyperdynamic phases of septic shock. In the later hypodynamic phase, hypothermia, pale mucous membranes, and signs of circulatory collapse are seen. The leukogram can vary from leukopenic to leukocytosis. Evidence of organ failure may be evident (liver, kidneys), and a coagulation profile may reveal disseminated intravascular coagulopathy. Blood cultures should be performed.

Dogs and cats with hypoadrenocorticism often have a waxing and waning history. In addition to hypoglycemia, biochemical analysis may reveal azotemia, hypercalcemia, hyponatremia, and hyperkalemia. A reverse stress leukogram (lymphocytosis, eosinophilia) can be seen.

Rarely a dog or cat presents with an uncommon cause of hypoglycemia. Glycogen storage diseases are rare and most commonly seen in animals less than 1 year old. Polycythemic patients present with dark mucous membranes, weakness, polyuria, polydipsia, and seizures, and have a packed cell volume greater than 65%.

TREATMENT

The goal of therapy is to increase serum glucose concentrations by administering intravenous dextrose. All patients with clinical signs should be treated. Patients that are able to eat (alert, not vomiting) should be fed as a part of their therapy. Some causes of hypoglycemia necessitate treatment of an underlying cause, and some warrant long-term therapy. Diagnostic testing must be performed to identify the underlying cause of the hypoglycemia.

Intravenous 50% dextrose at 1 to 4 ml/kg diluted 1 : 1 with sterile water delivered over a 15-minute period typically is given as an initial treatment for severe hypoglycemia. Patients with an insulinoma may have an increase in insulin secretion in response to the dextrose infusion, thus driving the blood glucose lower. Frequent feedings of foods high in complex carbohydrates may be better for these patients. If this is unsuccessful, a dextrose infusion may be better than an intravenous bolus of dextrose. Infusions of 2.5% or 5% dextrose solutions can be delivered at a rate that maintains a blood glucose high enough to eliminate clinical signs of hypoglycemia. Some patients may need dextrose concentrations of 10% or higher. Potassium supplementation should be used as needed based on maintenance requirements or laboratory values.

Insulinomas can be treated surgically (with partial pancreatectomy) or medically. There is no location predilection for the tumor in the pancreas. Medical management includes frequent feedings, prednisone or prednisolone (0.25 mg/kg orally twice daily), diazoxide (5 to 30 mg/kg orally twice daily, start at low end of dosage), and octreotide (10 to 40 μg subcutaneously two or three times daily). Toy breed dogs and young puppies and kittens should be fed frequent meals high in complex carbohydrates. A bottle of corn syrup should be available in case a hypoglycemic event occurs. Hunting dogs should be fed a meal before hunting and offered snacks every 2 to 4 hours while hunting. If these dogs still have hypoglycemic events, they should not be allowed to hunt anymore. If the patient is in a late term of pregnancy, cesarean section to remove the puppies is necessary. Polycythemia warrants therapeutic phlebotomy, and chemotherapy (hydroxyurea) may be needed for long-term control.

Monitoring

It can be difficult to monitor the glycemic status of these patients because of the production of counterregulatory hormones. Single or intermittent measurement of blood glucose is not recommended. Monitoring the blood glucose every 2 hours gives a better indication of the trends in glucose control. The target blood glucose is 60 to 150 mg/dl. Mental and neuromuscular status should be monitored frequently throughout the day because these are early signs of an oncoming hypoglycemic event. Patients with sepsis must be monitored very closely for signs of multiple organ failure syndrome, acute respiratory distress syndrome, and disseminated intravascular coagulopathy. Patients with hypoadrenocorticism should be monitored as previously described. Packed cell volumes should be monitored daily in polycythemic patients. Other monitoring should be based on the patient's underlying disease.

CONCLUSION

Stabilizing and treating an animal with a metabolic and endocrine emergency is a challenge. The presenting signs and symptoms can vary.

These animals need continual monitoring and assessment of their response to treatment. Often changes in the therapy are needed throughout the treatment. Understanding the role of fluid and drug therapy in stabilizing the metabolic and endocrine emergency is a crucial part of successful patient care.

BIBLIOGRAPHY

Chew DJ, Nagode LA, Carothers M: Disorders of calcium: hypercalcemia and hypocalcemia. In DiBartola SP, ed: *Fluid therapy in small animal practice,* Philadelphia, 1992, WB Saunders.

Chew DJ, Nagode LA, Rosol TJ et al: Utility of diagnostic assays in the evaluation of hypercalcemia and hypocalcemia: parathyroid hormone, vitamin D metabolites, parathyroid hormone–related peptide and ionized calcium. In Bonagura JD, ed: *Kirk's current veterinary therapy,* ed 12, Philadelphia, 1995, WB Saunders.

Crenshaw KL: Monitoring treatment of diabetes mellitus in dogs and cats. In Bonagura JD, ed: *Kirk's current veterinary therapy,* ed 13, Philadelphia, 2000, WB Saunders.

Feldman EC, Nelson RW: Complications associated with insulin treatment in diabetes mellitus and hypercalcemia and primary hyperparathyroidism in dogs. In Bonagura JD, ed: *Kirk's current veterinary therapy,* ed 13, Philadelphia, 2000, WB Saunders.

Feldman EC, Nelson RW: Diabetic ketoacidosis, hypocalcemia and primary hypoparathyroidism, and disorders of the parathyroid glands. In Feldman EC, Nelson RW, eds: *Canine and feline endocrinology and reproduction,* Philadelphia, 1996, WB Saunders.

Fox LE: The paraneoplastic disorders. In Bonagura JD, ed: *Kirk's current veterinary therapy,* ed 12, Philadelphia, 1995, WB Saunders.

Greco DS, Peterson ME: Feline hypoadrenocorticism. In Kirk RW, ed: *Current veterinary therapy,* ed 10, Philadelphia, 1989, WB Saunders.

Hardy RH: Hypoadrenal gland disease. In Ettinger SJ, Feldman EC, eds: *Textbook of veterinary internal medicine,* Philadelphia, 1995, WB Saunders.

Kintzer PP, Peterson ME: Hypoadrenocorticism in dogs. In Bonagura JD, ed: *Kirk's current veterinary therapy,* ed 12, Philadelphia, 1995, WB Saunders.

Leifer CE: Hypoglycemia. In Kirk RW, ed: *Current veterinary therapy,* ed 9, Philadelphia, 1986, WB Saunders.

MacIntire DK: Emergency treatment of diabetic crisis: insulin overdose, diabetic ketoacidosis and hyperosmolar coma, *Vet Clin North Am Small Anim Pract* 25:639, 1995.

Meleo KA, Caplan ER: Treatment of insulinoma in the dog, cat, and ferret. In Bonagura JD, ed: *Kirk's current veterinary therapy,* ed 13, Philadelphia, 2000, WB Saunders.

Nelson RW: Diabetes mellitus and insulin-secreting islet cell neoplasia. In Ettinger SJ, Feldman EC, eds: *Textbook of veterinary internal medicine,* Philadelphia, 1995, WB Saunders.

Nichols R, Crenshaw KL: Complications and concurrent disease associated with diabetic ketoacidosis and other severe forms of diabetes mellitus. In Bonagura JD, ed: *Kirk's current veterinary therapy,* ed 12, Philadelphia, 1995, WB Saunders.

Peterson ME: Hypoparathyroidism and other causes of hypocalcemia in cats. In Kirk RW, Bonagura JD, eds: *Kirk's current veterinary therapy,* ed 11, Philadelphia, 1992, WB Saunders.

Peterson ME, Kintzer PP, Kass PH: Pretreatment clinical and laboratory findings in 225 dogs with hypoadrenocorticism, *J Am Vet Med Assoc* 208:85, 1996.

Rumbeih WK, Kruger JM, Fitzgerald SD et al: Use of pamidronate to reverse vitamin D_3–induced toxicosis in dogs, *Am J Vet Res* 60(9):1092, 1999.

Rumbeih WK, Fitzgerald SD, Kruger JM et al: Use of pamidronate to reduce cholecalciferol-induced toxicosis in dogs, *Am J Vet Res* 61(1):9, 2000.

Waters CB, Scott-Moncrieff JCR: Hypocalcemia in cats, *Compend Contin Educ Pract Vet* 14:497, 1992.

Chapter 19

Urologic Emergencies

Urologic emergencies can result from trauma or disease. Animals that present with abdominal trauma from automobile collisions, fights, or physical abuse should be examined for kidney or bladder damage. Trauma also can occur during treatment for urologic emergencies. Overly aggressive palpation of the bladder or cystocentesis can cause the bladder to rupture. Improper catheterization techniques can cause urethral tears. The veterinary technician must understand the proper techniques for placing urinary catheters and the problems that can occur.

Urinary obstruction is common in small animals. It is most common in male cats and specific breeds of dogs. Immediate treatment is necessary to prevent further complications, which can lead to renal failure and possibly death.

Renal failure can be acute or chronic. Acute renal failure may be caused by ischemic or physiologic events, nephrotoxins, or diseases. Chronic renal failure is caused by progressive congenital disease or by renal disease that was acquired through life. Appropriate treatment depends on the cause and stage of the renal failure.

Stabilization and maintenance of the patient with a urologic emergency are based on an understanding of the signs associated with the various problems that can occur and the types of treatment that can be successful. These animals may need surgical intervention and medical management.

Equipment List

- Basic supplies needed for stabilization
  - Intravenous catheters
  - Fluid therapies
  - Quick assessment tests (packed cell volume, blood glucose, total protein, blood urea nitrogen)
  - Electrolyte analyzer
- Saline for flushing obstructions
- Rigid urinary catheters in multiple sizes (3.0 French, 3.5 French, 5-10 French)
- Flexible Foley (balloon on distal end) catheters for long-term bladder drainage in multiple sizes (5-14 French)
- Flexible feeding tubes (3.5 French) for cats
- Urinary collection system (sterile systems available with one-way valves or empty intravenous fluid bags and administration lines can be used)
- Drug therapies for renal failure
  - Furosemide
  - Mannitol
  - Cimetidine
  - Famotidine
  - Sucralfate

URINARY OBSTRUCTION

Urinary obstruction is the inability of urine to flow normally from the body. An obstruction can either be partial or complete, resulting from a physical or functional condition of urinary outflow. A physical obstruction is caused by a space-occupying object in the urethra, urinary bladder, ureters, or renal pelvis (Figure 19-1). Examples of these include urethral plugs, uroliths, tumors, and blood clots. Uroliths are composed of very organized crystals of phosphate, urate, cystine, and oxalate. Uroliths often are caused by a

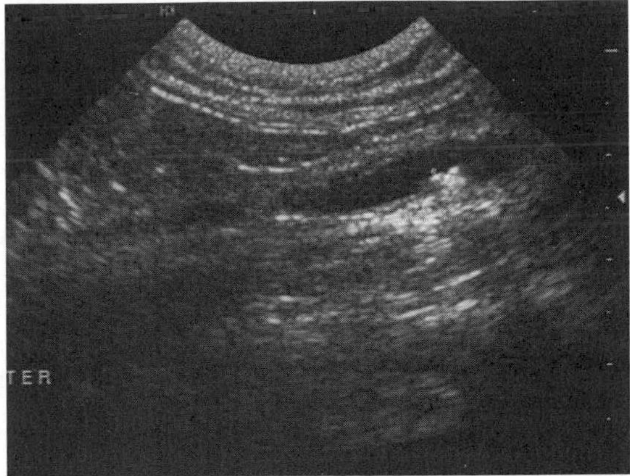

Figure 19-1

Ultrasound depicting a urinary obstruction caused by a stone in the urethra of a cat.

congenital abnormality in the metabolism or excretion of these minerals. Functional obstructions usually are abnormalities such as congenital strictures or damage to the nerves that control micturition; such nerve damage can result from a traumatic event.

Urinary obstructions can be found in dogs or cats, both male and female. Urinary calculi are the more common causes of outflow obstruction in male dogs and male cats. Whereas in dogs obstruction is caused by organized uroliths, in cats the debris is much less organized and usually forms a urethral plug at the tip of the penis. The blockage in the male dog usually is found in the bladder neck or the urethra. Whether physical or functional in nature, urinary obstructions must be treated immediately because they can lead to renal failure and possibly death.

The Blocked Cat

Physical obstructions in cats can be caused by a urethral plug composed of mucos and crystalline material. This condition is most common in male cats because the lumen of the urethra is small throughout its length and even smaller at the tip of the penis. The urethral plug generally is found at the tip of the penis, where the debris becomes trapped. Female cats rarely have urethral obstructions because of their shorter urethra and wider urethral lumen. Small clumps of crystals, tiny calculi, blood clots, and mucus can pass more easily during urination. Untreated urinary obstructions in the cat can lead to severe metabolic changes and death.

Clinical Presentation. Cats presenting with urethral obstruction may be alert or depressed depending on the duration and degree of obstruction. Owners may notice episodes of stranguria (straining to urinate) or pollakiuria (passing small amounts of urine frequently) and longer periods in the litter box. They may also find the cat urinating in unusual places outside the litter box. Hematuria (blood in the urine) also may be present in varying amounts depending on the amount of inflammation and irritation. Cats may appear restless and uncomfortable and lick continuously at the tip of the penis. These signs may be perceived by owners as signs of constipation.

Cats with complete obstruction have a distended, painful bladder on palpation. Palpating the bladder may cause the cat to cry out and may induce straining to urinate and the passing of a few drops of blood-tinged urine.

Prolonged obstruction leads to depression, dehydration, vomiting, a low body temperature, and fluid volume and serum electrolyte imbalances caused by an acute onset of uremia.

Diagnostics. A series of diagnostic tests can be performed to determine the severity of an obstruction. If the cat is stable, the bladder can be compressed carefully to check for resistance in urine outflow. It is very important not to put excessive or localized pressure on the bladder because it can rupture. Compressing the bladder can dislodge a urethral plug if it is at the tip of the penis, and normal outflow can be obtained.

If resistance is excessive and urine outflow is not adequate, a urinary catheter and irrigation of the urethra may be necessary to dislodge the plug back into the bladder. Before placing the urinary catheter, if the cat is very alert and active, it may be necessary to sedate the cat with ketamine and valium or propofol. Place an intravenous catheter and check for azotemia and serum electrolyte imbalances. An electrocardiogram (ECG) should be obtained to identify cardiac arrhythmias caused by hyperkalemia. If a urinary catheter cannot pass easily into the bladder because of a urolith, plug, swelling, or stricture in the proximal urethra, further diagnostic tests including ultrasound or radiographic imaging, including contrast, may be indicated to define the lesion.

Cystocentesis can be performed on a palpable bladder to collect urine for urinalysis and culture or to provide decompression if the bladder cannot be catheterized. This specimen allows a more accurate assessment of bacteria, cells, and crystals and the presence of blood or protein, specific gravity, and pH in the bladder. A cystocentesis should be performed with the cat in a ventral-dorsal position. The cat should be well restrained to prevent movement and possible trauma.

The collection site should be free of hair and prepared aseptically with soap and water and alcohol or a dilute solution of a tincture of benzalkonium chloride. A sterile 23- to 22-gauge needle 1 to 1.5 inches long (depending on the size of the animal) is attached to a 5-cc or 10-cc sterile syringe. A larger needle should not be used because it can cause leakage from the bladder wall. The bladder is then palpated and immobilized to direct needle insertion and to ensure an adequate volume for collection. The needle is inserted into the ventral midline about midway between the pelvis and dome of the bladder, with the tip of the needle pointing caudally at a 45-degree angle. If urine collection is unsuccessful because of misinsertion of the needle, the needle should be removed and both the needle and syringe should be replaced before the procedure is repeated.

Upon presentation, if the cat appears very depressed or dehydrated and has a low body temperature, blood work should be performed immediately. These results determine the rest of the diagnostic workup and in what order treatment should be initiated because the cat has begun to show signs of uremia.

Treatment. Treatment begins almost in conjunction with the diagnostic procedures and the efforts to relieve the obstruction. If the cat is showing signs of depression or dehydration and has a low body temperature, it is probably uremic, and an intravenous catheter should be placed and therapy should be started to correct fluid volume deficits, metabolic acidosis, and identified electrolyte disturbances. An ECG should be evaluated for evidence of arrhythmias and hyperkalemia. Hyperkalemia can cause bradycardia, diminished P waves, widened QRS complexes, and increased T waves (Figure 19-2). If abnormalities are recognized, sodium bicarbonate or dextrose with or without regular insulin can be administered to drive potassium into the cells and transiently correct the hyperkalemia and cardiac disturbances. Metabolic acidosis also should be treated with

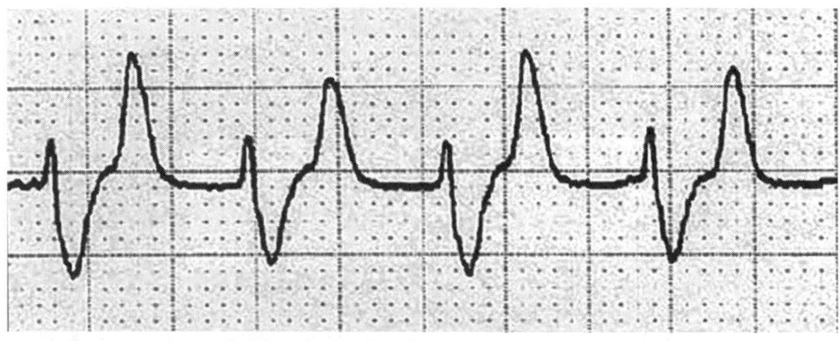

Figure 19-2

Electrocardiogram showing hyperkalemia in a severely uremic animal.

intravenous sodium bicarbonate if serum pH is less than 7.2 or the base deficit is greater than 10. Intravenous fluids should be given at a rate of 40 to 60 ml/kg/hr to correct existing fluid deficits. It is best to use 0.9% sodium chloride to minimize potassium administration.

Catheterization. The decision to use an indwelling urinary catheter should be made with an understanding of the rationale and therapeutic goals in mind. Catheters should not be placed haphazardly because they can cause injury, induce urinary tract infections, cause urethral strictures, and potentially rupture the bladder. The therapeutic goals of urinary catheterization are to document the rate of urine formation in critically ill patients, prevent reobstruction during the first 24 hours after the initial obstruction has been relieved, and keep the bladder decompressed to facilitate reestablishment of normal bladder wall contractility. A cystocentesis can be performed with a 22-gauge or smaller needle to relieve excessive pressure while attempts of urinary catheterization are implemented.

The following supplies should be assembled before insertion of an indwelling urinary catheter:

Equipment List

A sterile, soft, flexible catheter. For maximum benefit, the catheter should bc the largest diameter and most flexible that will pass readily through the urethra. This prevents urine leaking around the catheter insertion site. If urine is leaking from the site, the rate of urine production and the amount of urine collection cannot be calculated accurately. The preferred catheters are a 5-French feeding tube and urethral catheter (Sovereign) or a 3.5-French infant feeding catheter (Mallinckrodt Medical, St. Louis, Missouri).

Betadine ointment.

Cotton-tipped swabs.

Suture: 3-0 Ethilon (Ethicon, Inc.).

1-inch tape.

Antiseptic soap or Betadine surgical scrub (The Purdue Fredrick Company, Norwalk, Connecticut).

Small sterile urinary collection bag (Sherwood Medical, St. Louis, Missouri).

Sterile connecting adapters (Sherwood).

Sterile K-Y jelly (Carter Products, New York) or 2% lidocaine jelly (Abbott Laboratories, North Chicago, Illinois).

Sterile gloves.

12-cc syringe with a solution consisting of 4 ml Betadine and 250 ml sterile water.

Sterile needle holder and soft tissue thumb forceps.

Sterile drapes.

Cable ties and cable tie gun (Cole-Parmer, Vernon Hills, Illinois).

Placing the Male Cat Urinary Catheter. An indwelling urinary catheter should be placed aseptically to prevent a urinary tract infection as follows:

1. With the cat in a ventral-dorsal position, clip the hair from the prepuce and from a small area on the perineum around the preputial orifice.
2. Clean the preputial orifice with antiseptic soap and water or flush the orifice with Betadine solution.
3. Retract the prepuce to extrude the penis. Gently prepare the tip of the penis with antiseptic soap and water using soft cotton balls.
4. Place a sterile barrier drape under the penis to prevent contamination of the catheter with hair.
5. Put on sterile gloves.
6. Lubricate the sterile urinary catheter with sterile K-Y jelly or lidocaine jelly.
7. Retract the penis caudally to straighten the urethra, insert the catheter into the tip of the penis, and advance the catheter gently and carefully into the bladder using an aseptic technique.
8. Once the catheter is in the bladder, urine should flow into the catheter. Cap the catheter opening and allow the prepuce to return to a normal position.
9. Apply 1-inch tape to the catheter (making a butterfly around the catheter with the tape).

Place two stay sutures on opposite sides of the prepuce, and suture each flap of the butterfly to its corresponding stay suture.

10. Apply Betadine ointment with cotton-tipped swabs to the urethral orifice.
11. Using a sterile adapter, connect the catheter to a urinary drainage bag.
12. Make sure all joints are tight and secured with cable ties to prevent them from disconnecting or leaking.
13. Tape the extension tubing to the tail to prevent traction on the prepuce.
14. Place the collection bag lower than the patient so urine will flow only into the bag. If urine does not flow properly, it will increase the risk of urinary tract infection.

Placing the Female Cat Urinary Catheter. The list of preparatory supplies are the same as listed for male cats with the exception of a 3.5-French infant feeding tube, a nasal speculum or otoscope, and a light source.

The sedated cat is placed in sternal recumbency with the hind legs hanging over the edge of the table, and the tail is retracted back toward the head. Once the patient is positioned, the following procedure is recommended:

1. Clip hair from the vulvar area.
2. Gently clean the vulvar area with antiseptic soap.
3. Using a sterile syringe, gently flush the vestibule with a 1:60 dilution of Betadine solution.
4. Place a barrier drape around the perivulvar area.
5. Put on sterile gloves.
6. Lubricate the urinary catheter with sterile K-Y jelly or lidocaine jelly.
7. Gently insert a nasal speculum or otoscope in the vagina and locate the papilla and urethral orifice, insert the catheter into the urethra, and gently pass it into the bladder.
8. Once the catheter is in the bladder, it should fill with urine. Cap the catheter closed.
9. Attach 1-inch tape to the catheter, making a butterfly. Place two stay sutures on opposite sides of the vulva, and suture each flap of the butterfly to its corresponding stay suture.
10. Attach a sterile urinary collection system.
11. Attach the extension tubing to the tail to prevent tension on the catheter while allowing enough slack for a full range of tail movement.
12. Make sure all connections are secure and tight.

Managing Indwelling Urinary Catheters. Once an indwelling catheter has been placed, the cat must be monitored and the urinary catheter must be maintained properly. After the catheter is placed, the cat may undergo a postobstructive diuresis in which fluid administration must match the rate of urine production. The amount of a 0.9% NaCl solution to administer can be estimated from the urine produced during the previous 2 hours; fluid input must equal urine output. While the diuresis is occurring, serum electrolytes should be measured every 2 to 4 hours in a severely ill animal and every 6 to 8 hours in a stable patient. Cats should be weighed accurately every 12 hours to document net fluid balance. Serum potassium may drop quickly during the postobstructive diuresis, and potassium supplementation may be needed to prevent hypokalemia. Guidelines for parenteral potassium supplementation used at the Veterinary Medical Teaching Hospital intensive care unit at the University of California at Davis are listed in Table 19-1.

Cats with cardiac problems may not tolerate fluid administration and may be predisposed to

TABLE 19-1 Guidelines for Parenteral Potassium Supplementation

Plasma Protein K^+	KCl (Added to qs Fluids)
≥3.5	Do not add KCl.
3.0-3.5	20 mEq/L.
2.5-3.0	30 mEq/L.
2.0-2.5	40 mEq/L.
<2.0	50 mEq/L.

fluid overload. Auscultate the chest for heart murmurs or gallop rhythms, listen for lung sounds and possible crackles, and monitor changes in central venous pressure (CVP) when fluid is given. Continuous ECG recording is useful to monitor heart rate and rhythm and to detect potassium oversupplementation.

Urine output should be measured and recorded every 2 hours, and hematuria or excessive sediment should be noted.

For cats with prolonged obstruction, serum electrolytes and venous blood gases should be measured every 1 to 12 hours to detect ongoing electrolyte and acid-base abnormalities. Blood glucose concentrations should be measured every 1 to 4 hours if the cat is being treated with dextrose and insulin, and the packed cell volume (PCV) and total protein (TP) concentration should be measured in animals receiving fluid therapy every 6 hours. Azotemia (blood urea nitrogen [BUN], serum creatinine) should be documented every 6 hours. Obtunded cats must be turned every 4 hours.

Other medications that may be indicated are antibiotics to prevent urinary tract infections from the indwelling catheter, phenoxybenzamine to decrease urethral resistance, and bethanechol to manage atonic bladder by increasing detrusor muscle contractility. Corticosteroids should not be used in these patients because they can impair the immune system and make the patient susceptible to bladder infections.

The patient's bladder should be palpated every 4 to 6 hours to assess its volume. If the bladder is not emptying, the catheter and urinary collection system should be checked for kinks or plugs. If none are noted, the bladder may be compressed carefully to dispell urine. If the bladder remains distended, the catheter may be obstructed and should be flushed retrograde with sterile saline. Hydrogen peroxide, antiseptic soap and water, a 1:60 dilution of Betadine solution, and Betadine ointment are used to maintain urinary catheters:

1. Drain the urinary bag only every 2 to 4 hours to maintain a semiclosed urinary collection system. Do not disconnect the urinary catheter from the drainage bag.
2. Add 10 cc hydrogen peroxide to large urine bags and 5 cc to small urine bags whenever the urinary bag is drained. (Remember to subtract this volume from the total urine collected.) Do not use peroxide if urine chemical tests are to be performed on the collected urine or if hematuria is present. Blood in the urine will cause the peroxide to bubble up into the system. This may cause pressure inside the bag, which will lead to urine reflowing back into the bladder.
3. Cleanse the prepuce or vestibule with antiseptic soap and water.
4. Flush the sheath or vestibule with diluted Betadine solution.
5. Apply Betadine ointment with cotton-tipped swabs to the sheath or vulvar opening.

Urinary catheter care should be performed three times a day to prevent urinary tract infections and to monitor catheter function. The catheter should be kept clean at all times and free of fecal contamination.

Response to Treatment. At the Veterinary Medical Teaching Hospital at the University of California at Davis, the indwelling urinary catheter usually is removed after the first 24 hours of treatment if there are no complications such as hematuria or atonic bladder. The next 24 hours are devoted to careful monitoring of the cat for urine production and ability to void urine. If production is normal, all other clinical signs are stable, and the cat is eating and drinking normally, it can be sent home. The owner is instructed to watch the cat for straining to urinate and frequent trips to the litter box. They should observe the amount of urine produced and note whether blood is present.

The cat's diet must be monitored. Dietary recommendations include feeding canned food to increase water intake and feeding acidifying diets (e.g., Hill's Prescription Diet C/D, Waltham pH Control, Iams, Low pH/S, and CNM UR), which are low in phosphate and magnesium, to decrease the production of stuvite crystals.

The cat may also be continued on antimicrobials to reduce the incidence of urinary tract infections secondary to catheterization, phenoxybenzamine to reduce internal urethral sphincter tone, propantheline to decrease spasm of the urethra, and bethanechol to increase detrusor muscle tone.

If the patient does not void urine for 24 hours after catheter removal, a new indwelling catheter is placed and indwelling catheter procedures are started again. Recatheterization usually is attempted three times. If normal urine voiding is not achieved after the third catheterization, the urethra may be damaged and the prognosis is guarded.

Because urinary obstructions are most common in male cats, a urethrostomy, in which the penile urethra is amputated, may be performed as a salvage procedure to provide urethral patency. The urethrostomy removes the narrowest, scarred portion of the urethra to expose a larger urethral lumen, which usually prevents future obstruction.

The Blocked Dog

Urinary obstruction in the male dog usually results from a physical blockage of urinary outflow by a urolith; in the female dog the causes usually are associated with bladder tumors.

Functional outflow obstruction occurs secondary to a traumatic event affecting the nerves that control the detrusor muscles of the bladder for micturition.

Urinary calculi are the most common causes of male dog outflow obstruction, followed by scarring in the urethra and bladder neck tumors. Usual sites of obstruction are in the mid- to distal end of the penile urethra (Figure 19-3).

Uroliths form in urine supersaturated with minerals, which precipitate to form microaggregates. These aggregates can fuse together, forming stones of a variety of shapes, sizes, and composition that can build in the kidney or bladder and move down the urinary tract. Some examples of these mineral aggregates are magnesium ammonium phosphate (struvite), calcium oxalate, silica, and purines. Many different minerals can form uroliths, so when a urolith is removed from a site of obstruction, it should be analyzed to determine its composition. The exact composition of the stone dictates the course of medical or surgical treatment.

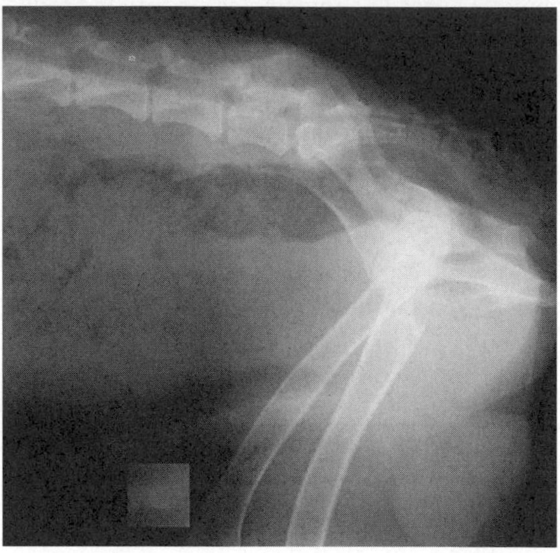

Figure 19-3
Urinary obstruction in the penile urethra of a male dog.

Clinical Presentation. Signs of urinary obstruction vary greatly and depend on the degree and location of the obstruction. Urethral obstruction can be associated with dysuria or anuria. If obstruction has been complete for a long time, there can be signs of uremia including depression, dehydration, and vomiting. The dog also may have a distended or turgid bladder. When an obstruction is located in the bladder, the dog may present with signs similar to those of cystitis. Hematuria can be present, and micturition can be characterized by the frequent passage of small amounts of urine. Ureteral obstruction can lead to hydronephrosis and cause cranial abdominal pain.

Diagnosis. The diagnosis of urinary obstruction is established on the basis of a complete history and physical examination and a series of diagnostic tests to determine the location and severity of the obstruction. If the dog has signs of uremia, a complete blood cell count (CBC) and serum chemistry profile should be performed to identify fluid, acid-base, and electrolyte imbalances. A cystocentesis can be performed to collect a sterile sample for urinalysis and culture and to alleviate bladder distention. The technique is similar to that

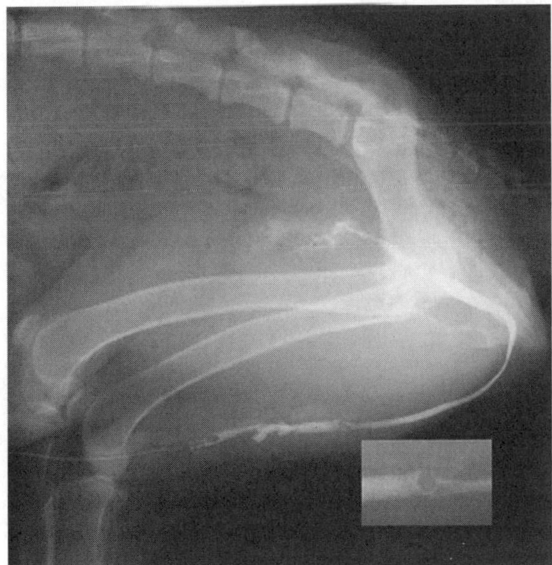

Figure 19-4

The use of a contrast medium to diagnose a urinary obstruction in the penile urethra of a male dog.

described for the cat. In large-breed dogs cystocentesis can be performed more easily in a standing position or lateral recumbency as long as the bladder is palpable and the procedure is performed aseptically. Once the urine is obtained, a careful analysis of the crystals can aid in determining urolith composition.

Urethral obstruction should be suspected if a urinary catheter of appropriate size cannot be passed up the urethra into the bladder.

Radiographic evaluation and ultrasound can be useful in diagnosing obstructions of the kidney ureters, bladder, or urethra. The use of contrast medium may help determine whether the obstruction is intralumenal or extralumenal (Figure 19-4).

Treatment. If the dog is weak, hypotensive, dehydrated, and uremic, treatment should be initiated to correct these conditions before the obstruction is corrected. An intravenous catheter should be placed and therapy should be started to correct fluid volume deficits, metabolic acidosis, and electrolyte disturbances. An ECG should be used to monitor cardiac arrhythmias and evidence of hyperkalemia.

Catheterization. Once the patient is stabilized, passage of an indwelling urinary catheter should be attempted to relieve the obstruction. If a catheter cannot be passed into the bladder because the urolith is blocking the urethra, urohydropropulsion can be used in an attempt to push the stone or stones back into the bladder.

When urine outflow has been established, an indwelling urinary catheter may be placed to keep the urethra from reobstructing.

Equipment List for Indwelling Urethral Catheter Insertion

Sterile soft flexible catheter such as a male infant feeding catheter sizes 5, 8, or 10 French (Mallinckrodt Medical, St. Louis, Missouri). Foley catheters for female dogs sizes 5, 8, and 10 French (Sherwood, St. Louis, Missouri).
Betadine ointment
Cotton-tipped swabs
Suture: 3-0 Ethilon (Ethicon, Inc.)
1-inch tape
Antiseptic soap or Betadine scrub (The Purdue Fredrick Company, Norwalk, Connecticut)
Sterile urinary collection bag (Sherwood)
Sterile connecting adapters (for the male urinary collection system) (Sherwood)
Sterile K-Y jelly (Carter Products, New York) or lidocaine jelly 2% (Abbott Laboratories, North Chicago, Illinois)
Sterile gloves
12-cc syringe with a solution of 4 ml Betadine and 250 ml sterile water
Sterile needle holder and soft tissue thumb forceps
Sterile barrier drape
Vaginal speculum and light source for female patient
Cable ties and cable tie gun (Cole-Parmer, Vernon Hills, Illinois)

Male Urinary Catheter Insertion

1. Place the dog in lateral recumbency.
2. Clip hair from the prepuce and around the preputial orifice.
3. Clean the preputial orifice with antiseptic soap and water.
4. Retract the sheath to expose the entire shaft of the penis. Disinfect the tip of the penis

with tincture of zephrine or chlorhexadine solution.

5. Put on sterile gloves.
6. Lubricate the sterile urinary catheter with sterile K-Y jelly or lidocaine jelly.
7. Insert the lubricated catheter into the urethra using an aseptic technique and gently pass retrograde along the urethra into the bladder.
8. Once the catheter is in the bladder, urine should fill the catheter. Cap the catheter opening and allow the prepuce to return to a normal position.
9. Apply tape to catheter using 1-inch tape to make a butterfly. Place two stay sutures on opposite sides of the prepuce, and suture both flaps of the butterfly to the stay sutures.
10. Using a sterile adapter, connect the catheter to a urinary drainage bag.
11. Make sure all joints are cable tied together to prevent them from disconnecting or leaking.
12. Tape the tubing to the hind leg or tail to prevent traction on the prepuce.

Female Urinary Catheter Insertion

1. Clip hair from vulvar area.
2. Gently clean the vulvar area with antiseptic soap or Betadine solution.
3. Using a sterile syringe, gently flush the vestibule with a 1:60 dilution of Betadine solution.
4. Put on sterile gloves.
5. Lubricate a sterile Foley catheter with sterile K-Y jelly or lidocaine jelly.
6. Gently insert a gloved finger, sterile speculum, sterile laryngoscope blade, or sterile otoscope into the vagina. Locate the papilla and urethral opening and insert the catheter.
7. Once the catheter is inserted, fill the balloon of the Foley catheter with the indicated amount of sterile water.
8. Gently retract the catheter to ensure that the balloon is within the bladder.
9. Attach a sterile urinary collection system.
10. Apply a piece of 1-inch tape around the hind legs. Tape the catheter or tubing to the tape on the leg or tail, allowing enough slack for the animal to stand and walk without tension on the catheter.
11. Make sure all connections are cable tied together to prevent leaking.

Urohydropropulsion. The disposition of the animal may necessitate sedation or general anesthesia for this procedure. If the animal is an anesthetic risk because of a uremic crisis, a topical application of lidocaine and a small dose of analgesia may be adequate to keep the animal comfortable.

With the animal in lateral recumbency, inject a liberal quantity of a 1:1 mixture of sterile saline solution and aqueous lubricant through a flexible catheter into the urethral lumen to facilitate movement. Have an assistant insert an index finger into the rectum and firmly occlude the lumen of the pelvic urethra by applying digital pressure. Inject sterile saline into the urethra through the catheter, and as the pressure builds up rapidly, release the pressure to the pelvic urethra. Pressure should be maintained in the urethral lumen by forcing more saline forward after the assistant has released digital pressure. This technique should force the fluid and usually the urethroliths into the urinary bladder. Sometimes the urolith returns quickly to the bladder, but it may be necessary to repeat the procedure a couple of times to get the urolith to reach the bladder.

Response to Treatment. Once urine outflow has been established, management is directed at surgical or medical removal of the uroliths and medical therapy to prevent reoccurrence.

Struvite is the most common mineral detected in canine uroliths. The urine must be supersaturated with magnesium, ammonium, and phosphate for struvite uroliths to form. In contrast to cats, struvite urolith formation in dogs generally is associated with urinary tract infections with urease-producing microbes, which cause alkalization of the urine. Resolution of the urinary tract infection with antibiotics is the foundation of therapy. Dietary modifications that reduce phosphorus and magnesium excretion and urinary acidification are recommended. Hill's Prescription Diet S/D is one such diet that is low in protein, phosphorus, and magnesium. Surgical removal of existing uroliths is the preferred method of treatment, but medical dissolution with antibiotics and dietary modification has been advocated and may be indicated in animals with recurrent disease or those who are poor surgical risks.

Ammonium urate uroliths are most common in dalmatians and are managed medically. They can be managed with dietary modifications that reduce urine concentrations of uric acid and ammonium and hydrogen ions. The diet should be a purine-restricted nonacidifying diet that does not contain supplemental sodium (Hill's Prescription Diet U/D or Hill's Prescription Diet K/D). Besides diet changes, xanthine oxidase inhibitors (Allupurinol) are given to block uric acid formation in the serum and urine. The urine should be alkalinized by the administration of sodium bicarbonate or potassium citrate orally to achieve a urine pH of 7.0. Documented urinary tract infections are treated with appropriate antibiotics.

Calcium oxalate uroliths are managed very differently. Surgery appears to be the most effective treatment because they are very difficult to dissolve. Some dietary modifications can be effective. A diet moderately restricted in protein, calcium, oxalate, and sodium such as Hill's Prescription Diet U/D may be considered to help prevent recurrences. Ideally, the diet should not be restricted or supplemented with phosphorus or magnesium. Attempts should be made to alkalinize the urine.

Some dog breeds are more susceptible to urolith production than others, and some breeds are predisposed to particular urolith types. According to the Minnesota Urolith Center, where extensive studies of canine uroliths were performed, the following uroliths were matched to a particular breed of dog. Calcium oxalate uroliths were prominent in male dogs, especially miniature schnauzers, Lhasa apsos, Yorkshire terriers, miniature poodles, and shih tzus. Struvite uroliths were more common in female dogs, possibly because of the higher prevalence of urinary tract infections. Common breeds associated with these uroliths are the miniature schnauzer, bichon frise, shih tzus, Yorkshire terriers, Lhasa apsos, cocker spaniels, and miniature poodles. Uroliths composed of purines were found mostly in male dogs, dalmatians, Yorkshire terriers, and English bulldogs. These breeds have normal serum uric acid concentrations but high urine uric acid concentrations.

RENAL DISEASE

Renal failure is the inability of the kidneys to perform their numerous functions of excretion, metabolic regulation, and hormone production. As the disease progresses, the animal begins to show signs of multiple-organ dysfunction, a syndrome called uremia. Conventional and specialized treatments are available. If the disease is treated early and aggressively, the kidney can regenerate and recover. If left untreated, the patient will deteriorate and eventually die.

The Kidney

The kidneys are located in the lumbar region of the abdomen, enveloped in peritoneum and loosely attached to the body wall.

Each kidney is made up of a variety of structures that are responsible for several functions, such as fluid regulation, electrolyte balance, excretion of metabolic waste products, and hormone production.

The functional unit of the kidney is the nephron. It is made up of a glomerulus, proximal tubule, loop of Henle, distal tubule, and collecting duct. As blood passes through the kidney, an ultrafiltrate is formed containing water and very small molecules. This filtrate is later modified by the nephron to form final urine. Water balance and electrolyte balance are maintained in these tubules and nitrogenous waste is excreted.

The kidneys also produce the hormones erythropoietin, renin, and calcitriol. Erythropoietin is responsible for producing red blood cells, renin is involved in controlling blood pressure, and calcitriol stimulates calcium absorption from the small intestine.

Renal Failure

When the kidneys are injured, resulting in their inability to maintain excretory function, they are considered to be in failure. Renal failure can be an acute or chronic condition.

Acute renal failure (ARF) is a sudden decrease in renal function, usually less than a week. ARF is classified as either prerenal, intrinsic renal parenchymal (functional element), or postrenal. Prerenal ARF is a functional consequence of reduced blood flow to the kidneys and is completely reversible with restoration of adequate renal perfusion. It can be caused by hemorrhage, vomiting, diarrhea, dehydration, poor fluid intake, and systemic diseases such as heart failure. Intrinsic ARF results from damage to the cellular structure of the kidney by ischemic or toxic events. Postrenal ARF results from an obstruction or diversion of the outflow of urine from the animal. Obstructions can be located in the urethra, bladder, ureter, or renal pelvis, and urine can be diverted into the abdominal cavity or soft tissue with rupture of the ureters, bladder, or urethra. All of these conditions are potentially reversible if diagnosed early and treated aggressively, and they constitute a urologic emergency.

Chronic renal failure (CRF) develops over an extended period of time, usually several months to years. The renal injury is not reversible, but in its early stages, the animal can be supported with proper diet and medication, and it is rarely considered an emergency condition.

Causes of Intrinsic Acute Renal Failure. ARF most commonly results from ischemic or physiologic (prerenal) events, nephrotoxins, or other diseases. Ischemic injury occurs with profound or prolonged decreases in renal blood flow. Prolonged ischemia causes the epithelial cells of the kidney to be deprived of oxygen, lose cellular function, and die.

Ischemia

Shock
- Hypovolemic
- Hemorrhagic
- Septic

Decreased cardiac output
- Heart failure

Renal thrombosis

Nephrotoxins

Organic compounds such as ethylene glycol (antifreeze) and pesticides.

Antimicrobials such as cephalosporins, aminoglycosides, and tetracyclines.

Anesthetics.

Heavy metals such as lead.

Analgesics or nonsteroidal antiinflammatory drugs including aspirin and phenylbutazone.

Snake venom.

Other conditions causing ARF are infectious diseases such as leptospirosis, bacterial infections including pylonephritis, immune-mediated diseases such as glomerulonephritis, and systemic conditions such as hypercalcemia.

Clinical Presentation of ARF in Animals. The presenting complaints typically are vague and nonspecific for renal disease and may include the following:

- Anorexia
- Vomiting
- Listlessness
- Diarrhea
- Halitosis
- Ataxia
- Seizures
- Known toxin exposure
- Oliguria, anuria, or polyuria

The physical examination may demonstrate the following:

- A normal body condition and hair coat, which helps differentiate ARF from CRF.
- Dehydration or overhydration. Dehydration is most commonly from a decrease in fluid intake, vomiting, or diarrhea; overhydration may be seen if the animal has been given parenteral fluids.
- Oral ulceration or necrosis of the tongue.
- Halitosis.
- Hypothermia or fever. Most uremic animals have low body temperature proportional to their azotemia, but if the condition is caused

by infection, the temperature may be elevated. A normal temperature in a uremic animal may suggest the presence of fever and infection.

Scleral injection.

Nonpalpable urinary bladder.

Tachypnea.

Bradycardia.

Large, painful, firm kidneys.

Causes of Chronic Renal Failure. Because this injury to the kidney is long-standing, there is little or no potential for repair. Surviving nephrons compensate maximally for those that have been lost. As the CRF progresses and renal function deteriorates, the animal becomes polyuric and progressively azotemic and eventually develops uremia. CRF results from congenital diseases that progress or from renal diseases acquired through life. The animal may be able to compensate for the loss of renal function initially, but over time, as more renal function is lost, the signs of renal failure materialize.

Clinical Presentation of Patients with CRF. Some telltale signs of CRF include weight loss, prior episodes of illness, polyuria, polydypsia, pale mucous membranes, small, irregular kidneys, low body temperature, and poor hair coat and body condition.

Diagnosis of Acute and Chronic Renal Failure. The diagnosis of renal failure is confirmed with laboratory tests that document the extent of renal impairment and distinguish between ARF and CRF. These tests may include the following:

A CBC may reveal changes in hematocrit depending on hydration levels. If the renal failure is caused by an infectious state, an increase in the white blood cell count will be seen. A CBC can distinguish regenerative from nonregenerative anemia. Anemia usually is not present in ARF but is present in CRF.

A chemistry panel demonstrates progressive increases in serum urea nitrogen, creatinine, phosphate, and potassium. Serum bicarbonate usually is decreased, and serum calcium may vary. The chemistry panel also helps determine whether other organ systems are involved.

Urine specimens should be obtained by cystocentesis to prevent contamination by the lower urogenital tract and to provide a clearer interpretation. In ARF, urine specific gravity ranges from 1.007 to 1.017, representing an inability to concentrate urine. A more concentrated urine predicts a prerenal component. Mild proteinuria usually is present. Casts, white blood cells (WBCs), red blood cells (RBCs), bacteria, and crystals usually are present. The presence of calcium oxalate crystals suggests ethylene glycol toxicity.

Radiographs typically reveal normal to large kidneys with smooth contours or may show small, irregular kidneys in animals with decompensated CRF. Ultrasound may confirm ethylene glycol toxicity, which appears as brightness of the cortex secondary to calcium oxalate crystal deposition. It can further define the shape and size of the kidneys and alterations in intrarenal architecture.

Renal biopsy confirms the diagnosis of ARF and may establish its cause. Renal histopathology can define the severity of the disease and its potential reversibility. It is an excellent indicator distinguishing between ARF and CRF. It is an invasive procedure with inherent risks such as hemorrhage and further renal damage.

Ethylene glycol levels should be assessed in cases of known antifreeze exposure or when calcium oxalate crystals are present in the urine of an animal with ARF.

Leptospirosis titers must be evaluated in animals with ARF. Leptospirosis is highly suspected in young dogs with ARF of unknown origin. Animals presenting with signs of systemic infection including fever and an increase in WBCs also must be evaluated for this disease. Leptospires are spirochetes that infect humans and animals. Urine from the infected host is the common source of contamination. The staff working with these animals should wear gloves and use other measures to prevent contamination.

Treatment of ARF. Once the diagnosis of ARF or CRF has been established, the goals of treatment are to minimize further injury to the kidney, quickly correct renal hemodynamics, and reestablish water and solute balances. The sooner treatment is implemented, the greater the chances for renal regeneration and recovery.

If a patient presents after a nephrotoxin has been ingested, gastric lavage should be instituted or vomiting induced, and activated charcoal should be administered within 30 to 60 minutes to absorb any residual toxin. When the toxin has been identified, specific treatments or antidotes can be given to reverse the effects. For example, ethanol or methylpyrazole is given to treat ethylene glycol toxicity.

ARF treatment can be divided into three areas: fluid therapy, drug therapy, and nutritional support.

Fluid Therapy. Animals with ARF can be dehydrated because of vomiting, diarrhea, and anorexia or overhydrated if they are anuric and have no way to excrete excessive fluid loads. If a fluid deficit is present, fluid volume to be replaced is calculated by multiplying the estimated percentage of dehydration by the body weight in kilograms. Fluids should be given intravenously through a peripheral or central venous catheter. It is preferable to use a jugular catheter because other diagnostic sampling or testing can be performed easily through this site. During the period of rehydration, the animal should be monitored to determine urine output and detect signs of overhydration. Changes in body weight, arterial pressure and CVP, PCV, and total solids. If blood losses also are detected, transfusion should be given to restore PCV and blood pressure.

Animals who are oliguric or anuric must be monitored closely because they have a greater potential of becoming fluid overloaded, hypertensive, and edematous.

Drug Therapy. If oliguria or anuria persists, additional treatment is needed to induce diuresis. Some agents used to induce diuresis are furosemide (Lasix, Hoechst) and mannitol (Osmitrol, Baxter). These drugs often are used in combination to enhance diuresis. Urine output should improve within 1 to 2 hours if treatment is likely to be effective.

Blood pressure should be monitored with changes in fluid balance. Blood pressure can be measured indirectly by oscillometric techniques or ultrasonic Doppler. Normal blood pressure of the dog should be 148 mm Hg systolic, 87 mm Hg diastolic, and 102 mm Hg mean. Normal blood pressure of the cat should be 125 mm Hg systolic, 75 mm Hg diastolic, and 100 mm Hg mean. Systemic hypertension develops from either fluid overload or uremia and may warrant antihypertensive therapy to prevent retinal detachment and cerebral hemorrhage.

Animals with ARF also have severe hyperkalemia and acidosis. Hyperkalemia is the most life-threatening electrolyte abnormality associated with ARF. Acidosis may resolve with fluid therapy, but if serum bicarbonate is less than 15 mEq/L, treatment with sodium bicarbonate should be initiated. Blood gases and total CO_2 should be reevaluated to determine whether additional therapy is needed.

Hyperkalemia can cause cardiac disturbances such as bradycardia, ventricular tachycardia, and fibrillation. ECG changes include peaked T waves, loss of P waves, and wider QRS complexes. If the ECG changes are severe, immediate therapy is needed to decrease serum potassium. Sodium bicarbonate helps correct serum potassium concentrations by exchanging intracellular hydrogen for extracellular potassium. The effects on the heart can be counteracted with calcium gluconate, which antagonizes the cardiotoxicity of high serum potassium concentrations. Glucose and insulin can be given in an emergency to promote the shift of potassium into the cells, where it is safe. If this therapy is used, it is very important to monitor for hypoglycemia.

Gastrointestinal complications such as vomiting, diarrhea, anorexia, and severe ulceration of the gastrointestinal tract and mouth are some of the most common signs of ARF. Vomiting can be controlled by histamine blockers such as cimetidine, ranitidine, or famotidine. Gastrointestinal protectives such as sucralfate can be given to promote gastric ulcer healing. Oral ulcerations are managed effectively by rinsing the mouth frequently with a 0.1% chlorhexidine solution.

Nutritional Support. Many animals with ARF cannot tolerate oral food intake because of vomiting, nausea, or ulcerations. Their diet should be low in protein, phosphorus, and sodium while providing adequate amounts of calories, vitamins, and minerals. The basal energy expenditure (BEE) in kilocalories per day can be determined by the formula 70 × body weight in kilograms to the 75th power. If an animal is critically ill, multiply the BEE by 1.5. If the animal is under minimal stress and has a low activity level, the BEE is multiplied by 1.25. When the patient is catabolic or has a very severe disease, the BEE should be multiplied by 1.75 to 2.0.

Animals that will not eat enough can be fed by a nasal gastric tube or through a percutaneous endoscopically placed gastric tube (PEG). Feeding can be achieved by blending therapeutic diets (Hill's Prescription Diet K/D, Waltham Low Protein Diet) or by using formulated liquid diets (Renal Care). PEG tube feeding should be provided 3 or 4 times daily. Each meal should not exceed one half the animal's stomach volume (60 ml/kg in cats, 90 ml/kg in dogs).

Response to Treatment. Appropriate therapy should improve renal hemodynamics and water and solute imbalances as predicted by a decrease in azotemia, normalization of serum potassium and serum bicarbonate, control of vomiting, resolution of oral and gastric ulceration, and a stabilization of body weight.

If medical management fails to increase urine production and the clinical complications associated with ARF cannot be controlled, alternative approaches must be initiated to stabilize the animal.

Treatment of CRF. CRF is irreversible and progressive. There is no cure, but medical management and dietary management can minimize the progression of CRF.

Fluid Therapy. In CRF, urine production is increased. Therefore, to maintain fluid balance and prevent dehydration, water consumption must be increased either orally, subcutaneously, or intravenously. Some owners are able to give their pets fluids subcutaneously while they are at home.

Drug Therapy. Animals with prolonged CRF become progressively azotemic and eventually develop uremia. Laboratory tests reveal changes in the serum blood chemistry, CBC, and fluid and electrolyte balances. These can include increases in serum bicarbonate, increases in serum phosphorus concentrations, and a nonregenerative anemia caused by the failure of the kidney to synthesize erythropoietin. Blood pressure monitoring can reveal systemic hypertension.

Metabolic acidosis can be treated with oral sodium bicarbonate. Hyperphosphatemia can be controlled with a dietary phosphate restriction and oral phosphate binders (aluminum hydroxide). Nonregenerative anemia can be supported with blood transfusions of compatible red packed blood cells or recumbinant human erythropoietin (Epogen, Amgen). Epogen stimulates RBC production.

Systemic hypertension can be treated with a combination of sodium-restricted diets (e.g., Hill's Prescription Diet K/D) and antihypertensive drugs such as enalapril, hydralazine, or diltiazem. Treatment depends on the severity and causes of the systemic hypertension.

Nutritional Support. Dietary therapy plays an important role in managing CRF. Some of the benefits of appropriate diet for animals with CRF include preventing clinical signs of uremia, minimizing the excess or loss of electrolytes and minerals, slowing the progression of CRF, and maintaining adequate nutrition.

Diets should be low in protein, phosphorus, and sodium. Examples of renal diets are Hill's Prescription Diet K/D, Waltham Low and Medium Protein Diets, and Purina CNM NF. The diets should be fed according to the animal's caloric needs. Appropriate measures should be taken if the animal is showing signs of an acute onset of uremia such as vomiting and anorexia.

Response to Treatment. The animal with CRF should be reevaluated at regular intervals to check for therapeutic response. Monitoring these animals regularly allows treatment of the changing needs that develop over time. If conservative medical management cannot support the patient with CRF, alternative treatments are available.

Alternative Treatments. When conventional therapy fails to restore renal function, or the clinical consequences of uremia, hemodialysis or renal transplantation must be considered.

Hemodialysis. Hemodialysis is a sophisticated renal replacement therapy instituted on a temporary or permanent basis when conventional therapies fail. In ARF, dialysis is initiated at an early stage to stabilize the animal and provide excretory supplementation until renal injury is repaired and adequate renal function returns. Hemodialysis also can be used in combination with conventional medical therapy in animals with severe CRF that cannot be managed with medications and diet alone (Figure 19-5).

Hemodialysis incorporates an artificial kidney or dialyzer to reduce the azotemia and correct life-threatening fluid, electrolyte, and acid-base imbalances. The artificial kidney uses a biocompatible membrane that removes nitrogenous waste products, excess water, and other solutes from the animal's blood down gradients from high to lower concentrations without permitting diffusion and ultrafiltration of larger constituents such as blood cells and proteins.

To perform hemodialysis, a special double-lumen catheter is surgically placed into the external jugular vein for access to the animal's blood for delivery to the dialysis machine. Blood is carried to and from the dialysis delivery system and dialyzer by extracorporeal tubing. Liters of blood, many times the total blood volume of the

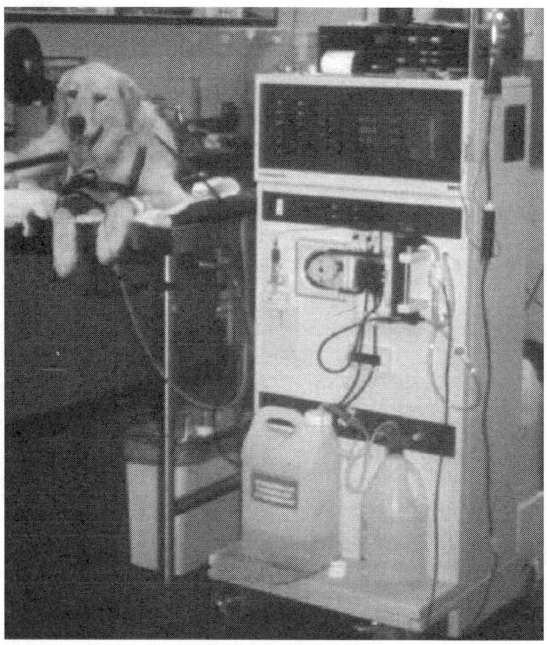

Figure 19-5

Animal receiving hemodialysis therapy.

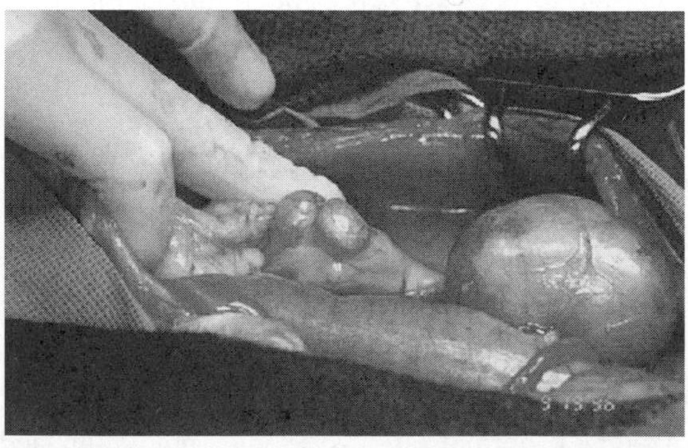

Figure 19-6

Kidney transplant. The left organ is a diseased kidney; on the right is the newly transplanted kidney. (Photograph courtesy of Dr. Lili Aronson, University of California Davis, Veterinary Medical Teaching Hospital, 1997.)

animal, are processed to normalize the serum creatinine and the blood urea nitrogen, concentrations of electrolytes, and water balances.

Many therapeutic options are available for animals with ARF. If treatments are initiated early enough, the chances of kidney regeneration and recovery increase. The animal may go on to lead a normal life with or without supportive care and nutritional management for many months to years.

Renal Transplantation. Renal transplantation can be used to treat cats with ARF or CRF if regeneration and recovery of the existing kidneys is unlikely (Figure 19-6).

The owners of the transplanted animal must be dedicated to treating their pet for life with medications to prevent donor kidney rejection. These medications are immunosuppressive drugs that are combined for optimum effect, such as cyclosporine and prednisone. Transplant recipients must be examined periodically to assess their renal function and cyclosporine levels. Transplanted patients can lead a normal life, and the new kidney can function for many years.

CONCLUSION

Treatment of the urologic emergency depends on the stage of disease or degree of trauma that has occurred. Monitoring equipment and blood analyzers must be available.

The veterinary technician plays a very important role in treating these patients by recognizing the progression of symptoms in the declining patient and understanding the tools used to evaluate the patient's condition.

BIBLIOGRAPHY

Cowgill LD: Renal failure, acute. In Tilley LP, Francis WK, Smithe JP, eds: *The five minute veterinary consult, canine and feline,* Baltimore, 1997, Williams & Wilkins.

Cowgill LD, Langston CE: Role of hemodialysis in the management of dogs and cats with renal failure, *Vet Clin North Am Small Anim Pract* 26(6):1347, 1996.

Finco DR: Obstructive uropathy and hydronephrosis. In Osborne CA, Finco DR, eds: *Canine and feline nephrology and urology,* Baltimore, 1995, Williams & Wilkins.

Lees GE: Management of voiding disability following relief of obstruction. In August JR, ed: *Feline internal medicine,* ed 2, Philadelphia, 1994, WB Saunders.

Ling GV: *Lower urinary tract diseases of dogs and cats. Diagnosis, medical management and prevention,* St Louis, 1995, Mosby.

Osborne CA, Kruger JM, Lulich JP, et al: Feline lower urinary tract disease: relationships between crystalluria, urinary tract infections and host factors. In August JR, ed: *Feline internal medicine,* ed 2, Philadelphia, 1994, WB Saunders.

Osborne CA, Lulich JP, Bartges JW, et al: Canine and feline urolithiasis: relationships of etiopathogenesis to treatment and prevention. In Osborne CA, Finco DR, eds: *Canine and feline nephrology and urology,* Baltimore, 1995, Williams & Wilkins.

Polzin D, Osborne C, Adams L: Nutritional management of chronic renal failure, *Semin Vet Med Surg (Small Anim)* 5(3):187, 1990.

Chapter 20

Reproductive Emergencies

Emergencies of the reproductive tract occur most often in the female animal during pregnancy or estrus. The pregnant patient creates a unique challenge because many lives can be threatened at one time.

The male animal also is susceptible to diseases or trauma of the reproductive tract. In both male and female patients, stabilization and treatment depend on disease severity, age, and breeding potential.

Equipment List

Oxytocin
Calcium gluconate
Antimicrobials
50% Dextrose
Antibiotics
Lubricant
Doxapram
Naloxone
Ear syringe for suction
Small endotracheal tubes
Feeding tubes (3.5, 5 French)
Towels
Hemostats
Tincture of iodine
Incubator
Small bottles and different sizes and shapes of nipples

REPRODUCTIVE EMERGENCIES IN THE FEMALE

Dystocia is defined as abnormal labor or birth. Normal parturition is the delivery by the bitch or queen of full-term healthy puppies or kittens, respectively, without outside assistance of any sort. Dystocia occurs in almost all breeds of dogs and is not uncommon. Dystocia in cats is not a common occurrence except in purebred cats such as Persians. Dystocia is common in breeds with large heads and wide shoulders.

Stages of Parturition

The demarcation between the three stages of labor is not always clear cut. The onset of stage 1 is heralded by increased maternal behavior. The dam displays nesting behavior, restlessness, panting, and shivering, and she may seek seclusion. Vomiting may be observed. Lactation and a transient temperature drop of approximately 2° F, in conjunction with luteolysis, occurs 24 to 36 hours before stage 1. Toward the end of stage 1 the cervix is dilated. The duration of the first stage is approximately 12 to 24 hours.

Increased strength and frequency of uterine contractions, visible abdominal contractions, and movement of the fetus through the cervix into the vagina are indicative of stage 2 parturition.

The time between the onset of straining and the delivery of the first fetus varies, but it should be less than 1 hour. Both resting and straining phases occur between individual deliveries. The resting phase may last up to 3 hours. It may take up to 30 minutes of maximum straining before subsequent fetuses are delivered. The size of the litter and the quality of the labor are factors in the length of time between delivery of the first and last fetus. The time from the first to the last birth is variable and can be as long as 24 hours, but this is undesirable. Stage 3 is the delivery of the allantochorion (placenta). This stage actually is interspersed with stage 2. Passage of the allantochorion may occur after each fetus or after two or three fetuses. The dam should be monitored for delivery of an allantochorion for each fetus. Retained allantochorion can lead to endometritis. Stages 2 and 3 alternate until all fetuses have been delivered. A green to reddish brown vaginal discharge can occur for up to 2 weeks after whelping, and light spotting can occur for 8 weeks.

Dystocia

Dystocia should be suspected when the dam experiences prolonged gestation. Dystocia can be characterized as active straining for more than 60 minutes without delivery of a fetus, resting without straining for more than 4 hours between deliveries with known retained fetuses, intermittent weak contractions for more than 2 hours, or maternal or fetal stress.

Causes. The causes of dystocia can be maternal or fetal. Maternal causes include uterine inertia or anatomic abnormalities. Uterine inertia is poor strength or frequency of myometrial contraction efforts. It can be caused by an inherited predisposition, overstretching (large litters), insufficient stimulation (small litters), systemic disease (obesity, hypocalcemia, hypoglycemia, septicemia), age-related changes, exhaustion, stress, and anxiety. Anatomic abnormalities include narrowing of the pelvic canal (congenital, neoplasia, or trauma related), uterine malposition, and developmental abnormalities of the genital canal. Fetal causes of dystocia include abnormally large, malpositioned, or dead fetuses.

Diagnosis. The normal variations of parturition make recognizing dystocia difficult. Diagnosis and therapy are based on thorough history and physical examination. In addition to the normal patient history, an obstetric history (Box 20-1) must be obtained.

As part of the physical examination, a digital examination (using aseptic technique) should be performed to ascertain the presence and position of a fetus in the birth canal. Bone or soft tissue abnormalities of the pelvis or vaginal vault (strictures, masses) also should be noted during the digital examination.

Diagnostic aids such as radiography and ultrasonography and Doppler examination of the fetal heart may help in decision making. Radiographs can reveal the presence, number, size, location, and possible viability of fetuses. Spinal collapse and malposition, intrafetal gas patterns, and overlapping cranial bones are suggestive of past fetal death (Figure 20-1). Assessment of the abdomen and pelvis also is aided by radiography. Ultrasonography can detect fetal movement, heartbeats, and heart rate, which is useful in assessing fetal stress.

Box 20-1 Questions to Ask as Part of an Obstetric History

- Is this the first litter? If not, have there been problems with previous litters?
- How long has it been since the last mating? Was any ovulation timing done?
- Did stage 1 of labor occur? How long did it last?
- Has an amnion or fetus been seen at the vulva? How long ago was this observed?
- How long has the straining lasted? Did it produce a neonate? What was the length of time between neonates?
- What was the condition of the neonates at birth?
- Any vaginal discharge? If so, what color and consistency?
- Have all the placentas been accounted for?

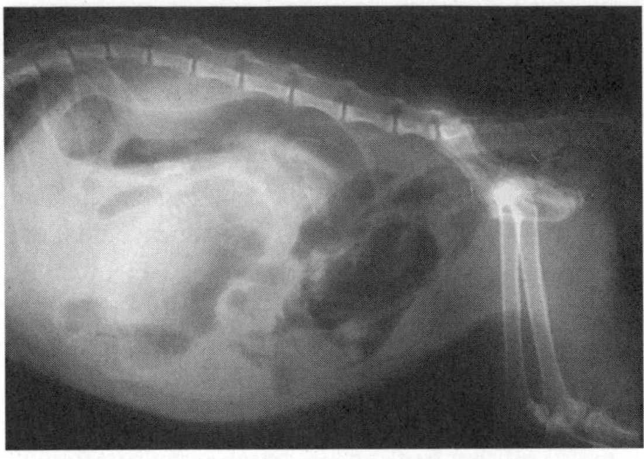

Figure 20-1

There is evidence of a fetus within the pelvic canal with air surrounding the fetus. There are three additional fetuses with evidence of abnormal position, suggesting fetal death.

Treatment. Management options depend on several factors. These factors include the value of the offspring and dam, the owner's wishes, and the availability of personnel and equipment. Three treatment options are available: medical intervention, manual manipulation, and surgical management.

Medical intervention may be as simple as administering a tranquilizer to calm a stressed dam. After obstruction has been ruled out and the quality of uterine contractions assessed, ecbolic agents may be given to stimulate uterine contractions. Oxytocin is the most common ecbolic agent used. The emergence of fetal monitoring in the veterinary patient is beginning to be seen. Fetal monitors help to guide medical therapy by revealing the frequency and strength of contractions. One of the benefits of fetal monitoring is a reduction in the amount of oxytocin given. Lower dosages (0.25 to 0.5 U/dog intramuscularly) have been used in the bitch with success. Previously, recommended dosages for oxytocin ranged from 1.1 to 2.2 U/kg intramuscularly. Oxytocin overdose can lead to tetanic uterine contractions, which can result in impaired placental blood flow. Calcium gluconate or dextrose can be administered when hypocalcemia or hypoglycemia has been confirmed and uterine inertia is a problem. If the initial dose of oxytocin is ineffective, calcium gluconate can be administered (even if serum calcium is normal) subcutaneously 15 to 20 minutes before subsequent oxytocin doses. Intravenous calcium should be given with caution, and heart rate and rhythm should be monitored. Intravenous calcium administration should be slowed or discontinued if bradycardia and arrhythmias develop. It has been suggested that calcium gluconate be given subcutaneously 15 minutes before oxytocin administration and that intravenous calcium be reserved for cases of eclampsia. (Personal Communication with Autumn P. Davidson, DVM, Dip. ACVIM.) It is believed that the oxytocin will stimulate contractions and the subsequent dose of calcium will strengthen them.

In the case of obstructive dystocia caused by fetal malposition or slightly oversized or dead fetuses, manual manipulation may be of benefit. Vaginal manipulation may be attempted digitally or by careful use of instruments. Obstetric instrumentation is difficult to use except in very large dogs. Lubrication may help, but the veterinarian must proceed cautiously to avoid injuring the fetus or dam.

Surgical intervention is needed in the case of uterine inertia that is unresponsive to medical therapy or obstructive dystocia that cannot be corrected by manipulation. If a cesarean section is to be performed, an anesthetic protocol should be selected that provides adequate analgesia, muscle relaxation, and sedation or narcosis to the dam with minimal depression or compromise to the fetuses. Steps should be taken to minimize anesthesia time, such as clipping and prepping the dam and surgeon before anesthetic induction. Fluid support should be provided to the patient so as to prevent hypovolemia. Hypotension may be a problem when the patient is placed in dorsal recumbency. Hypotension may be caused by compression of the caudal vena cava by the gravid uterus. If hypotension is a problem, the patient can be repositioned so that it is tilted slightly toward the surgeon. Hypoxia is a potential problem because the diaphragm is impinged by the abdominal contents. Once the neonates are delivered, the technician may be responsible for resuscitation. Resuscitation includes removing fetal membranes, clearing the airway with gentle suction, administering oxygen by a small face mask, or stimulating breathing with intramuscular doxapram or naloxone (if opioids are used). The umbilical stumps are tied off and swabbed with a tincture of iodine solution. The neonates should be placed in a prewarmed environment (incubator) until they can be placed with the dam. Routine postoperative care is provided to the dam.

PYOMETRA

Pyometra is an infection in the uterus that is most common in middle-aged to older bitches and queens during diestrus, 45 days after estrus. It can also be seen up to 10 weeks after estrogen therapy for mismating in bitches and in cats or dogs receiving progestins. It is caused by hormonally (progesterone or exogenous estrogens) induced changes.

Clinical Presentation. Patients may be depressed and septic or clinically normal. Clinical signs include lethargy, anorexia, dehydration, vomiting, diarrhea, polyuria, polydipsia, and vaginal discharge (with open pyometra). Clinical signs may be subtle in cats. Because of their grooming habits, vaginal discharge may not be seen.

Diagnosis. Diagnostic workup may include complete blood cell count, chemistry, urinalysis (do not attempt a cystocentesis if pyometra is suspected), cytology of discharge and culture, blood gases, and electrolytes. Additional diagnostic techniques include radiography and ultrasonography. Leukogram may show a leukocytosis with or without a left shift, or it may be normal. Nonregenerative anemia and hyperglobulinemia are common. Prerenal azotemia may be attributed to endotoxins elaborated by coliforms. Vaginal cytology and culture may be helpful in diagnosing pyometra and selecting antibiotics. Blood gases and electrolytes will help in developing a fluid therapy plan.

Radiography is used to confirm the presence of an enlarged uterus. Loss of abdominal detail may suggest peritonitis secondary to uterus rupture. Ultrasonography is used to differentiate pyometra from pregnancy or hydrometra.

Treatment. Treatment options are based on the condition, age, and breeding value of the animal. Pyometras can be surgically (treatment of choice) or medically managed. Medical management in the case of open pyometras involves prostaglandin administration. Patients receiving prostaglandin therapy should be observed in the hospital. Transient side effects such as anxiety, vomiting, diarrhea, tachypnea, and tachycardia may be seen shortly after prostaglandin administration. The therapeutic index of prostaglandins is narrow. All patients should be treated with intensive fluid therapy, antibiotics, and supportive care.

UTERINE TORSIONS

Uterine torsions are very uncommon in the dog and in the cat. A partial or complete torsion can occur during pregnancy. Possible causes include jumping or running late in the pregnancy, active fetal movement, premature contractions, partial abortions, or abnormalities of the uterus.

Clinical signs may include pain, collapse, and abdominal distention. Severe hemorrhage can occur if the uterine artery is damaged.

It is often difficult to differentiate between uterine torsion and dystocia. Radiographs may indicate a large fluid- or air-filled tubular structure in the abdominal cavity. Many times it is not diagnosed until surgery. Ovariohysterectomy is recommended.

MALE REPRODUCTIVE EMERGENCIES

ACUTE BACTERIAL PROSTATITIS

Acute bacterial prostatitis is acute inflammation of the prostate gland with gram-positive or gram-negative bacteria. The infection commonly results from bacteria ascending through the urethra. The bacteria also can be introduced through the bloodstream or reproductive tract. Older, intact male dogs are most commonly affected.

Clinical signs include lethargy, fever, dehydration, purulent or bloody discharge from the urethra, and caudal abdominal pain. The dog may walk with a stiff gait and arched back because of the pain. A diagnosis usually is made based on the examination, routine laboratory evaluation, and response to treatment. Caudal abdominal radiographs may show an enlarged prostate. Evaluation of the prostatic fluid including culture and cytology would be another tool for diagnosing bacterial prostatitis. It is very difficult to obtain prostatic fluid from a dog experiencing this painful disease because ejaculation is necessary. Prostatic washes are an option but must be performed very carefully because of the risk of sepsis.

An antimicrobial is chosen based on the urine culture and administered for 4 to 6 weeks. Stabilization and fluid therapy may be necessary for more severe cases. Castration is recommended once the animal is stabilized.

Prostatic Abscess

Prostatic abscess occurs in dogs with an acute or chronic form of prostatitis. Clinical signs include lethargy, fever, vomiting, dysuria, abdominal pain, and urethral discharge. The animal may also present with signs of shock if the abscess has ruptured. A prostatic abscess can be confirmed by the use of radiography, ultrasonography, and prostate fluid analysis.

Surgical drainage of the prostatic abscesses or prostatectomy is performed once the dog has been stabilized. Castration also is recommended. Antimicrobials are continued postoperatively.

Paraphimosis

Paraphimosis, the inability to retract the penis within the prepuce, most commonly occurs after copulation. Treatment includes cleaning and lubricating the penis before attempting to replace it manually into the prepuce. Hyperosmotic agents (50% dextrose) applied on the penis may help decrease swelling. Sedation may be needed. Surgical intervention may be necessary if the penis cannot be returned to the normal position or if the penile vessels have been thrombosed.

Testicular Torsion

Testicular torsion is most common in dogs with retained testicles. Clinical signs include acute abdominal pain, anorexia, vomiting, and occasionally collapse. A dog with scrotal testes will present with a stiff gait and testicular swelling if a testicular torsion is present. Treatment involves excision of the testicle.

CONCLUSION

It is important to understand the breeding potential of the animal with a reproductive emergency. Owners must understand the treatment options and relative risks. The veterinary technician can provide information to help the owner make the best decision for the patient.

BIBLIOGRAPHY

Gaudet DA, Kitchell BE: Canine dystocia. *Compend Contin Educ Pract Vet* 1985; 7(5).

Grotter AM: Diseases of the ovaries and uterus. In Birchard SJ, Sherding RG, eds: *Saunders manual of small animal practice,* Philadelphia, 1994, WB Saunders.

Macintire DK: Emergencies of the female reproductive tract. In Kirby R, Crow DT, eds: *Veterinary clinics of north america,* Philadelphia, 1994, WB Saunders.

Chapter 21

Ocular Emergencies

The eye is a sensitive organ that when irritated, can cause much discomfort to the animal. This discomfort may cause the animal to rub and scratch at the area. A mild inflammation or infection may change to a serious condition in a short period of time. When an owner calls with a concern involving a pet's eye, the animal should be seen to rule out a serious condition and provide pain relief as soon as possible. All brachycephalic breeds should be seen as soon as possible when any signs of blepharospasm are present.

Problems can occur in various parts of the eye. The globe, eyelids, cornea, anterior chamber, and lens are the areas covered in this chapter (Figure 21-1).

Equipment List

OptiVisor for magnification
Tonopen for glaucoma
Mannitol
Topicals
- Ophthaine
- Nonsteroidal antiinflammatory drugs (Volteron)
- Steroid (prednisolone acetate)
- Combination steroid and antibiotic (Maxitrol)
- General antibiotic
- Atropine 1%
- Phenylephrine 2.5%

Suture materials
- 4-0 or 5-0 silk with P-3 or G-3 needle
- 8-0 Vicryl

Surgical pack with the following instruments
- Nasolacrimal cannula (23 gauge)
- Bishop Harmon dressing forceps
- Barraquer cilia forceps
- Troutman-Barraquer cornea utility forceps
- Hartman curved hemostatic mosquito forceps
- Barraquer eye speculum (pediatric and adult sizes)
- Catalano needle holder, curved with or without lock (8-0 Vicryl)
- Westcott curved or straight tenotomy scissors
- Stevens straight tenotomy scissors
- Derf needle holder

GLOBE

Exophthalmos, an enlargement of the globe, is seen with glaucoma, intraocular tumors, panophthalmitis, retrobulbar mass, and proptosis.

Glaucoma can present with dilated pupils, corneal edema, and conjunctival congestion, and the pupillary light reflex may or may not be present. Glaucoma can be caused by inherited predisposition, trauma, anterior luxating lens or infection (Figure 21-2, Color plate 4).

Treatment begins by determining whether vision is present and whether the glaucoma is a chronic or acute condition. If it is chronic and vision is not apparent, pain relief is the goal. Pain relief is accomplished medically or surgically. Medical therapy can include topical drugs that increase the uveoscleral outflow of the aqueous humor (Xalatan) and Alphagan increases uveoscleral outflow and decreases production of aqueous humor. Other topical drugs (Timoptic, Trusopt) and oral medications (Methazolamide) are used to

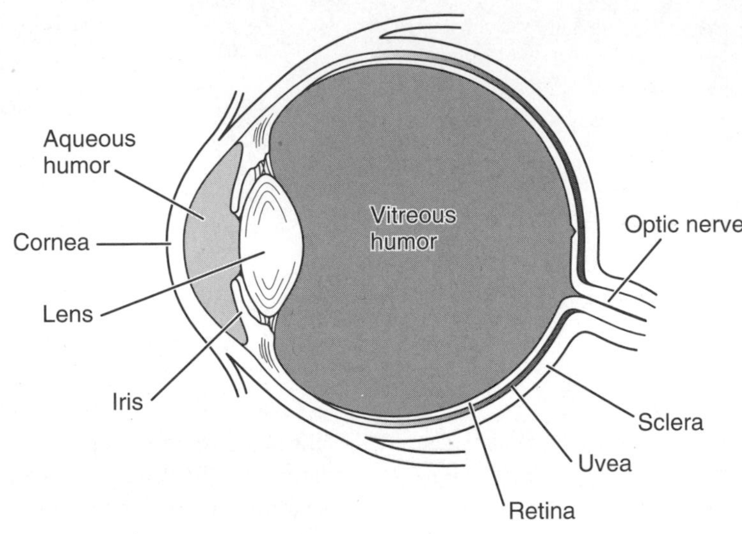

Figure 21-1

Diagram of the eye.

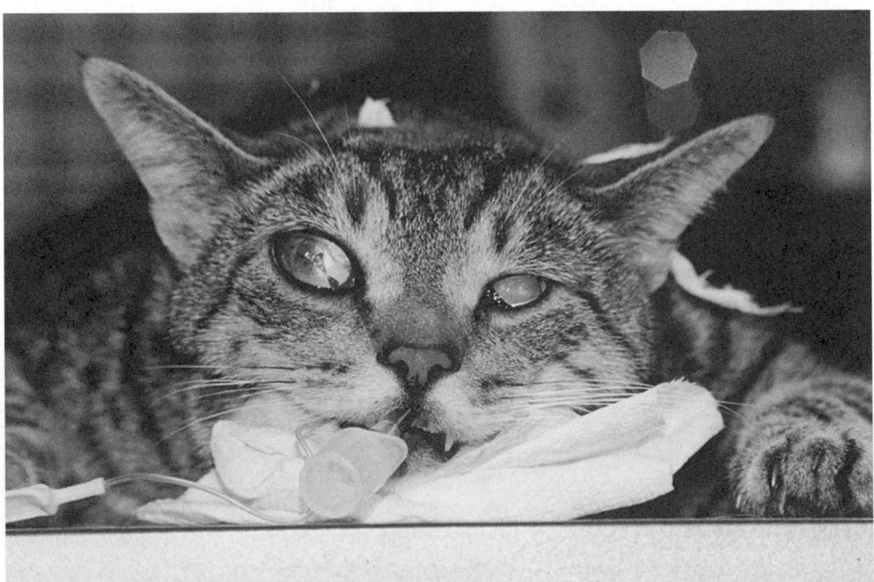

Figure 21-2

A cat with buthalmia (enlargement and distention of the globe) in the right eye caused by glaucoma.

decrease fluid production. Surgical procedures used to relieve the pain in the blind eye include enucleation, ciliary body ablation, and intrascleral prosthesis (Table 21-1).

If the glaucoma is acute, the vision may be saved with immediate treatment. Mannitol is administered intravenously (1 g/lb) to shrink the vitreous humor. Topical drugs are used concurrently. Laser or surgical treatment may be necessary:

- Cyclophotoablation (laser therapy) and gonio implants are used to decrease intraocular pressure.
- Surgical removal of the lens is an option to relieve the pressure and preserve vision if a luxated lens is the cause of the glaucoma.

Intraocular tumors may present as an acute onset of pain. Hyphema, melanois (a change in the iris, most common in cats), buthalmia, inability to retropulse the eye, and medial or lateral strabismus are other signs associated with tumors. Pupillary light response may or may not be present. Cats may present with a history of a previous trauma to the affected eye, sometimes years earlier, and have a sudden onset of these signs. Treatment usually involves orbital enucleation or exenteration to relieve pain.

Panophthalmitis is inflammation of all structures or tissues of the eye. It presents as an acute onset of pain, conjunctival congestion, or hypopyon (pus in the chamber). Panophthalmitis can be a secondary sign of a systemic illness, especially if hypopyon is present. Aggressive oral and topical antibiotic therapy is necessary. Antiinflammatory medications also are used. Enucleation often is necessary to relieve the pain.

Retrobulbar mass can be caused by trauma, tumors, or abscess. Skull radiographs, chemistry profiles, and a complete blood cell count are performed, try to determine the underlying cause. The protrusion of the globe, inability to blink, and inability to retract the eye are common presenting signs. Once the underlying cause is determined, treatment can begin. The cornea must be protected from drying with a lubricating ointment.

Proptosis, the forward displacement of the globe, may present with conjunctival hemorrhage and/or hyphema. The common causes include trauma or tumors. Intravenous dexamethasone is used to decrease inflammation in the optic nerve. The eye can be replaced with or without a lateral canthotomy. Then a temporary tarsorrhapy is performed to protect the cornea. Topical antibiotic is used to protect the cornea. Oral antibiotics and cortisone are continued after surgical intervention. Lids are closed for 2 weeks minimally, and an Elizabethan collar is used to prevent rubbing. Lateral strabismus may be observed after proptosis.

Enophthalmos, the backward displacement of the globe into the orbit, presents with a retracted eye, prolapse of the third eyelid, blepharospasm, miotic pupil, or epiphoria. Corneal ulcers, a foreign body, Horner syndrome, acute glaucoma, trauma, and entropion are possible causes of this condition. It is important to determine the underlying cause if possible. Topical anesthetic (Ophthaine) is used to relieve the blepharospasm. Horner syndrome should be suspected if there is no relief with the topical anesthetic.

Horner syndrome involves the sympathetic nervous system. The sympathetic nerves are located very shallow under the skin, and consistent pressure applied to this area, as by a choke collar, can damage these nerves. Drops of 2.5% to 10% phenylephrine are used to test for this disorder. If there is a positive response, the pupil dilates, the third eyelid goes down, and the eyeball comes forward. If the underlying disorder is not determined, this treatment can be used as needed. Some animals recover without treatment, but when the underlying disorder is determined, it must be treated appropriately.

EYELID

The animal with entropion, the inward displacement of the lid, presents with squinting, third eyelid protrusion, epiphoria, and blepharospasm. There is an inherited form and a spastic form of entropion. The spastic form usually is caused by trauma or corneal ulceration. If a corneal ulcer is present, enophthalmia can result from pain, relaxing the eyelids to cause entro-

TABLE 21-1 Common Medications Used for Ocular Emergencies

Drug	Effect	Treatment Protocol
Acetylcytine 10% (topical)	Assists in stopping collagenic activity.	1 drop every hour on melting ulcers, usually mixed with equal amount of an antibiotic.
Alphagan	Increases uveoscleral outflow and reduces production of aqueous humor.	TID
Atropine 1% (topical)	Dilates pupils, relieves pain, prevents synechia.	1 drop as needed to dilate; effect is long lasting.
Cosopt	Combination of timolol and Trusopt (less expensive than both drugs alone).	TID
Dexamethasone (intravenous)	Decreases inflammation of optic nerves, uvea, anterior chamber.	0.25 mg/lb.
Gentocin (topical)	Antibacterial medication.	1 drop TID or QID up to every hour for severe ulcer.
Mannitol (intravenous)	Decreases pressure by shrinking vitreous humor.	1 g/lb IV given slowly over 20-30 min. If solution is crystallized, dissolve crystals by immersing bottle in hot water.
Maxitrol (topical)	Controls inflammatory response; steroid/antibiotic combination.	1 drop every 2-8 hr depending on severity of infection.
Methazolamide (oral)	Decreases fluid production.	0.25-0.5 mg/lb BID.
Muro 128 Ointment 5%	Assists in attachment of new epithelial cells.	Apply every 8 hr for ulcers. Always apply 30-60 min after any other medication.
Mydriacyl 1% (topical)	Dilates pupils. Short acting (4-6 hr).	Can be toxic to the epithelium. Use 1-3 drops only as needed to relieve pain to perform necessary tests.
Ophthaine (topical)	Anesthetic; relieves blepharospasm.	Can be toxic to the epithelium. Use 1-3 drops only as needed to relieve pain to perform necessary tests.
Optimmune ointment	Tear stimulant.	Apply ¼ inch TID.
2.5% Phenylephrine (topical)	Dilates pupils. Usually for Horner's syndrome PRN to bring third eyelid down.	SID or BID.
Pred Forte 1% (topical)	Controls inflammatory response.	1 drop every 2-8 hr depending on severity of inflammation.
Propine 0.1%	Decreases aqueous production and enhances outflow.	TID
Timolol/Timoptic (topical)	Decreases fluid production.	1 drop every 8 hr.
Trusopt (topical)	Decreases fluid production. Topical does the same as the oral methazolamide.	1 drop every 8 hr.
Vira A ointment	Antiviral medication.	¼ inch every 6 hr. Decreases weekly.
Viroptic (topical)	Antiviral medication.	1 drop every 6 hr initially. Usually decreases weekly.
Diclofenac (Voltaren) (topical)	Nonsteroidal antiinflammatory drug.	1 drop BID.
Xalatan (topical)	Increases uveoscleral outflow of the aqueous humor. Human drug used only at bedtime, when pressure usually rises. May cause severe miosis and may have to be discontinued. Can be used SID or BID.	

pion. Treatment for spastic entropion includes temporary tacking of the eyelids and applying lubricating ointment. Antibiotic ointment may be necessary if an infection is present.

Age is an important factor in the inherited form of entropion. Many dogs grow out of the defect, and surgical intervention in young dogs is to be avoided if possible. Temporary eyelid tacking may be necessary until the animal is fully grown (Table 21-2).

Ectropion, the outward displacement of the lids, can cause epiphoria and mucopurulent discharge. Horner syndrome, enophthalmia caused by trauma, and lagophthalmos can cause this condition. Ectropion is an inherited disorder. Lubricating ointment is used to protect the corneal surface, and an Elizabethan collar is placed to prevent further trauma.

Meibomian gland abscess or adenoma (chalazion) is the chronic or acute swelling of one or more meibomian glands along the upper and lower eyelids. Crusting or bleeding along the eyelids may be observed. Inflammation caused by an abscess or benign growth of the glands is a common cause of this condition. Treatment includes lancing the swelling if an abscess is present and surgical excision of the growth if a tumor is present. Topical antibiotic ointment follows the surgical intervention, and an Elizabethan collar is placed on the animal to prevent rubbing.

Symblepharon is the adhesion of the conjunctiva to the lid and the eyeball. This condition occurs in utero and is caused by a virus (herpes, calici, chlamydia). Treatment includes surgical correction by removing the conjunctiva from the corneal surface and treating the underlying virus with an ophthalmic ointment (VIRAA Ophthalmic Ointment, Viroptic Ophthalmic Solution).

Cherry eye, or prolapsed gland of the third eyelids, can appear very red and irritated. Trauma and breed predisposition are the common causes of this condition. The gland can be replaced manually after the use of a topical anesthetic. Cortisone ointment (Maxitrol) controls the inflammatory response. Surgical intervention may be necessary if it continues to prolapse. Removing the gland is not recommended because of the risk of keratoconjunctivitis sicca. Suturing it in place is preferred.

CORNEA

Corneal ulcers can cause epiphoria, blepharitis, mucopurulent discharge, and photophobia. Ulcers can be superficial, recurrent, collagenase, desmetocele, or viral. They occur when the cornea has been irritated by chemicals, foreign bodies, ectopic cilia, or trauma. Breed predisposition also can be a factor. Treatment varies according to the type of ulcer present. An Elizabethan collar should be placed and other necessary measures taken to prevent further trauma for all types of ulcers (Figure 21-3, Color plate 5).

Superficial ulcers are commonly treated with an antibiotic solution or ointment (e.g., Gentocin opthalmic solution or ointment or triple-antibiotic ointment).

Recurrent erosions present as chronic ulcers that did not respond to previous therapies. Additional treatment or medication is needed. A grid keratectomy usually is necessary. Topical and general anesthesia may be needed before the procedure. First, a cotton swab is used to debride the ulcer, then a 25-gauge needle is used to make a grid. This allows attachment of new epithelial cells to the cornea. A sodium chloride ointment (Muro 128 ophthalmic ointment) can be used to promote attachment of new epithelial cells.

Collagenase ulcers, or melting ulcers, are the most difficult to treat. Brachycephalic breeds are commonly affected. The cornea is made of collagen, and the ulcer produces a collagenase that eats through the cornea. Intensive medical therapy is necessary. Serum can be used from the patient as an eyedrop to stop the collagenic activity. Acetylcysteine and Gentocin are also used hourly to stop collagenic activity in some cases. A nonsteroidal antiinflammatory drug (Voltaren) may be necessary if uveitis is present. Conjuntival grafting is performed if the medical therapy fails.

Desmetocele is an ulcer that has progressed to the last layer of the cornea. The cornea will rupture if it progresses. Topical therapy may be indicated if blood vessels are present and there is no leakage. Medical therapy must be attempted with caution. Sometimes just a sneeze will rupture the cornea. A

TABLE 21-2 Breed Predisposition for Ocular Disease

Dogs	
Akita	Entropion
Alaskan malamute	Glaucoma
American Staffordshire terrier	Entropion
Australian cattle dog	Anterior luxating lens
Basset hound	Glaucoma, entropion, ectropion
Beagle	Glaucoma, cherry eye
Belgian sheepdog	Pannus
Belgian tervuren	Pannus
Bloodhound	Entropion, ectropion, cherry eye
Border collie	Anterior luxating lens
Boston terrier	Glaucoma
Bouvier des Flandres	Glaucoma
Boxer	Ectropion, corneal ulcers
Brachycephalic breeds	Corneal ulcers
Brittany spaniel	Anterior luxating lens
Bulldog (English)	Entropion, ectropion, cherry eye
Bull mastiff	Glaucoma, entropion, ectropion
Burmese mountain dog	Entropion
Cairn terrier	Glaucoma
Chesapeake Bay retriever	Entropion
Chinese shar-pei	Glaucoma, anterior luxating lens, entropion, cherry eye
Chow chow	Glaucoma, entropion
Clumber spaniel	Entropion, ectropion
Cocker spaniel	Glaucoma, entropion, ectropion, cherry eye
Dachshund	Pannus
Dalmatian	Glaucoma, entropion
English springer spaniel	Entropion
English toy spaniel	Entropion
Flat-coated retriever	Entropion
German shepherd	Pannus
Golden retriever	Glaucoma, entropion
Gordon setter	Entropion, ectropion
Great Dane	Glaucoma, entropion, ectropion
Greyhound	Pannus
Irish setter	Entropion
Japanese chin	Entropion
Labrador retriever	Entropion, ectropion
Lhasa apso	Cherry eye
Mastiff	Entropion, ectropion
Newfoundland	Entropion, ectropion, cherry eye
Norwegian elkhound	Glaucoma
Old English sheepdog	Entropion
Pekingese	Entropion
Pomeranian	Entropion
Pug	Entropion
Rottweiler	Entropion
Saint Bernard	Entropion, ectropion

TABLE 21-2 Breed Predisposition for Ocular Disease—cont'd

Dogs—cont'd	
Samoyed	Glaucoma
Shih tzu	Entropion, ectropion
Siberian husky	Glaucoma, entropion
Smooth fox terrier	Glaucoma
Terriers	Anterior luxating lens
Tibetan spaniel	Entropion
Viszla	Entropion
Weimaraner	Entropion
Welsh springer spaniel	Glaucoma
Wire-haired fox terrier	Glaucoma, anterior luxating lens
Yorkshire terrier	Entropion
Cats	
Burmese	Corneal sequestrum, keratoconjunctivitis sicca
Himalayan	Corneal sequestrum
Persian	Corneal sequestrum
Siamese	Corneal sequestrum

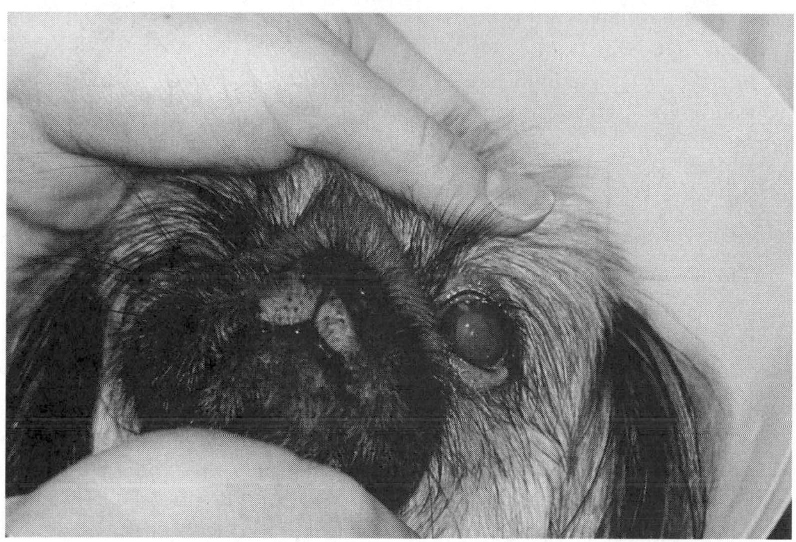

Figure 21-3

A Pekinese with conjunctival hyperemia, with mucopurulent discharge in the left eye caused by a corneal ulcer.

topical antibiotic, acetylcysteine 10% (stops collagenic activity), and atropine 1% (dilates pupil and relieves pain) are commonly used for the medical treatment. Surgery is recommended to preserve vision and prevent rupture of the eye. Surgical correction may include conjunctival grafting or corneal scleral transposition.

Viral ulcers commonly occur in cats with a history of upper respiratory infection. Treatment includes a systemic antibiotic for a bacterial infection and topical antiviral medications (VIRAA ophthalmic ointment, Viroptic ophthalmic solution).

Keratoconjunctivitis sicca (KCS) can cause purulent discharge, blepharitis, and a dull cornea. Thickened eyelids may result from rubbing. Cats may present with very mild signs, but Burmese cats are more susceptible. Cherry eye removal, conjunctivitis, congenital defects, anesthesia, drug therapy (i.e., sulfa drugs), and hypothyroidism can cause this. Treatment involves stimulating tear production with topical ointments (Optimmune) and maintaining moisture with artificial tears several times daily.

Keratitis can cause a cloudy or pigmented cornea and blepharitis. Chronic exposure, KCS, virus, lagophthalmos, pannus, trichiasis, distichia, and facial nerve paralysis can cause this condition. The underlying problem must be determined and treated appropriately.

Pannus, the superficial vascularization of the cornea with infiltration of granulation tissue, is most common in certain breeds. It is believed to be an immune-mediated disease. Depigmenting of the third eyelid, granulation tissue, superficial blood vessels, and pigment on the cornea are common presenting signs. Optimmune ophthalmic ointment and corticosteroids are used to treat pannus.

A corneal foreign body can cause acute blepharospasm, epiphoria, and conjunctival hyperemia. The object usually can be removed with topical anesthetic. A small-gauge hypodermic needle or ophthalmic surgical forceps are used for this procedure. The ulcer is treated with topical antibiotics, and an Elizabethan collar is placed around the patient's head to prevent further damage. If the injury is deep, Acetylcysteine 10% may be needed.

Corneal sequestrum occurs when an area of the cornea has become sequestered. Brown or black areas can be seen on the cornea; epiphora and blepharospasm also can be observed. The animal usually has a history of corneal injury. It can also be caused by a virus or breed predisposition in cats. Topical therapy is used to prevent infection and lubricate the eye. Surgical excision is usually necessary to remove sequestered tissue.

ANTERIOR CHAMBER

Uveitis, inflammation of the vascular layer of the eye, can cause blepharospasm, miosis, iritis, iris color change, photophobia, hypopyon, and epiphora. It can be idiopathic or caused by a virus, systemic illness, or trauma. It is important to diagnose and treat any underlying problems. Topical therapy can include nonsteroidal or steroidal antibiotics or a combination thereof.

Hyphema, blood in the anterior chamber, can cause blepharospasm, epiphora, and glaucoma. Trauma, retinal detachment, iris tumors, and ciliary body bleed are possible causes. Topical cortisone can be used if the cornea is intact. Intravenous dexamethazone and intraocular injection of tissue plasmin activator is used to break up clots and reduce the chance of adhesion. Oral steroid therapy and topical therapy are continued until the clot is absorbed and the intraocular structures can be viewed.

LENS

Anterior lens luxation can cause corneal edema, blepharospasm, and lethargy. The resulting glaucoma causes severe pain in acute cases. Breed predisposition, trauma, and glaucoma are the most common causes of this condition.

Mannitol 20% 1 g/lb intravenously over 30 minutes can be used to relieve intraocular pressure. Mydriatics (Mydriacyl 1%, Murocoll 2 ophthalmic solution) can be used to dilate the pupil and allow the lens to fall behind the iris. Antiinflammatories and antiglaucoma medications also may be needed to control the pressure. It may be necessary to remove the lens to restore vision and relieve pressure and the inflammatory reaction in the acute cases.

Cataracts can cause epiphora, uveitis, blepharospasm, hypopyon, miosis, a white pupil, and vision loss in acute cases. Trauma, diabetes, and chronic uveitis are possible causes of this condition; cataracts can also be hereditary or age related.

The goal in acute onset is to control the reaction caused by the changing lens. Medications can control the reaction caused by the cataract but will

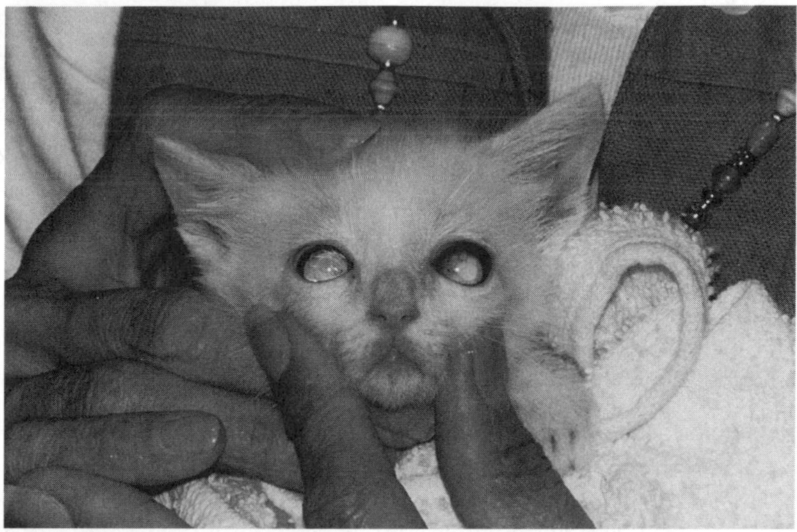

Figure 21-4

A kitten with congenital cataracts in both eyes.

not cure the condition. Topical steroids and nonsteroidal medications are used to control lens-induced uveitis. Mydriatics are used to dilate the pupil and prevent synechia. The cataract is removed once the lens-induced uveitis is controlled (Figure 21-4, Color plate 6).

Nuclear sclerosis is the hardening of the nucleus of the lens. It is characterized by a graying of the lens and may be confused with cataracts. Depth perception and limited visual capabilities in various lighting may be observed. There is no treatment for this condition.

CONCLUSION

It is not easy to determine the severity of an ophthalmic emergency over the phone. If the animal is experiencing pain around or on the surface of the eye (as evidenced by squinting, epiphora), it must be seen. A mild infection can quickly turn into a severe problem if the animal rubs or scratches the area. Pain relief is important.

Many problems of the eye are a secondary sign of a primary infection. Other tests should be run to determine whether there are any other underlying problems. (It is true that the eyes may be the window to the soul.)

The emergency facility must be equipped to deal with eye problems. Instruments used only for eyes should be stored in a separate pack; ointments and eyewash also should be available. Pain relievers and restraints are used to prevent the animal from damaging the eye after treatment. A variety of Elizabethan collars should be available to meet the needs of each patient.

BIBLIOGRAPHY

Chrisman CL: *Problems in small animal neurology,* Malvern, Pa, 1991, Lea & Febiger.

Ocular disorders presumed to be inherited in purebred dogs, 1996, American College of Veterinary Ophthalmologists.

Physician's desk reference for ophthalmology, ed 27, Philadelphia, 1999, WB Saunders.

Chapter 22

Neurologic Emergencies

In general, neurologic emergencies fall into two categories: perceived emergencies and true veterinary emergencies. Almost every veterinarian and technician has experienced a frantic call from an owner late at night whose healthy young pet has had its very first seizure lasting for less than a minute. Certainly, this is not a life-threatening emergency. The pet should be seen by a veterinarian the next morning, but a single short seizure in an otherwise healthy pet does not warrant an emergency visit. On the other hand, a seizure that lasts longer than 3 to 4 minutes or several seizures occurring within a short period of time truly is a veterinary emergency. These situations warrant immediate medical care at an emergency clinic. Prolonged or consecutive seizures can cause permanent neurologic damage and can result in hyperthermia, disseminated intravascular coagulation, and death. The distinction between these two situations is important in dealing with neurologic veterinary emergencies, not only to help minimize the cost of veterinary emergency care but also to provide appropriate attention to true emergencies.

Clinical neurology relies to a great extent on the physical examination to help locate the portion of the nervous system with an abnormality. This is in stark contrast, for example, to diseases of the liver, kidney, or blood, for which multiple ancillary laboratory or imaging procedures often are needed to determine the site of disease. This difference allows veterinarians to diagnose and treat neurologic emergencies rapidly.

The neurologic examination, the hallmark of clinical veterinary neurology, involves a systematic approach to evaluate the central and peripheral nervous system. The neurologic examination is outlined in Box 22-1). Accurate observations of the patient with a neurologic disorder are crucial in a busy emergency veterinary clinic, so veterinary technicians must understand the neurologic examination.

Equipment List
Pleximeter
Hemostats
Bright light source
Safety pin
Indirect or direct ophthalmoscope
Valium (injectable form)
SoluMedrol (Methylprednisolone sodium succinate)

SEIZURES

Veterinary emergency clinics often deal with cats, dogs, and to a lesser extent other species such as ferrets and birds with seizure disorders. To help these patients rapidly, the ability to understand and recognize a seizure is essential.

The veterinary literature includes excellent definitions of seizures. A contemporary definition, "the clinical manifestation of a paroxysmal cerebral disorder resulting from a transitory disturbance of brain function," has been offered by LeCouteur and Schwartz-Porsche. The event "tends to appear suddenly out of a background of normality and then disappears with equal abruptness." The definition

Box 22-1 Components of the Neurologic Examination

Mentation
Gait
- Paresis: lower versus upper motor neuron
- Ataxia: cerebellar, vestibular, general proprioception

Postural reactions: includes hopping, hemiwalking, proprioceptice placing, wheelbarrowing
Spinal reflexes
- Commonly evaluated reflexes:

Forelimbs	*Hindlimbs*
Flexor*	Flexor*
Extensor carpi radialis*	Patellar*
Biceps	Cranial tibial*
Triceps	Gastrocnemius
Cross-extension	Cross-extension

- Other reflexes:
  - Cutaneous trunci (sometimes called paniculus)
  - Perineal

Tone (e.g., limb, anal), pain, and muscle atrophy
Cranial nerves

*Most reliable reflexes.

of a seizure probably should be expanded to include both the telencephalon (cerebral hemispheres) and the diencephalon (thalamus and hypothalamus), which together embryologically are called the prosencephalon. Seizures can originate in either the telencephalon or the diencephalon.

Physiologically, seizures are thought to be associated with hyperexcitable neurons that suddenly depolarize in the prosencephalon. These neurons may have a disturbance caused by a structural abnormality, such as a brain tumor, brain trauma, inflammation, infection, or a congenital abnormality or may result from some metabolic or toxic disturbance in the cell or the surrounding parenchyma. The net result is a sudden uncontrollable electrical discharge of neurons. These neurons may then enlist surrounding neurons to recruit a larger portion of the brain into abnormal action. The location of these electrically discharged cells determines the abnormal clinical signs seen in a seizure. For example, if the affected cells are located unilaterally in the motor cortex, there may be abnormal tonic-clonic movements on the contralateral side of the body.

A great deal of effort has been devoted to classifying seizures in veterinary medicine, as has been done in human neurology. Very briefly, seizures have been divided into partial and generalized seizures. Partial seizures reflect a limited set of neurons being affected and sometimes are called focal or local seizures. In contrast, general seizures occur when there is synchronous electrical discharge of both sides of the prosencephalon. Unfortunately, this classification scheme, unlike the counterpart in human medicine, adds little to our understanding of the cause of a particular patient's seizure activity. Also, in veterinary medicine this classification scheme does not appear to help in selecting the best anticonvulsant therapy or treatment for a particular patient.

Terms used by clients to describe a seizure are varied. They include *epilepsy, fits,* and *convulsions*. The term *epilepsy* is somewhat problematic because even among veterinary neurologists it has different meanings. Probably the most widely accepted definition of *epilepsy* is a nonprogressive, intracranial disorder that induces recurring seizures. This definition assumes that the cause of the seizure is nonprogressive. Causes of epilepsy include genetically determined primary brain disorders and inactive, nonprogressive brain disorders that have resulted in a seizure focus. Idiopathic epilepsy is a disorder for which the exact cause or mechanism for the seizure is unknown, and it is not progressive.

Seizures often are confused with other clinical entities by many owners. The veterinarian and veterinary technician must accurately and quickly distinguish seizures from other diseases that occur episodically and suddenly. Some of the syndromes most commonly confused with seizures are listed in Box 22-2.

A systematic approach is imperative to identify the cause of seizures. A method to determine the cause of seizure activity is shown in Figure 22-1. This method distinguishes patients with normal and abnormal neurologic examinations and takes into consideration the fact that most patients admitted to emergency clinics either are having or have just had a seizure at the time of admission. The postictal period is the time after a seizure or group of seizures, during which the animal may be disoriented, unresponsive, confused, or restless. Many animals are temporarily blind. Some are very agitated or aggressive. Usually this transient period lasts for a few seconds to several hours after the seizure, but some dogs and cats have postictal periods that last for 1 to 2 days. The important thing to remember about the postictal period is that the results of the neurologic examination may not represent the patient's true neurologic state. Many patients have abnormal findings during this period that do not persist once the animal has recovered from the postictal period. Therefore, conclusions about the neurologic examination should be drawn once the animal is completely recovered. Also, medications used to stop seizure activity (valium and other medications) will influence the neurologic examination. Therefore, conclusions about the cause of a seizure should be reached after the sedative effects of medication have worn off.

Box 22-2 Episodic Syndromes Sometimes Confused with Seizures

- Cataplexy and narcolepsy
- Syncope
- Behavioral abnormalities
  - Obsessive-compulsive behaviors
- Vestibular diseases
- Myasthenia gravis
- Pain
  - Neck pain from intervertebral disc disease
- Metabolic disturbances
  - Polycythemia or hyperviscosity syndromes
  - Portosystemic shunts
  - Addison's disease
- Polymyopathies and neuropathies

In Figure 22-1, causes of seizures in a pet with a normal neurologic examination fall into three general categories. The first, idiopathic epilepsy

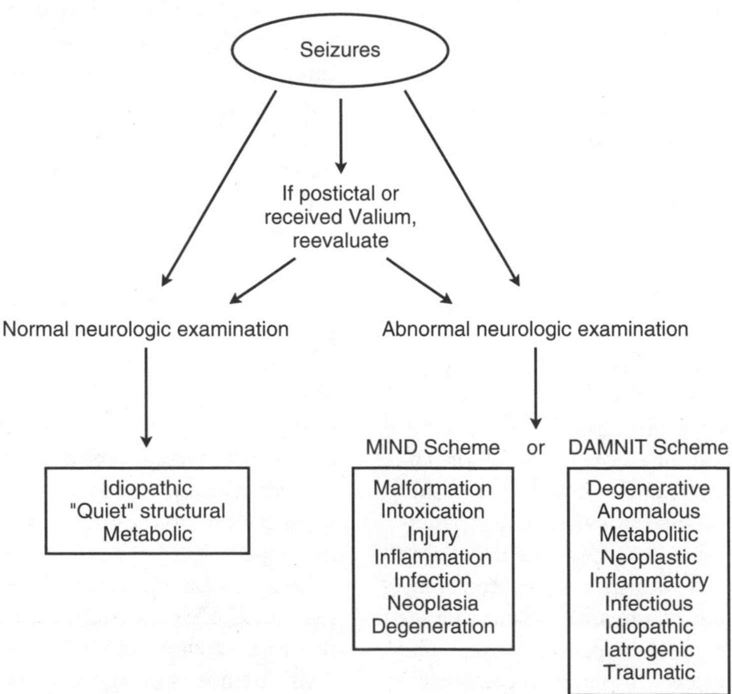

Figure 22-1

Algorithm to help determine the cause of seizure activity.

occurs in dogs usually between 1 and 6 years of age. These patients do not have abnormalities detectable by diagnostic workup. Idiopathic epilepsy is a diagnosis of exclusion.

Quiet structural causes of seizures are diseases that affect portions of the brain that do not have readily apparent abnormalities on the neurologic examination. For example, a brain tumor or a granuloma in the olfactory bulbs or frontal lobes of the brain can cause seizures without causing abnormalities in the neurologic examination. Quiet structural causes of seizures often warrant further diagnostic procedures such as collection of cerebrospinal fluid and advanced imaging techniques such as computer-assisted tomography or magnetic resonance imaging. Likewise, patients with seizures caused by metabolic diseases, such as a portosystemic shunt or insulinoma, often have normal neurologic examinations. These diseases often are detected when laboratory results are analyzed.

If abnormal results are found on neurologic examination in a patient not in the postictal period and not having just received medication to stop seizures (such as valium), two acronyms are helpful to remind clinicians and technicians of broad categories of diseases that can cause seizures. The acronym MIND represents the following categories: malformation, intoxication, injury, inflammation, infection, neoplastia, and degeneration. The DAMNIT acronym stands for degenerative, anomalous, metabolic, neoplastic, inflammatory, infectious, idiopathic, iatrogenic, and traumatic.

Treatment and Diagnostic Procedures

Treatment of seizures in an emergency veterinary clinic should be directed at stopping seizure activity. This is paramount in patients with status epilepticus, a seizure lasting more than 3 to 4 minutes, or in a patient having cluster seizures (more than 3 to 4 seizures in 30 to 40 minutes or a group of seizures over a 12- or 24-hour period of time). A specific treatment depends largely on whether the animal is taking antiepileptic drugs and usually has good seizure control or whether the patient is presenting with seizures for the first time. Box 22-3 describes a step-by-step approach for the initial treatment and diagnosis for a first-time seizure.

In patients presenting in status epilepticus or with cluster seizures that have previously been on anticonvulsants and have a definitive cause for seizure activity or those that are considered idiopathic epileptics, the treatment protocol in Box 22-4 should be followed. These patients usually do not need the extensive battery of blood tests that a patient who has just recently started to seizure needs. If it has been an extended period of time or if the intensity or severity of seizures has changed, it may be necessary to repeat some of the blood work.

Monitoring and Care of Patients with Seizures

Once the initial emergency of cluster seizures or status epilepticus is resolved, the most important thing in seizure management is to remember to give maintenance anticonvulsants. Phenobarbital can be given intravenously, intramuscularly, orally, or rectally. Potassium bromide can be given either orally or rectally. In the anesthetized patient, both medications can be loaded rectally. To do this, use a red rubber polyethylene feeding tube and large syringe, making sure to flush the catheter with water after administering the medication to ensure that the patient receives the entire dose. A tomcat polyethylene catheter or teat cannula also can be used, but they are much shorter and the medication can spill from the anus. In addition, treatment of the anesthetized patient should include the following:

- Turn patient every 6 hours, alternating the side of recumbency, to prevent atelectasis and bed sores.
- Lubricate the eyes to prevent corneal ulcers.
- Express the bladder two or three times daily to prevent stretching of the bladder muscles. Consider placing a closed, indwelling urinary catheter.
- Maintain intravenous access via an intravenous catheter. Also consider maintenance IV fluids, if indicated.
- Give anticonvulsants as indicated.

Box 22-3 Treatment and Diagnosis in Patients Not Previously Diagnosed with a Seizure Disorder and Presenting with Cluster Seizures or Status Epilepticus

1. Place intravenous catheter.
2. Draw blood for initial data base to include the following:
   - Blood glucose
   - Electrolytes
   - Packed cell volume and total protein
   - Peripheral blood smear
   - Complete blood cell count
   - Chemistry profile
   - Urinalysis
   - Lead levels (if indicated)
   - Serology for infectious diseases (if indicated)
3. Give intravenous drugs to stop seizures.
   - Diazepam (Valium) (usually first choice).
     - Dosage: 0.25-1.0 mg/kg, repeat up to three times.
     - Quick dosing suggestions
       - Small dog = 2.5-5.0 mg, repeat up to three times.
       - Medium dog = 5.0 mg, repeat up to three times.
       - Large dog = 10-20 mg, repeat up to three times.
       - Cats = 2.5 mg, repeat up to three times.
     - After stopping seizures, give constant-rate infusion of diazepam if necessary. Give amount of diazepam used to stop initial seizure in a solution of 1.2 ml lactated Ringer's/lb/hr.
   - Pentobarbital (if not responsive to valium).
     - Dogs: 1-8 mg/kg IV slow and to effect.
     - Cats: 1-4 mg/kg IV slow and to effect.
     - Not necessary to completely anesthetize with pentobarbital as long as it stops the seizure.
     - Anesthesia induced with pentobarbital may not totally stop seizure activity (as revealed by electroencephalogram) but will prevent life-threatening hyperthermia and disseminated intravascular coagulation.
   - Other drugs to consider include the following:
     - Propofol
     - Thiopental
4. Give maintenance anticonvulsant medications.
   - Loading doses. These are the calculated dosages needed to quickly achieve therapeutic serum concentrations.
     - Phenobarbital: 4 mg/kg IV, PO, IM, or PR every 6 hr for 24 hr (total dosage = 16 mg/kg). Can go as high as 30 mg/kg over the first 24 hr. Stop loading if very groggy, especially in the cat.
     - Potassium bromide: 100-150 mg/kg every 12 hr for four doses or 2 days. Can give PO or PR. If necessary, can load much more rapidly by giving 300-600 mg/kg all at once. Total loading dose should not exceed 600 mg/kg.
   - Maintenance doses.
     - Phenobarbital: 1.0-4.0 mg/lb two to three times daily PO.
     - Potassium bromide 25-80 mg/kg/day.
       - Use higher dosage if not on phenobarbital concurrently.
       - Usually give divided total dose twice daily, but not necessary.
     - Maintenance medication is essential in the anesthetized patient.

Box 22-4 Treatment and Diagnosis in Patients Previously Diagnosed with a Seizure Disorder and Presenting with Cluster Seizures or in Status Epilepticus

1. Place intravenous catheter.
2. Draw blood for initial data base to include the following:
   - Blood glucose
   - Electrolytes
   - Packed cell volume and total protein
3. Give intravenous drugs to stop seizures.
   - Diazepam (Valium) (usually first choice).
     - Dosage: 0.25-1.0 mg/kg, repeat up to three times.
     - Quick dosing suggestions
       - Small dog: 2.5-5.0 mg, repeat up to three times.
       - Medium dog: 5.0 mg, repeat up to three times.
       - Large dog: 10-20 mg, repeat up to three times.
       - Cats: 2.5 mg, repeat up to three times.
     - After stopping seizures, give constant-rate infusion of diazepam if necessary. Give amount of diazepam used to stop initial seizure in a solution of 1.2 ml lactated Ringer's/lb/hr.
     - Pentobarbital (if not responsive to valium)
       - Dogs: 1-8 mg/kg IV slow and to effect.
       - Cats: 1-4 mg/kg IV slow and to effect.
       - Not necessary to completely anesthetize with pentobarbital as long as it stops the seizure.
       - If anesthetized with pentobarbital, may not totally stop seizure activity (as revealed by electroencephalogram) but will prevent life-threatening hyperthermia and disseminated intravascular coagulation.
     - Other drugs to consider include the following:
       - Propofol
       - Thiopental
4. Continue with the maintenance drugs, usually phenobarbital or potassium bromide.
5. Consider starting other anticonvulsants if maintenance drugs are not controlling seizures adequately.
6. Obtain anticonvulsant blood levels to adjust dosing.

- Monitor carefully for seizure activity.
- Monitor vital signs carefully (thermoregulation, respiration, cardiovascular perfusion).

SPINAL CORD TRAUMA

Spinal cord trauma is very common in veterinary medicine. In general, cord trauma is divided into intrinsic and extrinsic causes. Intrinsic causes include extrusion and protrusion of disc material and fractures secondary to bone diseases such as neoplastic or nutritional disorders. Extrinsic causes of spinal cord trauma include fractures, luxations, and subluxations secondary to traumatic events. This would include automobile accidents, gunshot wounds, and, much less commonly, animal abuse or bite wounds inflicted by another animal.

A schematic of the vertebral column is shown in Figure 22-2. The diagram depicts three basic structures: the bony vertebral column, the intervertebral disc (between the ventral portions of two consecutive vertebrae), and the spinal cord (between the dorsal and ventral portions of the bony vertebrae).

By far the most common cause of intrinsic trauma to the spinal cord is intervertebral disc disease. As shown in Figure 22-2, the intervertebral discs are located between two consecutive vertebrae from the second cervical vertebrae through the caudal vertebrae of the tail. Under normal circumstances the intervertebral disc acts

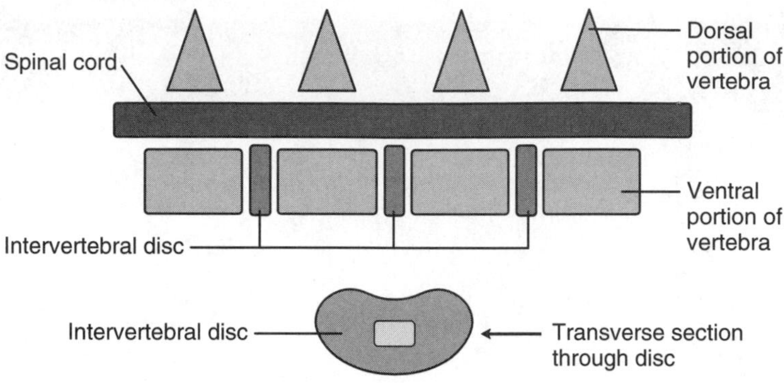

Figure 22-2

Schematic sagittal section of a vertebral canal.

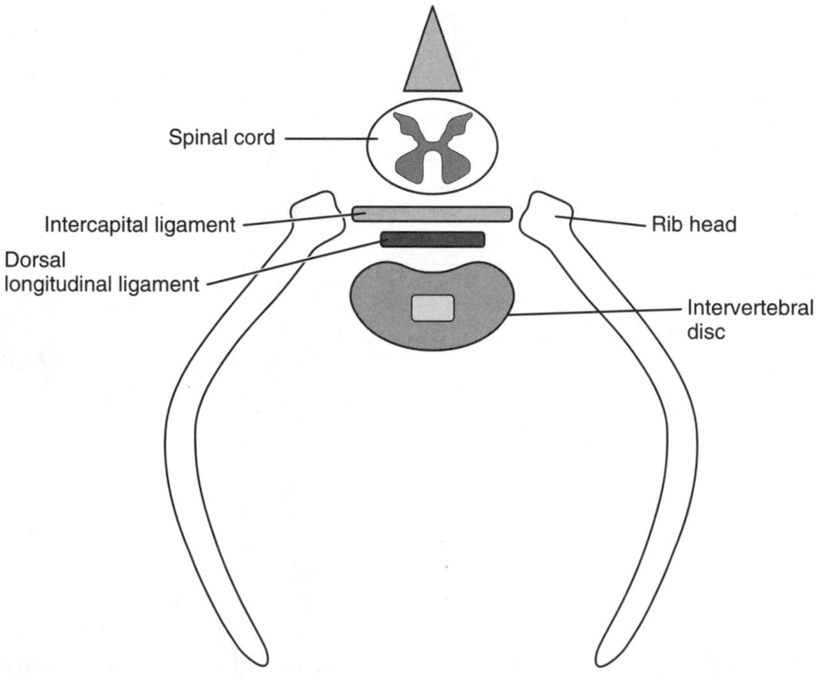

Figure 22-3

Schematic transverse section through the T4-5 intervertebral space. Note the presence of intercapital ligament and thick dorsal longitudinal ligament.

as a cushion to absorb concussive energy along the vertebral column.

The intervertebral disc is composed of an outer fibrous material, the annulus fibrosus, and an inner gel-like material, the nucleus pulposus. The annulus fibrosus can rupture, allowing the nucleus pulposus to extrude dorsally to impinge on the spinal cord or dorsolaterally to put pressure on the nerve roots. This can result from external trauma or intrinsic factors. In certain breeds of dogs called chondrodystrophic breeds (e.g., dachshund, Lhasa apso, and basset hound), the nucleus pulposus degenerates and the annulus fibrosus weakens. When this occurs, the disc can no longer absorb energy and ruptures through the annulus fibrosus, compressing the dorsally located spinal cord, even under minimal stress. The nucleus pulposus is displaced dorsally because the annulus fibrosus is thinnest dorsally, and the nucleus pulposus takes the path of least resistance. The most common location for a disc to rupture is at the T13-L1 space. Several hypotheses have been proposed to explain this. Anatomically the dorsal longitudinal ligament is thinner in this region. Also, there is no intercapital ligament between rib heads to provide extra support. Finally, there is greater mobility and less muscular support in this region than in the thoracic region. Figures 22-3 and 22-4 illustrate the anatomic differences that can explain the increased frequency of disc extrusions at the T13-L1 intervertebral space.

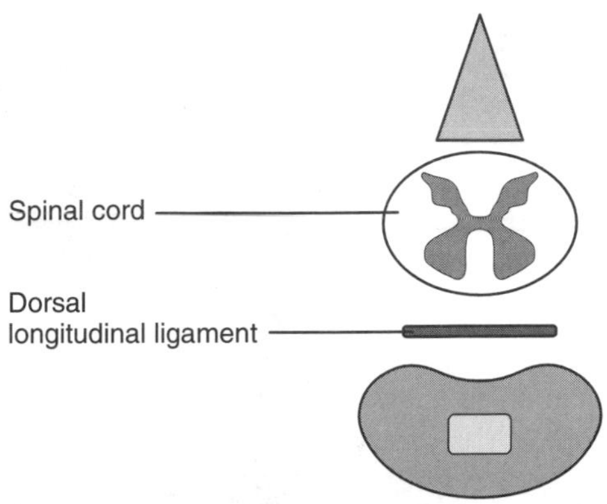

Figure 22-4

Schematic transverse section through the T13-L1 intervertebral space. Note the very thin dorsal longitudinal ligament and the absence of rib heads and intercapital ligament.

The types of injuries and forces on the vertebral canal most commonly associated with external trauma are shown in Figure 22-5. Flexion alone usually results in extrusion of disc material into the spinal cord. The resulting clinical signs vary from mild paresis to complete paralysis and destruction of the spinal cord. A combination of compression and flexion forces, the type of injury most commonly seen in automobile accidents, usually results in a wedge fracture of the ventral portion of a vertebrae. The compressive force occurs when the dog or cat tries to get out of the way of the automobile. The back end of the animal is hit by the bumper of the vehicle while the forelimbs are caught firmly on the ground. The vertebral canal often is quite stable in this type of injury. The majority of damage to the spinal cord occurs at the time of impact, and the resulting clinical signs vary. A third type of injury and force causing spinal cord trauma is that associated with concurrent flexion and rotation of the vertebral column. If rotation is the predominant force, the resulting injury probably will involve a luxation and fracture of the vertebrae. If the majority of force is flexion of the vertebrae, the injury probably will be luxation of the vertebral column. These types of injuries often are very unstable, and careful management is needed to prevent further damage to the spinal cord. In addition, the spinal cord trauma in these injuries often is very severe.

The site of the spinal cord injury must be localized accurately. Many times, even with severe vertebral fractures, the exact location of the injury is not apparent on physical examination, and a complete neurologic examination is needed. The neurologic examination is done to prevent further injury to the spinal cord while providing other life-saving treatments. In addition, it helps define specific sites to image with techniques such as radiography, myelography, or computed tomography.

For all practical purposes the spinal cord can be divided into four regions (Figure 22-6). Spinal cord injury prevents information about the location of the limbs and trunk in space, proprioception, from getting to the brain. In addition, descending upper motor neuron fibers from the brain, which are responsible for tone, movement, and strength, can also be affected by a spinal cord injury. Interference with these descending upper motor neuron fibers results in increased tone and hyperreflexia as well as weakness. The conduit of these descending

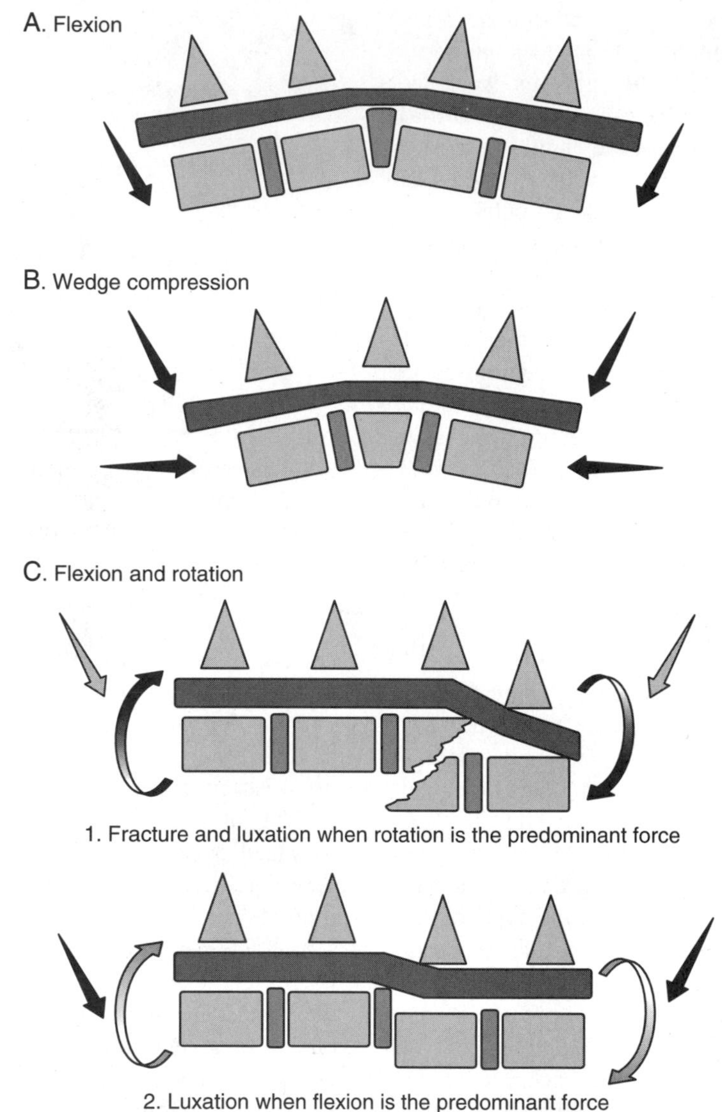

Figure 22-5

Types of injury and forces associated with trauma to the vertebral canal (arrows indicate direction of force).

upper motor neuron fibers from the spinal cord to the muscles of the limbs is the lower motor neuron system. Injury of the lower motor system, from the cell body in the ventral gray horn of the spinal cord to the nerve root, peripheral nerve, neuromuscular junction, and muscle results in decreased tone, hyporeflexia, and weakness. Lower motor neuron diseases usually do not affect the ascending proprioceptive fibers, so postural reactions (e.g., hopping, proprioceptive placing) are often not affected. The common clinical sequelae to a T13-L1 disc extrusion are shown in Figure 22-6. Clinical signs are limited to the hindlimbs and include paresis (weakness) or paralysis, hypertonia and hyperreflexia, and postural reaction deficits.

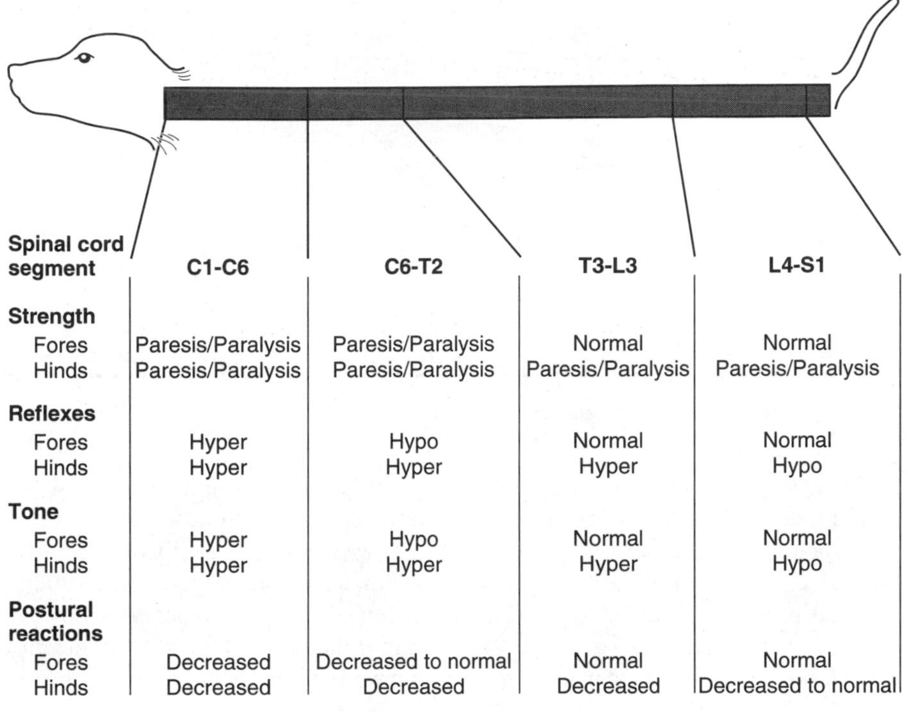

Spinal cord segment	C1-C6	C6-T2	T3-L3	L4-S1
Strength				
Fores	Paresis/Paralysis	Paresis/Paralysis	Normal	Normal
Hinds	Paresis/Paralysis	Paresis/Paralysis	Paresis/Paralysis	Paresis/Paralysis
Reflexes				
Fores	Hyper	Hypo	Normal	Normal
Hinds	Hyper	Hyper	Hyper	Hypo
Tone				
Fores	Hyper	Hypo	Normal	Normal
Hinds	Hyper	Hyper	Hyper	Hypo
Postural reactions				
Fores	Decreased	Decreased to normal	Normal	Normal
Hinds	Decreased	Decreased	Decreased	Decreased to normal

Figure 22-6

Neurologic findings associated with injury of a particular spinal cord segment.

Some clinical exceptions to Figure 22-6 should be noted. Spinal shock is a syndrome that is seen with severe spinal cord trauma. Under most circumstances, when there is a spinal cord lesion at the T13-L1 spinal cord segments the resulting clinical signs include hypertonia and hyperreflexia of the hindlimbs. Occasionally, a patient that presents to a clinic within the first 12 hours of a severe spinal cord injury has the expected hyperreflexia. However, the hindlimbs are hypotonic. The exact mechanism for this paradox is not known. It is thought that for a brief period there is a temporary lack of facilitators to the extensor muscles, along with the expected lack of inhibition to the extensor muscles. The result is hypotonia in the hindlimbs for the first 12 to 36 hours. The hypotonia is replaced by the expected hypertonia at the end of this period of time.

The second exception is Schiff-Sherrington syndrome. Most technicians working in a busy emergency clinic have seen examples of Schiff-Sherrington syndrome. Like spinal shock, this condition occurs when there is a very severe spinal cord injury, usually within the T3-L3 spinal cord segments (Figure 22-7). Under these circumstances there is interference of the ascending, inhibitory fibers from the L1-L5 spinal cord segments to the spinal cord segments innervating the forelimbs. These ascending fibers are inhibitors to the extensors of the forelimbs. Normally these fibers help the hindlimbs and forelimbs coordinate movement. When there is severe spinal cord damage, this communication is interrupted. The result is severe extensor rigidity in the forelimbs.

Treatment

Treatment of a patient with a suspected vertebral fracture begins before arrival at the hospital. If a patient must be transferred from one hospital to

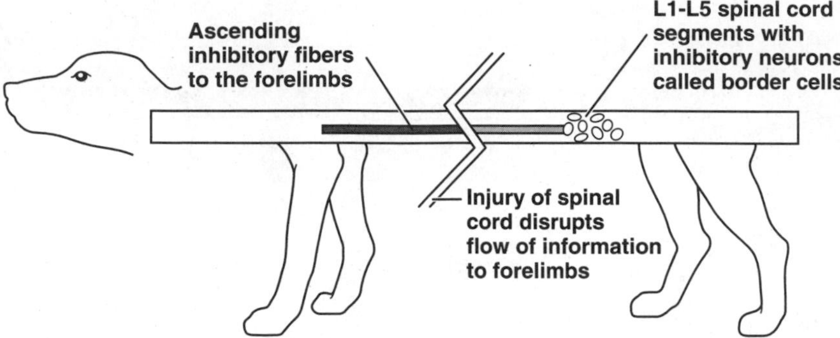

Figure 22-7

Schematic of anatomic pathway for Schiff-Sherrington syndrome.

another, it should be done with extreme care. When a client or referral veterinarian calls an emergency clinic, he or she should be instructed on how best to transport a patient with a suspected vertebral injury. This includes placing and carefully securing the animal on a flat, firm board such as a door or piece of plywood, warning owners that even the nicest pet may unexpectedly try to bite or scratch because of severe pain associated with a spinal column injury.

Once the injured patient arrives at the hospital, it is extremely important to limit any unnecessary movement. The patient should receive a complete physical and neurologic examination before the suspected vertebral fracture is addressed. Initial treatment is aimed at stabilizing the patient's respiratory and cardiovascular systems. If the animal is in pain, analgesics such as butorphanol (0.2 to 0.4 mg/kg intramuscularly, subcutaneously, or intravenously), oxymorphone (0.05 to 0.1 mg/kg intramuscularly or intravenously), morphine (0.5 to 2.0 mg/kg intramuscularly, subcutaneously, or intravenously), or buprenorphine (0.01 to 0.15 mg/kg intravenously or intramuscularly) can be administered. Care must be taken to not compromise respiration with any medication in a patient that may have trauma such as a fractured rib or damaged lungs because some drugs can cause respiratory depression. Also, diazepam (Valium) can be used as a sedative at a dosage of 0.2 to 0.4 mg/kg intravenously if the patient is overly anxious or is flailing.

Very little definitive clinical information is available about the use of steroids in spinal cord injury in veterinary medicine. The majority of literature reports experimental studies in cats that received different types and dosages of steroids and other antiinflammatory medications at the time of injury. The results of these studies vary with experimental procedure and often have conflicting findings. In human clinical studies involving spinal cord injury, methylprednisolone sodium succinate at a dosage of 30 mg/kg at initial presentation, followed by 5.4 mg/kg/hr in a constant-rate infusion for the next 23 hours has been shown to be beneficial if administered within 8 hours of the injury. No complete similar study has been done in veterinary medicine. However, most veterinary neurologists and neurosurgeons recommend this or a similar protocol for spinal cord trauma, including intervertebral disc extrusion and vertebral fractures. Some veterinary neurologists use an initial dosage of 30 mg/kg methylprednisolone sodium succinate followed by two boluses of 15 mg/kg at 2 and 6 hours after the initial bolus. Care must be taken to administer the methylprednisolone slowly, over 5 to 10 minutes. Failure to administer this drug slowly can result in vomiting or hypotension.

Although it is commonly used in practice, there is little experimental and no clinical evidence that dexamethasone is effective in spinal cord trauma in veterinary medicine; therefore methylprednisolone sodium succinate should be used when available.

In the absence of methylprednisolone sodium succinate, dexamethasone can be tried at a dosage of 0.5 to 1.0 mg/kg intravenously at initial presentation. It is believed that gastrointestinal side effects, such as gastrointestinal and colonic ulcers, are more common with dexamethasone than with methylprednisolone sodium succinate. Therefore, if dexamethasone is used for spinal cord injuries, concomitant gastroprotectant administration may be helpful.

Spinal cord injuries can be treated medically or surgically depending on the type and severity of the lesion. Medical management may involve a back or neck brace, cage rest, or drug therapy. Surgical intervention often involves some type of spinal cord decompression or vertebral column stabilization. Regardless of this decision, the initial emergency care is crucial for a positive outcome.

HEAD TRAUMA

Head trauma is common in the setting of emergency medicine, usually the result of being hit by a car. Other causes include blunt trauma from being hit by an object, falling from a height, or having an object fall on the animal. Regardless of the cause of the insult, head trauma results in the same pathophysiologic disorders as brain injury, so the same basic principles of treatment and care apply.

Initial Diagnosis

Most patients present to veterinary hospitals with a history of someone having seen the cause of trauma. Occasionally owners find their pets acting abnormally and have not witnessed the accident that caused the trauma. In this case, one can surmise that a traumatic incident has occurred based on finding abrasions on the head and face, bleeding from the mouth or nose (epistaxis), blood in the ears or in and around the eyes, or asymmetric pupillary size (anisocoria).

Animals present with a wide variety of neurologic signs that depend on the area of the central nervous system that is affected. Neurologic examination often is consistent with a disturbance in the prosencephalon. Most often animals demonstrate an altered state of mentation (dullness, stupor, or coma). Other observations include circling, aimless, propulsive wandering, or seizures. Abnormal pupil size and symmetry can be seen as well. Occasionally caudal fossa signs (cerebellum, pons, medulla, and caudal midbrain) predominate. In this situation, balance problems, abnormal eye movements (nystagmus), head tremors, or paralysis or paresis can occur.

It is critically important to perform a thorough neurologic examination on admission to identify the location of lesions. These abnormalities can be monitored serially to detect improvement or deterioration in status. Based on sequential examinations, further diagnostics and treatments can be implemented. The frequency of monitoring depends on the critical nature of the patient and degree of impairment.

Pathophysiology

The concussive forces that cause head trauma result in primary brain injury. Primary injury includes cerebral edema and intracranial hemorrhage. The intracranial hemorrhage can be epidural (between the calvaria and dura mater), subdural (between the dura mater and the arachnoid), subarachnoid (between the arachnoid and brain tissue), or intraparenchymal (within the brain tissue). In contrast to human patients, subdural hemorrhage is extremely rare in veterinary patients.

As a consequence of primary brain injury, secondary brain injury results. In people who suffer head trauma, this secondary injury is a major determinant of the outcome. Secondary brain injury can be divided into systemic or intracranial effects. Systemic secondary brain injury occurs as a result of hypotension (low blood pressure), hypoxia (low blood oxygen content), anemia, changes in blood glucose levels (either too high or too low), acid-base, or electrolyte disturbances. Intracranial secondary brain injury includes intracranial hypertension (raised intracranial pressure), cerebral edema, or a mass effect as a consequence of hemorrhage.

Serial Neurologic Monitoring

Integral to treatment is sequential monitoring. This monitoring allows the clinician to tailor treatment to the individual needs of the patient. The clinician relies on technicians to evaluate the patient's changing mental status.

The simplest parameter to evaluate is mentation. Mentation often is described as normal (alert and responsive), quiet, dull, stuporous (responsive only to painful stimuli), or comatose (unresponsive to stimuli). As the patient's condition deteriorates, mentation changes from normal to comatose.

In addition to mentation, pupil size and responsiveness must be evaluated. To fully understand the importance of anisocoria and pupillary light reactions (constriction of the pupil in response to light), an understanding of the neural control of the pupil is necessary. Pupil constriction begins with light stimulating the retina of the eye, resulting in stimulation of the optic nerve. This afferent limb (ascending into the central nervous system) of the reflex sends impulses to the midbrain, where the nervous control of the pupil is located (oculomotor neuron). The oculomotor nerve, after leaving the brain, stimulates the pupil to constrict in response to light. This reflex arch is under a degree of constant inhibition by nervous control from descending upper motor neurons from the prosencephalon.

Many patients with head trauma present with anisocoria. Changes in pupil size can be a result of trauma to the eye and surrounding structures, which often causes the pupil to be small, whereas trauma to the brain stem, where the innervation to the pupil originates, results in a widely dilated pupil that is unresponsive to light stimulation and does not constrict (pupillary light reflex).

Although anisocoria helps the clinician localize the traumatized region, evaluating pupillary changes from the initial status helps the clinician detect changes in intracranial pressure. As intracranial pressure increases, nerves that descend from the prosencephalon and inhibit the portion of the brain stem that causes pupillary constriction are inhibited. As a result, the oculomotor nerve is disinhibited and the pupils constrict. As pressure builds, the brain shifts inside the calvaria and begins to herniate, putting pressure on the origin of the oculomotor nerve in the brain stem and blocks its function. The pupils then become dilated and unresponsive.

Brain herniation is the final sequela to raised intracranial pressure. Brain herniation is a process by which intracranial pressure pushes the brain tissue out of its normal anatomic position. Brain tissue can herniate in several different ways, the most important of which is herniation out of the foramen magnum (the exit of the calvaria through which the spinal cord exits). As the brain herniates out the foramen magnum, it puts pressure on the fibers that descend through the spinal cord and thereby causes paralysis. Animals undergoing this process assume a posture called decerebrate rigidity. They are recumbent and opisthotonic (head and neck arched backward) and have both hindlimb and forelimb extensor rigidity. In addition, the herniating brain tissue puts pressure on the nervous control centers for breathing and causes respiratory depression and eventual cessation of breathing.

Treatment

Although the primary brain injury has already occurred, the goal of treatment is to thwart the effects of secondary brain injury and the consequences of raised intracranial pressure. The most crucial aspect of treatment is to treat all the needs of the patient and not to concentrate on brain-specific therapies. In general, addressing the patient's systemic needs will additionally address the needs of the central nervous system.

Hypotension has been shown to adversely effect outcome in people with head trauma. Hypotension results in cerebral ischemia (lack of blood flow). Mean arterial pressure is a major determinant of cerebral perfusion (blood flow). Cerebral perfusion equals the mean arterial pressure minus intracranial pressure. Therefore, maintaining a normal mean arterial pressure ensures adequate cerebral perfusion and prevents cerebral ischemia. Appropriate intravenous fluid administration is crucial in treating hypotension. Blood pressure monitoring can aid in addressing hypotension and tailoring fluid administration. Mean arterial blood pressure should be kept greater than or equal to 90 mm Hg.

Similarly, hypoxia can result in secondary brain insult and thereby worsen outcome. Many patients with head trauma suffer concurrent trauma to other organ systems. Appropriate red blood cell mass should be evaluated with packed cell volume and serially monitored. Additionally, red blood cells should be given to maintain adequate red blood cell counts. Chest trauma also can contribute to hypoxia because injuries such as pneumothorax, hemothorax, and pulmonary contusions impair ventilation and oxygenation. Patients with head trauma should always be evaluated for concurrent chest trauma. Chest injuries must be treated adequately. Supplemental oxygen should be administered if necessary. Proper oxygenation can be monitored by evaluating arterial blood gas analysis or pulse oximetry. Oxygenation saturation should be maintained between 98% and 100%.

Mannitol has long been used to reduce raised intracranial pressure and increase cerebral blood flow. It appears to work via two mechanisms. The first mechanism is by increasing intravascular volume and reducing blood viscosity and thereby increasing cerebral blood flow. This is accomplished immediately and seems to work best when mannitol is administered as a rapid intravenous bolus (over a 10- to 20-minute infusion).

The second mechanism of action is as an osmotic diuretic resulting in osmotic dehydration of the brain. The duration of this effect varies from 90 minutes to 6 hours and is slightly dose dependent at dosages ranging from 0.25 to 1.0 g/kg of a 25% solution. Mannitol administration can be repeated every 4 to 8 hours, with a maximum of three doses over 24 hours. Care must be taken when mannitol is given in the initial setting of resuscitation because dehydration can precipitate hypotension. Also, mannitol administration should be avoided when there is known bleeding within the cranial vault. Administration of mannitol during active hemorrhage will result in increased blood outside of vascular structures, thereby increasing intracranial pressure.

Like mannitol, furosemide can be given to help reduce intracranial pressure by causing diuresis and decreasing cerebrospinal fluid production. An initial dosage of 2 to 4 mg/kg intravenously is recommended. Furosemide often is given before mannitol to prevent an initial detrimental rise in intracranial pressure associated with the intravascular volume expansion from the mannitol administration. Like mannitol, furosemide should not be given to a dehydrated, hypovolemic, or hypotensive patient.

In cases of severe head trauma, mechanical ventilatory assistance sometimes is necessary. This is especially true in the setting of stupor or coma. It has long been advocated that during mechanical ventilation $Paco_2$ (partial pressure of arterial carbon dioxide) should be maintained between 25 and 30 mm Hg. Hypocapnea induces cerebral vasoconstriction and a resultant reduction in intracranial pressure by reducing the total volume of blood in the cranial vault. However, prolonged hypocapnea can exacerbate cerebral ischemia. Prophylactic hyperventilation less than or equal to 35 mm Hg should thus be avoided. However, hyperventilation should be used in established intracranial hypertension to reduce raised intracranial pressure rather than chronic prophylactic hypocapnea to prevent intracranial hypertension.

Steroids have been recommended in head trauma in the past. However, in people who suffer severe head trauma, steroids have been shown to lack efficacy and in some cases have been detrimental. Their use in human patients has been curtailed. In veterinary medicine, steroids are still used to a great extent, but there is no convincing evidence that they are beneficial with head trauma in veterinary patients. Steroids can be used as a last resort or in severely traumatized patients. Methyl-prednisolone sodium succinate at an initial rate of 30 mg/kg intravenously is used in severe head trauma. Tapering doses of 15 mg/kg are given at 2 and 6 hours.

Elevating the patient's head often is helpful in reducing the intracranial pressure by maximizing venous blood return from the brain to the heart.

This can be accomplished by placing a solid board under the patient and elevating the front 20 to 30 degrees. It is also important to make sure no blankets are compressing the jugular veins, which could decrease venous blood flow and increase intracranial pressure.

Patients with head trauma may experience severe pain or dementia. This may result in the patient flailing around in the cage, causing further head trauma and increased intracranial pressure. In these patients diazepam (Valium) should be used as a sedative at a dosage of 0.2 to 0.4 mg/kg intravenously. In addition, opioid analgesics can be used to provide pain relief.

Finally, head trauma must be approached with a standardized treatment regimen. Patients must be evaluated for central nervous system trauma as well as trauma to all other organ systems. Proper physiologic resuscitation is crucial. Brain-specific treatments must be supplemental to full resuscitation to all extracranial organ systems.

VESTIBULAR DISORDERS

Veterinary emergency clinics often see patients with vestibular disorders. Luckily, these diseases rarely are life threatening at the time of presentation.

Paramount to treating vestibular disorders is determining the location of the disturbance. For this reason, vestibular diseases are clinically divided into peripheral and central vestibular diseases. Peripheral vestibular disease implies that the neuroanatomic site is the vestibular portion of the vestibularcochlear cranial nerve and there are no signs of a brain stem disturbance. The anatomic site of central vestibular disease, in contrast, is the medulla, cerebellum, and pons. The vestibular signs associated with both peripheral and central vestibular disorders (i.e., head tilt and falling, leaning, or turning toward the side of the lesion) usually are identical. The other clinical signs are used to differentiate peripheral and central vestibular diseases. Table 22-1 indicates the clinical differences between peripheral and central vestibular disorders.

Differentiating between peripheral and central vestibular disease is important from a prognostic point of view. In general, central vestibular diseases carry a worse prognosis than peripheral vestibular diseases, but there are exceptions to this rule. For example, metronidazole toxicity and thiamin deficiency both are central vestibular diseases that have an excellent prognosis if recognized early. Similarly, a squamous cell carcinoma in the ear of a cat that causes peripheral vestibular disease has a very poor long-term prognosis. However, in general it is important to remember that central vestibular diseases have a poor prognosis and peripheral vestibular diseases have an excellent prognosis.

A few individual diseases should be mentioned. The first, idiopathic old dog (geriatric) peripheral vestibular disease, probably is the most common vestibular disease seen in an emergency clinic. This disease can affect dogs as young as 8 years old but is more common in dogs 12 years and older. The owners often believe that the

TABLE 22-1 Differences between Peripheral and Central Vestibular Disease

	Peripheral	Central
Postural reactions	Normal.	Abnormal.
Mental status	Normal.	May be depressed.
Cranial nerve deficits	7.	5-12.
Other nerves	Sympathetic.	—
Nystagmus	Fast phase is opposite the side of the head tilt, either horizontal or rotary.	Fast phase can be any direction. If vertical or changes direction, it is usually central.

dog has had a stroke because of the peracute onset and obvious neurologic signs. Dogs often have severe clinical signs including a head tilt with the fast phase nystagmus directed opposite the side of the head tilt, a severe vestibular ataxia, and no postural reaction deficits, all consistent with peripheral vestibular disease. During the first 24 hours it may be difficult to distinguish between central and peripheral vestibular disease because of the severity of the vestibular ataxia. The most important thing to know about this disease is that the majority of patients improve with supportive care. Some dogs have a persistent head tilt, but the vestibular ataxia gradually improves over 2 to 6 weeks. The exact cause of this syndrome is unknown, but it does not appear to be a stroke.

Feline idiopathic peripheral vestibular disease is another common vestibular syndrome. This is a disease of young to middle-aged indoor-outdoor cats. Indoor-only cats do not develop this syndrome. The majority of cats with this disorder are seen in July, August, and September. The disease is not recognized in large urban areas. As with the canine variety, all the clinical signs reflect involvement of the peripheral vestibular system. The exact cause of this syndrome is unknown. As with the dog, the majority of clinical signs in feline idiopathic vestibular disease resolve in 2 to 6 weeks.

Otitis media/interna (ear infection) is a common syndrome causing peripheral vestibular disease in both cats and dogs. Ear infections occur as a primary infection or secondary irritation from ear mites or an allergen. Regardless of the cause, it is important to recognize the neurologic signs associated with otitis media/interna. These include findings consistent with peripheral vestibular disease, facial paralysis, and possibly Horner's syndrome. The latter findings are associated with damage to the seventh cranial nerve and the sympathetic nerve respectively. Horner's syndrome is recognized by an elevated third eyelid; a small palpebral fissure, called ptosis; a sunken eye, called enophthalmia; and a small pupil, called miosis. If other cranial nerve abnormalities or postural reaction deficits are detected, the cause of the vestibular disease cannot be only otitis media/interna. Diagnosis of otitis is made by a good otic examination or other imaging modalities such as radiographs, computed tomography, or magnetic resonance imaging.

No specific treatment generally is needed for vestibular disorders in an emergency clinic. Patients with vestibular disorders usually are stable, and immediate attention and treatments often are not warranted. Patients sometimes are started on maintenance fluids because they are too nauseated to drink or eat. It may be necessary to pad a cage with extra blankets to keep the animal from harming itself by rolling or flailing in the cage. In the case of ear infections, patients are started on broad-spectrum antibiotics. Occasionally medication is needed to sedate an animal with severe vestibular signs. Usually diphenylhydramine at 2.2 mg/kg orally or intramuscularly twice daily is sufficient to cause sedation. Rarely, diazepam (Valium) may be necessary at 0.2 to 0.4 mg/kg intravenously or intramuscularly to gain the level of sedation needed. In general, steroids are not recommended for vestibular diseases in an emergency clinic setting for several reasons, including the ability of steroids to mask important clinical signs and laboratory findings necessary for an accurate diagnosis. Occasionally steroids can exacerbate clinical diseases such as otitis media/interna. If a patient's clinical signs deteriorate dramatically and become life threatening, it may be necessary to use steroids such as dexamethasone at an initial dosage of 0.5 to 10 mg/kg intravenously or methylprednisolone sodium succinate at 30 mg/kg intravenously. Dexamethasone often is associated with adverse gastrointestinal signs, so a gastroprotectant may be helpful when using dexamethasone. Although many patients with vestibular disease are nauseous, specific antiemetic drugs usually are not necessary for treating vestibular diseases in animals.

CONCLUSION

A neurologic emergency can result from many factors. Seizures and trauma-related neurologic disorders are common in veterinary practice. Understanding how to examine and assess the

airway, breathing, and circulation. These patients may arrive in various stages of toxicity. They may present with very mild clinical signs (e.g., anxiety) or very serious clinical signs (e.g., seizure or coma).

Attempt to get a thorough history from the owners. Then prevent further absorption of the toxin, administer an antidote if available, facilitate removal of absorbed toxin, and provide supportive therapy. The animal should be monitored until the intoxication has resolved.

PREVENTING FURTHER ABSORPTION

The route of exposure must be considered first. For ocular exposure, the eyes should be rinsed with large amounts of physiologic saline for 20 to 30 minutes. For chemical burns, the eyes can be treated with lubricant ointments and lid closure techniques. Corticosteroids may be beneficial and used only if the corneal epithelium is intact. The severity of ocular damage that can occur depends on the type of chemical that was in the eye and how quickly it was treated.

The animal that has been exposed to a toxin topically should be bathed only in a mild hand-dishwashing detergent. Solvents can disperse chemicals and increase the exposed area of the skin. Also, they change skin permeability. Topical ointments also should be avoided because they can enhance absorption of the chemical.

The person bathing the animal should wear protective clothing, including a mask and goggles, to avoid contamination. Bathing should continue until all toxin has been removed, rinsing frequently with large amounts of water. If the substance is a powder, the animal should be vacuumed before bathing.

Ingestion must also be considered in animals that arrive with a topical poisoning because of the grooming instinct. The animal that has ingested a toxin can be decontaminated by inducing emesis, performing gastric lavage, and administering adsorbents, cathartics, and enemas.

Rapid dilution of the toxin with large amounts of milk or water is not recommended because it may enhance the absorption of toxins into the gastrointestinal tract. Dilution is considered only for animals that may have ingested a corrosive substance.

Inducing emesis involves introducing a technique or substance to the animal so it will vomit. It is preferred over gastric lavage for removing stomach contents. Vomiting removes 40% to 60% of the chyme (semifluid mass of partially digested food that is passed from the stomach to the duodenum).

Several emetic substances are available. Emetics work by two different mechanisms: local gastric irritation or central nervous system stimulation. Some work by both mechanisms. Emetics are most effective when administered quickly and when there is some food in the stomach.

The most common emetics include syrup of ipecac, hydrogen peroxide, salt, liquid dishwashing detergent, and apomorphine.

Syrup of ipecac is obtained from plant roots and contains active alkaloids, emetine, and cephaeline, which act by local gastric irritation and stimulate the chemoreceptor trigger zone. Water should be given after it is administered. The recommended dosage is 0.5 to 1 tsp per 10 lb PO in the dog or 1 tsp PO for average size cat. Cats find the taste very objectionable, and diluting the dose 50:50 with water may assist in administration. Vomiting should occur within 30 minutes. Side effects have been observed most commonly when the fluid extract was used (it is no longer available) or with chronic usage. Side effects include cardiotoxicity, hemorrhagic diarrhea, and skeletal muscle weakness. Activated charcoal absorbs ipecac well and can be used if any side effects are observed.

Hydrogen peroxide (3%) induces emesis by gastric irritation. The recommended dosage is 1 TBS/20 lbs and can be repeated if emesis has not occurred within 10 minutes. This product is not a reliable emetic.

Salt acts as a pharyngeal stimulator and is not recommended because of the risk of sodium toxicity. It is also unreliable as an emetic.

Dishwashing detergent has been used primarily in humans and only in dogs experimentally. The recommended dosage for humans is 3 tablespoons detergent in 8 oz water. It is not adjusted by size. This should be used only if there is no alternative (i.e., hydrogen peroxide or syrup of ipecac) or if the owners cannot get the animal to the hospital quickly.

Apomorphine is considered the most reliable emetic. It is a morphine derivative that stimulates dopamine receptors in the chemoreceptor zone. This activates the vomiting center. The recommended dosage for apomorphine is 0.04 mg/kg intravenously or 0.08 mg/kg intramuscularly. The dosage for topical conjunctival or subcutaneous application is 0.03 mg/kg. It is poorly absorbed after oral administration. If using apomorphine topically on the conjunctiva, the conjunctiva should be rinsed thoroughly with physiologic saline after the animal vomits to alleviate some of the irritation that will occur. Side effects that can occur with apomorphine include lethargy or restlessness and protracted vomiting. Vomiting usually occurs within 10 minutes of intravenous injection and within 20 minutes of administration via other routes. Its use in cats is considered contraindicated by some.

Xylazine hydrochloride is an α_2-agonist that has sedative, analgesic, and muscle relaxant properties. It is commonly used as an emetic for cats. The dosage for cats is 0.44 mg/kg intramuscularly or subcutaneously. For dogs, the recommended dosage is 1.1-2.2 mg/kg intramuscularly or subcutaneously or 1.1 mg/kg intravenously. The animal must be monitored closely when this drug is used because of the possibility of increased respiratory depression and bradycardia. Vomiting usually occurs within a few minutes.

Vomiting should not be induced during a seizure or if the animal is comatose, dyspneic, hypoxic, or lacking normal pharyngeal reflexes. It also is contraindicated if the animal has ingested a caustic substance or a central nervous system (CNS) stimulant. Caustic substances can permanently damage the mucosa of the gastrointestinal system. If the toxin is a CNS stimulant, inducing vomiting may increase the risk of seizures. Do not attempt to induce vomiting in rabbits or rodents because they lack the natural ability to vomit.

Gastric lavage is the act of washing out the stomach. This technique is used primarily when inducing emesis is contraindicated or when a large amount of toxin has been ingested. It is most reliable and efficient when performed 2 to 4 hours after ingestion. It is not recommended for animals that have ingested a caustic substance or are having seizures.

GASTRIC LAVAGE TECHNIQUE

- A large-bore stomach tube and large amounts of tepid water are necessary for the lavage.
- The animal is lightly anesthetized so intubation with a cuffed endotracheal tube is possible. This reduces the patient's risk of aspirating any of the fluid.
- The tube is premeasured from the tip of the nose to the xiphode cartilage, lubricated, then introduced into the stomach. The stomach tube must be passed with care, and the lavage should be done with very little pressure. The stomach wall may be weakened by the toxin, and lavaging could push the toxin into the duodenum.
- Once the lavage has been completed, activated charcoal should be given.
- Kink the tube at the end before removal to prevent excess fluid from running into the mouth, which increases the risk of aspiration.

A gastrotomy or endoscopy should be considered in animals that have ingested a metal object (e.g., pennies, lead weights). This can be confirmed radiographically.

ACTIVATED CHARCOAL

Activated charcoal acts as an adsorbent. An adsorbent is a drug that inhibits gastrointestinal absorption of drugs, toxins, or chemicals by attracting and holding them to its surface. Activated charcoal decreases the amount of toxin released into the circulation because it contains large-bore molecules to which toxins bind. This does not inactivate the toxin by changing its chemical composition but prevents further absorption.

Several types of activated charcoal are available. The type chosen should be vegetable or petroleum in its origin. Animal-based charcoal should not be used. Charcoal is available in a suspension, tablets, and powder. Highly activated charcoal made from petroleum (SuperChar-Vet, Gulf Biosystems) has better adsorbent qualities than activated charcoal.

The suspension forms (Toxiban, Vet a Mix) can be administered orally or through a stomach tube. Toxiban with sorbitol also is available in suspension form. The sorbitol acts as a cathartic (charcoal treatment can cause constipation). Activated charcoal compressed in tablet form (B.C. Crowley and Requa Mfg.) was found to be approximately 25% less adsorptive than powders or suspension but sometimes is preferred because of its ease of administration. The powdered form must be made into a slurry before administration. The recommended dilution is 1 g activated charcoal in 5 to 10 ml water.

The dosage is 2 to 8 g charcoal per kilogram of body weight. It may be beneficial to administer the activated charcoal three to four times a day for 2 to 3 consecutive days for some intoxications.

Dairy products and mineral oil are known to decrease the adsorbent properties of activated charcoal. Mixing other types of food with activated charcoal can either enhance or reduce the efficiency of the charcoal. It can prevent the charcoal from interacting with the toxin or allow more time for the charcoal and drug to interact by decreasing gastric emptying. Many factors determine the effects of food may have on the charcoal. The amount and time of food ingestion and the amount and physical characteristics of the charcoal must be considered. In general, charcoal should not be mixed with food.

Administering charcoal can be a very messy procedure. Placing the animal in a tub and wearing protective clothing such as a mask, cap, and gown can save cleanup time.

CATHARTICS

Cathartics are used in conjunction with activated charcoal to assist in the elimination of the toxin and the toxin-bound charcoal. It can also decrease the incidence of charcoal-induced constipation. Cathartics should be used 30 minutes after activated charcoal treatment.

Sodium sulfate is the preferred cathartic because of its efficiency in evacuating the bowel. A recommended dosage is 250-500 mg/kg PO in the dog and 200 mg/kg PO in the cat. Cathartics containing magnesium have been reported to result in hypermagnesemia and CNS depression. Cathartics should not be used if the animal has diarrhea or if the toxin that has been ingested may cause diarrhea. Precautions must be taken in using cathartics in very old or very young animals.

WHAT TO DO WITH TOXINS ALREADY ABSORBED

Most toxins that are absorbed are excreted through the kidneys. Increasing kidney function through the use of diuretics has been suggested for animals that present with severe clinical signs, those that have ingested a potentially lethal dose, and those whose condition continues to deteriorate. The most common diuretics used are mannitol and furosemide. Renal function is monitored by noting urine output and performing regular laboratory tests. Proper hydration must be maintained throughout treatment. If urine output is below normal, then peritoneal dialysis must be considered.

ION TRAPPING

Ion trapping increases the excretion rate of the toxin. Most drugs are weak acids or weak bases. Many drugs cannot pass through a cell membrane unless they are in a nonionized form. The pH of a drug combined with the pH of the environment the drug is in determines how well it is ionized and absorbed. Weakly acidic drugs placed in an acidic environment do not ionize readily and absorb well. Weakly basic drugs absorb well in an alkaline environment. If a mildly acidic drug is in an alkaline environment or a mildly alkaline drug is in an acidic environment, it is readily ionized and unable to be absorbed. This is what traps it in its environment. The animal that has ingested a toxin that is reabsorbed by the kidneys can benefit from ion trapping by changing the pH of the urine. This helps prevent toxin reabsorption into the distal tubules. Urinary alkalinizers increase elimination of the weak acids, and urine acidifiers increase elimination of weak bases.

GASTROTOMY

A gastronomy or gastric endoscopy may be indicated if the animal has ingested metal objects such as pennies or lead weights.

SUPPORTIVE CARE

Supportive care depends on many factors, including the type of toxin, the amount of toxin, and the success of the initial stabilization and treatment. The supportive care can range from observing the animal for the night to assisting ventilation or controlling seizure activity by anesthetizing the patient.

SPECIFIC TYPES OF TOXICITIES

METHYLXANTHINES

Methylxanthines stimulate the heart and respiratory muscles and cause minor diuresis. Caffeine, theobromine, and theophylline can be found in coffee, tea, stimulants, medications, and chocolate.

Chocolate (Theobromine Toxicity). Theobromine is found in cocoa beans, cocoa bean hulls, chocolate, colas, and tea. The cocoa bean contains three methylxanthine compounds: caffeine, theophylline, and theobromine. Theobromine is toxic to dogs and cats. Cats are less likely to experience this type of toxicity because of their selective eating habits. The toxic dosage of theobromine is 250 to 500 mg/kg. Milk chocolate contains 44 mg/oz theobromine, and baking chocolate contains 390 mg/oz theobromine.

Clinical signs include anxiousness, vomiting, diarrhea, tachycardia, cardiac arrythmias, urinary incontinence, ataxia, muscle tremors, abdominal pain, hematuria, seizures, cyanosis, coma, and sudden death caused by cardiac arrhythmia.

Diagnosis is based on the history and clinical signs and the presence of xanthines in serum, plasma, tissue, urine, or stomach contents. Theobromine is stable in serum and plasma for 7 days at room temperature.

Treatment includes inducing vomiting if not contraindicated, gastric lavage, charcoal, and cathartics. It may be beneficial to induce vomiting even if the ingestion occurred more than 2 hours earlier because chocolate melts and forms a semisolid mass in the stomach. Diazepam may be necessary to control seizure activity and antiarrythmics to control arrhythmias. It is also recommended to catheterize the bladder frequently because methlyxanthines can be reabsorbed from the urinary bladder.

Caffeine. Caffeine can be found in coffee, tea, chocolate, colas, and stimulant drugs. The lethal dosage is 140 mg/kg. The clinical signs include vomiting, diuresis, restlessness, and hyperactivity. Tachypnea and tachycardia may be present. Ataxia, cyanosis, cardiac arrhythmias, and seizures also may be observed. Death is not common in caffeine toxicity but can result from cardiac collapse. Diagnosis and treatment are the same as for theobromine toxicity. Owners should be educated about the possible toxic effects of these common household items.

RODENTICIDES

Anticoagulants include warfarin, pindone, bromadiolone, brodifacoum, chlorphacinone, difethialone, diphacinone, coumafuryl, dicoumarol, and difenamarol, which are sold under various names and a variety of formulations.

These anticoagulants bind the vitamin K factor, which then inhibits the synthesis of prothrombin (factor II) as well as factors VII, XI, and X. The depletion of these factors slows all coagulation pathways. This effect can occur within 6.2 to 41 hours in a dog and is very dependent on the type of anticoagulant ingested.

The various types of anticoagulant rodenticides are classified as first-generation or second-generation rodenticides. The categorization is based on the rodenticide's ability to kill warfarin-resistant rats. A few first-generation rodenticides include warfarin, pidone, diphacinone, and chloraphacinone. They can depress the clotting factors for 7 to 10 days. The second-generation rodenticides (capable of killing warfarin-resistant rats) include brodifacoum and bromadiolone. These can depress the clotting factors for 3 to 4 weeks.

Animals usually are poisoned by directly ingesting rodenticides, but delay toxicosis also can occur, in which poisoning is induced when an animal eats something that has died from eating a rodenticide. It is uncommon but has been noted in cats or other animals that regularly consume rats and animals that may already be hypoprothrombic because of another disease process.

The lethal dosage varies with many factors, including the species of the animal that has been exposed, age, preexisting disease conditions such as renal failure or liver failure, number of ingestions, and concurrent drug (e.g., aspirin) use.

Clinical signs occur after the depletion of active clotting factors, which usually occurs 1 to 2 days after ingestion. Clinical signs include lethargy, vomiting, anorexia, ataxia, diarrhea, hemorrhage, melena, dyspnea, epistaxis, sclerol or subconjunctival hemorrhage, bruising, and pale mucous membranes. Sudden death may result from hemorrhage into the pericardium, thorax, mediastinum, abdomen, or cranium.

Diagnosis is based on the history of exposure to the toxin, prolonged bleeding times, and the response to vitamin K therapy, which usually occurs 24 to 48 hours after the initiation of therapy. Dye-colored feces may be present if a rodenticide has been ingested.

Treatment includes inducing vomiting (if not contraindicated) and administering activated charcoal, and cathartics. Whole blood transfusions may be necessary to replace clotting factors and red blood cells if the patient is anemic. Fresh frozen plasma (10 to 20 ml/kg) can be used for animals in need of the clotting factors but not red cells. Vitamin K (3 to 5 mg/kg) should be administered every 24 hours until toxic concentrations of the anticoagulant are no longer in the animal. Vitamin K will begin the synthesis of new clotting factors 6 to 12 after administration. Clotting factors should return to normal within 24 to 36 hours. Oral administration with canned dog food is the preferred route unless there is concern about gastrointestinal dysfunction or if activated charcoal has been administered. The fat in the dog food will increase the absorption rate. Subcutaneous administration is the next best route unless animal is hypovolemic. Intravenous administration may cause anaphylaxis, and intramuscular injections may cause hemorrhage.

The animal that arrives with a packed cell volume of more than 30% and mild clinical signs should be given vitamin K and observed.

Animals that have ingested brodifacoum or diphacinone (second-generation anticoagulants) should remain on vitamin K therapy for 21 days.

Cholecalciferol. Cholecalciferol is an active vitamin D_3 derivative used in the rodenticides Quintox, Rampage and Rat-Be-Gone. The baits contain 0.075% active ingredient and usually are in a cereal or pellet form. The mechanism of action is calcium reabsorption from the bone and intestine into the blood. There is then increased calcium absorption by the kidneys. Hypercalcemia (more than 11.5 mg/dl) is the result; if not treated appropriately, it will result in soft tissue calcification and nephrosis. Death is caused by hypercalcemic cardiotoxicity. The toxic dosage can range from 1 g/kg to 100 g/kg.

Clinical signs usually occur 12 to 36 hours after ingestion. They include anorexia, vomiting, muscle weakness, and constipation. They can progress to hypertension, ventricular fibrillation, seizures, polyuria, and polydipsia. Calcium deposits can be found on postmortem examination in soft tissues, aorta, tendons, and muscle if there has been long-term exposure.

The diagnosis is based on the history of exposure and the clinical signs. Most often it is discovered when a routine serum chemistry panel is performed and the serum calcium concentration is greater than 12 mg/dl.

Inducing vomiting and administering activated charcoal and cathartics are recommended if ingestion has occurred within 2 hours of presentation. Correcting the electrolyte balances with physiologic saline (not Lactated Ringer's solution because it contains calcium) intravenously is also recommended. The following drugs are commonly used to reduce and prevent hypercalcemia. Furosemide (5 mg/kg intravenously followed by 2.5 mg/kg orally three or four times a day) increases calcium excretion from the kidneys. Prednisone (2 to 3 mg/kg orally once or twice a day) helps decrease calcium reabsorption from the bone and intestines. Calcitonin also is administered (4 to 6 IU/kg subcutaneously every 2 to 3 hours initially) until serum calcium levels stabilize (less than 11.5 mg/dl). It is a peptide hormone that functions in hypercalcemia to lower the calcium concentration. This is accomplished by decreasing the calcium and phosphorus mobilization from bone and increase phosphate movement into the bone from extracellular fluid. Calcitonin also increases renal calcium and phosphorus excretion. Furosemide and prednisone treatment is continued for 2 to 4 weeks, and a low-calcium diet is recommended.

Bromethalin. Bromethalin is found in the rodenticides Assault, Vengeance, and Trounce. It is a pellet that is usually green or tan, sold in 0.75- to 1.5-oz packages. Bromethalin is an uncoupler of oxidative phosphorylation in the CNS. Cerebral edema and an increase in cerebrospinal fluid pressure results in decreased nerve impulse conduction, paralysis, and death. The toxic dosage in dogs is 4.7 mg/kg and in cats it is 1.8 mg/kg.

In a high-dose toxicity, clinical signs usually present within 24 hours of exposure, including excitement, tremors, and seizures. In a low-dose toxicity, clinical signs can be observed 1 to 5 days after ingestion. Tremors, depression, and ataxia are more common signs. The diagnosis depends on the history of exposure to the toxicant and the clinical signs on presentation.

Treatment includes decontaminating the intestinal tract if recent ingestion has occurred. Once the clinical signs have presented, the effectiveness of treatment is questionable. Mannitol and glucocorticoids have been used to decrease and control cerebral edema. Diazepam or phenobarbital is recommended for seizure control. The animals who have the greatest chance for survival are those who have ingested small amounts and have been treated aggressively with supportive care. Improvement may occur within 2 to 3 weeks in these cases.

Rodenticides are available in many different concentrations, formulations, and packaging. Many appear to be very similar because of their color and pellet or cereal property. It is imperative to determine the trade name as well as the chemical name of the rodenticide ingested, the concentration of the active ingredient, the largest amount the animal may have ingested, and the time interval since exposure before a proper treatment regimen can be determined.

Acetominophen

Acetaminophen is a common over-the-counter medication used for analgesia. It is available in capsules, tablets, and liquid. The common strengths of the drug in tablet form are 80 to 160 mg/dose for children and 500 to 1000 mg/dose for adults. In most species acetaminophen is biotransformed. Cats cannot biotransform acetaminophen because of reduced ability to form the specific enzyme glucuronyl transferase, which is needed to conjugate acetaminophen to glucuronic acid. The glucuronic acid binds to the drug, changing it to a nontoxic form. A toxic dosage for dogs is 160 to 600 mg/kg and in cats it is 50 to 60 mg/kg. If a cat is given two doses within 24 hours, death is almost inevitable. The most common cause of intoxication is owner administration.

Clinical signs can be observed 1 to 2 hours after ingestion. In cats they include vomiting, salivation, facial and paw edema, depression, increased respiratory rate, dyspnea, and pale mucous membranes. Cyanosis is another common clinical sign, usually observed 4 to 12 hours after acetaminophen ingestion. This occurs because of the methoglobinemia. Prognosis in cats is guarded to poor.

Dogs can present with lethargy, anorexia, vomiting, and abdominal pain. Dogs can recover spontaneously within 48 to 72 hours in moderate toxicity. More severe toxicity may result in hepatic necrosis, icterus, weight loss, hemolysis, and hemoglobinuria. Death usually occurs within 2 to 5 days after the presentation of clinical signs.

Diagnosis includes the history and presentation of clinical signs. Treatment of acetamenophin toxicity involves restoring the depleted glutathione stores and converting methemoglobin back to hemoglobin. Initially, vomiting should be induced if ingestion has been within 2 hours. Activated charcoal is not recommended because it may adsorb the antidote, acetylcysteine. Oxygen should be administered to cyanotic patients.

The drug used in acetominophen toxicity is acetylcysteine at 140 mg/kg orally every 8 hours. Intravenous acetylcysteine also is available in a sterile 10% to 20% solution. It should be diluted with saline or sterile water before intravenous or oral administration. It is given at a dosage of 70 mg/kg intravenously every 6 hours for seven treatments. Acetylcysteine is a glutathione stimulator that helps protect the liver.

Asorbic acid (30 mg/kg orally four times a day) is used for methemoglobinemia in affected cats. Blood transfusions also may be necessary to treat animals with a packed cell volume less than 15% or to aid in the treatment of methemoglobinemia. Supportive care including fluid therapy is necessary. Clinical response should be seen within 36 to 48 hours.

METALS

Lead is a common toxicity in companion animals. Cats are less likely to have this toxicity than dogs because of their selective eating habits. It is more common in dogs and cats less than 6 months of age because of their chewing habits and because the blood-brain barrier can be penetrated easily in immature animals.

The most common source for lead poisoning is lead-containing paint, which was used before the 1950s. Other sources include batteries, linoleum, plumbing supplies, ceramic containers that were not glazed properly, lead pipes, fishing sinkers, and shotgun pellets. Lead poisoning usually results from a recent exposure but can result from chronic exposure and accumulation. The most common signs involve the gastrointestinal and nervous systems.

Anorexia, vomiting, abdominal pain, diarrhea, megaesophagus, and constipation usually are observed before the neurologic signs. These signs are more commonly observed with high-level toxicity. Anxiousness, behavioral changes (e.g., whining or barking, continuous running or snapping), tremors, seizures, ataxia, opisthotonos, and blindness also are seen.

Diagnosis begins with a history and clinical signs. Blood smears containing large numbers of nucleated red blood cells, with increased numbers of cells with basophilic stippling and a packed cell volume of 30% or more supports the possibility of lead poisoning. To confirm the diagnosis, whole blood is submitted for lead levels. Concentrations of 35 μg/dl or more is supportive, but a concentration of 60 μg/dl is diagnostic.

Treatment includes removing any lead from the gastrointestinal tract, which may be accomplished through a magnesium or sodium sulfate cathartic, or surgery may be indicated if it is a lead object. The following chelators are commonly used to treat lead poisoning. Thiamine is given intramuscularly or subcutaneously at 2 mg/kg to alleviate the clinical signs. It can cause muscle soreness at the injection site. Commercial calcium EDTA is used to help remove lead from the body stores. It is given intravenously or subcutaneously 100 mg/kg/day divided into four daily doses for 2 to 5 days (10 mg EDTA in 1 ml 5% dextrose). This drug can cause renal toxicity and should not be used in anuric patients. Hydration must be maintained throughout this treatment to promote renal function and the proper excretion of the chelated lead. D-Penicilliamine is another drug commonly used as a chelation treatment in animals less severely affected by the lead poisoning or as a treatment after the calcium EDTA therapy. The recommended dosage is 110 mg/kg/day divided into three or four oral doses given 30 minutes before feeding for 1 to 2 weeks. Adverse side effects include vomiting, anorexia, and lethargy. If this occurs, the animal can be premedicated with dimenhydrinate (Dramamine) or the dosage can be reduced to 55 mg/kg/day orally divided into three or four doses.

Zinc toxicosis most commonly occurs after the ingestion of pennies, galvanized metal, and zinc oxide ointment. This toxicity is most common in dogs. Zinc oxide is used in many products, including diaper rash ointment, cosmetics, soaps, rubber, textiles, and electrical equipment. An animal with an acute toxicity after zinc oxide ingestion may present with severe vomiting, CNS depression, and lethargy. Subacute or chronic toxicity from elemental zinc may cause hemolysis, regenerative anemia, renal failure, vomiting, lethargy, diarrhea, pica, icterus, spherocytosis, and an inflammatory leukogram.

Diagnosis is based on the history of exposure and clinical signs. Foreign objects may be discovered by an abdominal radiograph. Serum zinc levels above the normal range of 0.06 to 0.2 mg/dl would confirm the diagnosis.

Treatment includes removing any metal object endoscopically or surgically. Stabilization and supportive care may include blood transfusions and fluid therapy. Chelation therapy with the use of calcium EDTA also should be implemented.

ETHYLENE GLYCOL

Ethylene glycol is one of the most common causes of poisonings in companion animals. It can be found in antifreeze used for automobile radiators, color film processing solutions, and other heat exchange fluids. The most common form ingested is drained radiator solution from automobiles. Animals like the sweet taste. The minimal lethal dosage of the undiluted product for the cat is 1.5 ml/kg. The minimal lethal dosage of undiluted product for the dog is 6.6 ml/kg. Ethylene glycol is converted in the liver into several metabolites that cause severe metabolic acidosis and acute renal failure.

The most common clinical signs observed within 12 hours after ingestion include CNS depression (the animal may appear intoxicated), vomiting, ataxia, lethargy, polydipsia, polyuria, seizures, coma, and death. Tachypnea and tachycardia may be observed 12 to 24 hours after ingestion. Severe lethargy, vomiting, diarrhea, oliguria, isosthenuria, azotemia, uremia, and death usually are observed 12 to 24 hours after ingestion.

Diagnosis begins with the history and presentation of clinical signs. An increase in serum osmolality, hypocalcemia, a high ion gap, and metabolic acidosis are considered a strong indication of ethylene glycol poisoning. Calcium oxalate monohydrate crystals can be observed on a urinalysis but cannot confirm ethylene glycol poisoning unless there are other clinical signs. This type of crystal also can be found in the urine of normal dogs and cats. It is also more common to see these crystals in dogs that have been poisoned with ethylene glycol than in cats.

Treatment includes inducing emesis and administering adsorbents if ingestion occurred within 3 hours of presentation. Sodium bicarbonate may be necessary to correct metabolic acidosis, and fluid therapy may be needed for diuresis and maintaining hydration. Ethanol and 4-methylpyrazole are used to inhibit ethylene glycol metabolism and prevent or reduce the effects of the renal phase. 4-Methylpyrazole is not effective in cats. The ethanol dosage in dogs is 5.5 ml 20% ethanol/kg intravenously every 4 hours for five treatments, then every 6 hours for four treatments. The ethanol dosage in cats is 5 ml 20% ethanol/kg intravenously every 6 hours for five treatments, then every 8 hours for four more treatments. The goal is to give enough alcohol to cause CNS depression but not semicoma. Animals treated with ethanol must be monitored closely. It reduces body temperature and can cause death if overdosed.

The 4-methypyrazole dosage for dogs is 20 mg/kg intravenously as a 5% solution for the first dose, then 15 mg/kg at 12 hours, 10 mg/kg at 24 hours, and 5 mg/kg at 36 hours. It has been shown to be more effective in dogs than ethanol and does not cause the negative side effects, as ethanol therapy does.

Peritoneal dialysis may also be necessary and beneficial in removing ethylene glycol and its metabolites from the body, especially if the animal is oliguric or anuric.

Snail Bait

Metaldehyde and methiocarb are two types of snail or slug killers. The baits are very palatable to dogs and cats. Metaldehyde's mechanism of action is unknown; methiocarb is a carbamate and parasympathomimetic. Both cause a rapid onset of severe neurologic symptoms that include hypersalivation, incoordination, muscle fasciculations, hyperesthesia, tachycardia, and seizures. Hyperthermia and severe acidosis also are common, and cats present with nygstagmus. Bradycardia, respiratory and neurologic depression, and pulse irregularities may be noted in severely affected animals.

Diagnosis is based on the history and presentation of clinical signs. The odor of acetaldehyde (resembles formaldehyde) in the stomach contents may be noted.

The treatment includes inducing emesis and administering adsorbents. Pentobarbital or other muscle relaxants may be necessary to control CNS hyperactivity. Supportive care includes correcting acidosis.

Garbage Toxicity

This is more common in dogs, and those that are allowed to roam freely are at greatest risk. Enterotoxemia can occur if the animal ingests decomposed food, carrion, or compost. The small bowel pH may rise above 6, which results in an absence of hydrochloric acid (achlorhydria). Hydrochloric acid promotes normal digestion and prevents multiplication of bacteria. Achlorhydria increases the risk of enterotoxemia. Common enterotoxin-producing bacteria associated with enterotoxicosis include *Streptococcus, Salmonella,* and *Bacillus* species.

Clinical signs can begin within minutes to a few hours after ingestion. The signs include anorexia, lethargy, vomiting, diarrhea, ataxia, tremors, and anxiousness. This can progress to endotoxic shock and death.

Diagnosis is based on the history and clinical signs. Treatment includes fluid therapy, broad-spectrum antibiotics, and intestinal protectants. Corticoid steroids should be administered in large dosages if endotoxic shock is present.

Insecticides

Pyrethrins and Pyrethroids. Pyrethrins are extracted from the *Chrysanthemum cineriaefolium* and other related plant species. They are commonly used in pet sprays, dips, shampoos, dusts, foggers, premise sprays, and yard and kennel sprays to control flea and tick infestation in dogs and cats.

Pyrethroids are synthetic compounds that vary significantly in structure and potency. They are most commonly found in pet sprays, dips, foggers, premise sprays, and yard and kennel sprays.

It is uncommon for toxicity to occur if these products are used according to the instructions on the labels. When they are used frequently in heavy applications or used on sensitive animals (more common in cats than dogs) or when an ingestion occurs, toxicity can result.

Common clinical signs include hypersalivation, vomiting, diarrhea, tremors, hyperexcitability, or lethargy in the early phase of the toxicity. It can progress to dyspnea, tremors, and seizures.

Diagnosis is based on the history and clinical signs. Treatment includes bathing the animal in a mild soap for topical exposures. Inducing vomiting and administering activated charcoal and cathartics are recommended for ingestion. Diazepam given intravenously (0.5 to 1 mg/kg intravenously, 5 to 10 mg to effect) may be necessary to control seizure activity, and atropine (0.02 to 0.04 mg/kg intramuscularly or subcutaneously) can be used to control hypersalivation.

Organophosphates. Organophosphates and carbamate insecticides inhibit cholinesterase activity. This interferes with autonomic nervous system function. These insecticides are highly fat soluble and are well absorbed from the skin and gastrointestinal tract. Carbamates are found in dusts, sprays, shampoos, and flea and tick collars. Organophosphates are commonly found in dips, pet sprays, dusts, yard and kennel sprays, premise sprays, and systemics. Toxicity usually occur after one of these preparations have been applied to the animal's skin or if the animal has licked the preparation off during grooming. Cats, animals that have been previously exposed to an anticholinesterase insecticide, and animals that are malnourished are more susceptible to this toxicity.

Clinical signs of carbamate and organophosphate poisoning may include excessive salivating, vomiting, diarrhea, muscle twitching to fasciculations, and miosis. Signs can progress to seizures, coma, respiratory depression, and death. Diagnosis is based on the history and clinical signs. The response to a dose of atropine (0.2 mg/kg) also supports the diagnosis.

Treatment of this toxicity includes washing the animal in a mild detergent if a topical exposure has occurred and administering activated charcoal if ingestion has occurred. Atropine also is recommended to control the muscarinic signs at a dosage rate of 0.2 to 0.4 mg/kg, half intravenously and half intramuscularly or subcutaneously. This dose can be repeated, being cautious not to induce an atropine intoxication, signs of which include tachycardia, ataxia, and lethargy. Pralioxime chloride is recommended for organophosphate poisoning. It reactivates cholinesterase that has been inhibited. The dosage is 20 mg/kg intramuscularly twice a day for several days or until clinical signs of the toxicity are no longer observed. Exposure to another anticholinesterase insecticide should be avoided until 4 to 6 weeks after recovery.

Plant Toxicity

Plant ingestion is most common in animals that are confined and in juvenile animals. Most toxicity occurs with the ornamental plants that are kept indoors. The severity of toxicity is very dependent on the type of plant, the part of the plant, and the amount that has been ingested. A sample of the suspected ingested plant should be identified by its scientific name if possible. Many ornamental plants contain different types of toxins, which can cause different clinical signs with varying degrees of severity. Many references can be accessed for this information. A local greenhouse, florist, or garden store may be able to assist in the identification if necessary.

The most common plants ingested by companion animals are from the Araceae family (i.e. dumb cane and split-leaf philodendron). These plants contain calcium oxalate crystals and histamine releasers. Common clinical signs include hypersalivation, oral mucosal edema, and local pruritus. More severe signs may be observed if a large amount of the plant has been ingested and can include vomiting, dysphagia, dyspnea, abdominal pain, vocalization, hemorrhage, gastritis, and enteritis.

The oral cavity should be rinsed with milk or water to remove the calcium oxalate crystals, and gastrointestinal decontamination and supportive care may be necessary. The prognosis for this toxicity usually is very favorable.

Another type of ornamental commonly used for landscaping that has been known to cause more severe toxicity in dogs and cats is the grayanotoxin-containing plants. The family Ericaceau contains the commonly known plants *Rhododendron* (rhododendron, azalea), *Kalmia* (lambkill, mountain laurel, bog laurel), and *Pieris* (Japanese pieres).

Signs occur within 2 to 6 hours after ingestion and can include vomiting, diarrhea, abdominal pain, CNS depression, weakness, dyspnea, tachypnea, hypotension, and pulmonary edema. Animals that have ingested these plants often are found dead. Occasionally, seizures are observed before death.

Treatment includes inducing emesis (if not contraindicated), activated charcoal administration, gastric lavage, and supportive care.

CONCLUSION

Animals are exposed to many toxins each day. This chapter has covered a few of the most common toxicities observed in veterinary practice. Many good reference materials focus on the various toxicities that can occur, and these should be available in every practice. Poison control center numbers also should be posted. The ASPCA National Animal Poison Control Center is a 24-hour service staffed by veterinarians and board-certified veterinary toxicologists. They can provide updated information on many species-specific responses to poisons and treatment protocols. For more information, call 1-900-680-0000 and 1-800-548-2423. There is a fee for these calls.

Veterinary technicians must educate owners during routine visits about the dangers of potential toxicity. The animals at greatest risk are juveniles and those that are allowed to roam without supervision. Preventive information can be provided through handouts or newsletters.

BIBLIOGRAPHY

Aronson L, Drobatz K: Acetominophin toxicosis in 17 cats, *J Vet Emerg Crit Care* 6(2):65, 1996.

Bailey EM, Garland T: Toxicologic emergencies. In Murtaugh R, Kaplan P: *Veterinary emergency and critical care medicine,* St Louis, 1992, Mosby.

Beasley VR, Dorman DC: Management of toxicosis. In Beasley VR: *The Veterinary Clinics of North America Small Animal Practice: Toxicology of Suspected Pesticides, Drugs and Chemicals,* Philadelphia, 1990, WB Saunders.

Dibartola S: *Fluid therapy in small animal practice,* Philadelphia, 1992, WB Saunders.

Dorman DC: Anticoagulant, colecalciferol and bromethalin based rodenticides. In Beasley VR: *Veterinary Clinics of North America: Small Animal Practice (Toxicology),* Philadelphia, 1995, WB Saunders.

Dorman DC: Diagnosing and treating toxicosis in dogs and cats, *Vet Med* 92(3):171, 1997.

Feller RG, Messonnier SP: *Handbook of small animal toxicology and poisonings,* St Louis, 1998, Mosby.

Firth A: Treatment of snail bait toxicity in dogs: literary review, *J Vet Emerg Crit Care* 2(1):25, 1992.

Forrester SD: Diseases of the kidney and ureter. In Leib M, Monroe W: *Practical small animal internal medicine,* Philadelphia, 1997, WB Saunders.

Garland T, Bailey M: Toxic ornamental and garden plants. In Bongara JD, Kirk RB: *Kirk's current veterinary therapy,* ed 12, Philadelphia, 1995, WB Saunders.

Hansen S: Management of adverse reactions to pyrethrin and pyrethroid insecticides. In Bongara JD, Kirk RB: *Kirk's current veterinary therapy,* ed 12, Philadelphia, 1995, WB Saunders.

Knight M, Dorman D: Selected poisonous plant concerns in small animals, *Vet Med* 92(3):260, 1997.

Kore A: Over-the-counter analgesic drug toxicosis in small animals, *Vet Med* 92(2):158. 1997.

Monroe W: Diseases of the parathyroid gland. In Leib M, Monroe W: *Practical small animal internal medicine,* Philadelphia, 1997, WB Saunders.

Murphy M: *A field guide to common animal poisons,* Ames, 1996, Iowa State University Press.

Murphy M: Toxin exposures in dogs and cats: pesticides and biotoxins, *J Am Vet Med Assoc* 205(3):414, 1994.

Nicholson S: Toxicology. In Ettinger S, Feldman E: *Textbook of internal medicine,* Philadelphia, 1995, WB Saunders.

Oliver J, Lorenz M, Kornegay J: Systemic and multifocal signs. In *Handbook of veterinary neurology,* Philadelphia, 1997, WB Saunders.

Owens JG, Dorman DC: Common household hazards for small animals, *Vet Med* 92(2):140, 1997.

Owens J, Dorman D: Drug poisoning in small animals, *Vet Med* 92(2):149, 1997.

Talcott PA, Dorman DC: Pesticide exposures in companion animals, *Vet Med* 92(2):167, 1997.

Wanamaker BP, Pettes CL: *Applied pharmacology for the veterinary technician,* Philadelphia, 1996, WB Saunders.

Section 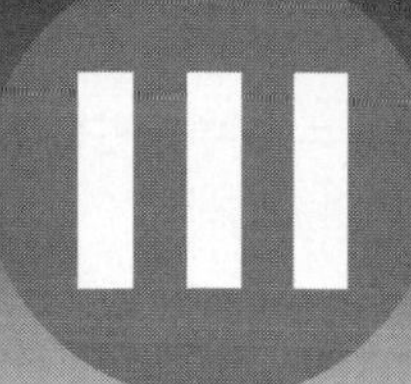

Work Schedules

Maintaining a 24-hour emergency team is very challenging, but it can be done successfully using proper scheduling techniques. This section describes how using different rotations and maintaining a routine to optimize sleep can help alleviate the stress of working overnight.

Chapter 24

The Art of Scheduling

People responsible for scheduling a team of 24-hour emergency and critical care technicians must consider many factors: how scheduling a specific person on a particular shift will affect his or her personal, physical, and emotional well-being; whether rotations are necessary; and what schedule will best fit the needs of the patients and doctors.

Emergency and critical care veterinary technicians must make an extra effort to take care of themselves to be efficient and productive shift workers. Applicants for positions in a 24-hour unit must understand that they may be expected to work one of the undesirable shifts. Many people agree to these arrangements without understanding how such schedules can affect them. The person responsible for the schedule must communicate and reevaluate each technician's progress during transitional periods. Likewise, veterinary technicians must notify their supervisors when having any difficulties working these shifts.

Shift lag is the term used for the negative effects of shift work. Manifestations of these effects can be emotional and physical. Irritability and moodiness are noted by coworkers and partners of shift workers. Overly emotional behavior and overreacting to problems also have been observed. Forgetfulness is another common occurrence. Sleep-awake disorders, gastrointestinal disorders, and cardiovascular disorders are the primary physical problems seen. Sleep deprivation has been noted as the primary cause of many of these problems.

SLEEP DEPRIVATION

The internal biological clock, or circadian rhythm, is reset each day by the light of the sun and the darkness of the evening. Those who work the late shift (also called the graveyard shift or night shift, 11 PM to 6 AM) are at the greatest risk because around 3 AM the body is at its lowest ebb and the daily biological clock is reset. This conflict is called circadian dysrhythmia. Those who work evenings and nights are continually readjusting this clock. The majority of people soon revert to a daytime schedule.

The most common complaint of people working various shifts is sleep deprivation. The average person needs 7.5 to 8.5 hours of sleep each day. The night shift worker averages 5 to 7 hours less sleep per week than the person who works the day shift. Over time this leads to serious physical problems.

Sleep-deprived people are more susceptible to colds, flu, and gastrointestinal problems. People who work nights are more prone to heart disease, accidents, and obesity.

Women who work rotating shifts may have more difficulty conceiving. Two European surveys found that women working irregular shifts were twice as likely to experience delays in conceiving. Miscarriages and low birth weights also were higher in women with unstable work schedules.

Depression and chronic fatigue also are common among night workers. If poor morale is affecting the staff, fatigue may be the cause.

Weight gain commonly affects shift workers because of the tendency to snack on unhealthful foods. It is difficult to attain a standard mealtime during these hours. Research has also suggested that sleep-deprived people have larger appetites. Boredom also can increase snacking during these hours.

Many studies have been done over the years to determine how to help people adapt to shift work. Twenty percent of all workers in the United States are involved in shift work (26% if part-time employees are included). Law enforcement, news publishing, emergency services and hospitals, food industry, printing, military, airlines, paper production, and railroads are the many industries affected. Our lives depend on people who are fully functional during our hours of sleep.

HELPFUL HINTS FOR DAY SLEEPING

A new night worker can try taking a 3-hour nap before the shift begins and sleeping right after the shift is over. The goal is to increase the sleep time after the shift and decrease it before the shift. This gradual change has worked for many.

There are ways for the night worker to become a successful day sleeper. It is important to keep the routine as consistent as possible.

Go to bed immediately after work. Resist the temptation to do anything because this stimulates the body clock to go into the day mode. Exercise should be planned after sleep. The shift worker should exercise at least five times a week to prevent heart disease and obesity.

Seek total darkness. This can be accomplished by using dark, heavy drapes or black plastic garbage bags over the windows to block any sunlight. A blindfold may be a good investment. Be vocal about the need for peace during these hours. Inform friends about sleep schedules, put a "Do Not Disturb" sign on the door, and wear earplugs if necessary. Night workers' sleep schedules should be posted so the staff can avoid calling them during those times, if possible. The supervisor of the night workers should avoid encroaching on their sleep time when scheduling meetings or performance reviews.

White noise has also been used as a sleep inducer and has been found to be very successful for some. White noise is acoustical or electrical noise in which the intensity is the same at all frequencies. Fans and bubbling fish filters are two examples. Tapes and machines made specifically for white noise also are available.

Many people sleep better in a cooler environment. Adjust the thermostat to a comfortable temperature.

Avoid using sleep inducers. Melatonin supplements are commonly used to help travelers avoid jet lag, sleep, and reset their body clocks. Melatonin is the sleep-inducing chemical released in the brain during the hours of darkness. The synthetic form may be helpful in assisting the body to adjust to the first few days of night shift work, but no studies have been done to evaluate the safety of chronic use.

Sleeping pills are not recommended because of the psychological addiction that may occur. Any such drugs should be used in moderation. It may be best to use them only on the first day after the first night back on the night shift.

It takes extra effort for the night worker to arrange a sleep schedule, but it is worth it. In the book *Restful Sleep,* Deepak Chopra writes, "the purpose of sleep is to allow the body to repair and rejuvenate itself. The deep rest provided during sleep allows the body to recover from fatigue and stress and enlivens the body's own self repair and homeostatic, or balancing, mechanisms." Invest in yourself and take the time to guarantee a routine of daily sleep periods.

WORKING THE NIGHT SHIFT

There are other ways to become a healthier and more productive night worker. Drink plenty of water. Dehydration was noted to be very common among shift workers. Avoid caffeinated beverages after midnight during the shift. Caffeine remains in the body for an average of 6 hours and can interfere with sleep and cause indigestion. One should cut back on caffeine slowly if accustomed to consuming large quantities. Withdrawal symptoms include headaches and nausea.

Plan to eat your biggest meal of the day during your lunch break on your night shift. It will help limit snacking throughout the shift. Bring plenty of healthful snacks for late-night cravings.

Exercising during the night shift has been proven to increase alertness and ability to sleep during the day. Take at least 20 minutes to do some aerobic exercise. Walking the animals during the shift may not be enough unless the case load of ambulatory animals is high. Walking up stairs or around the hospital may be necessary.

Bright light therapy for night workers is becoming very popular. It helps the body clock shift to an active mode by suppressing the secretion of the nighttime hormone melatonin. Bright lights also may enhance the effectiveness of serotonin and other neurotransmitters, which shift the circadian rhythm (10,000 lux therapy is the intensity suggested, which is 20 times the intensity of average indoor light). Three to six or more hours under bright lights increases alertness during the night shift and ability to sleep during the day. Practices can install these light sources, or light boxes can be purchased individually.

AFTER THE SHIFT

After your shift it is best to limit your exposure to sunlight and avoid eating a breakfast-type meal. Dark sunglasses can be used on the ride home.

If a person cannot adjust to the night shift, the only other solution may be a day shift. People in their mid-40s to early 50s have greater difficulty adjusting to these shifts. Researchers do not understand why. Because of the health risks, a person should not work nights for more than 6 years.

CREATING THE OPTIMAL SHIFT FOR THE EMPLOYEES

Scheduling is one of the greatest challenges a manager faces. What works for one person may not work for the others. It is also important to remember that a schedule that meets the needs of the employees may not meet the needs of the patients or doctors.

First, determine what person is best suited for what shift. Interview each veterinary technician and determine what will work best for them. Allow the staff to submit their own ideas. Let them know that their preference may not be possible, but you are willing to consider possibilities. Open and frequent communication promotes teamwork.

Discuss possible scenarios that may occur on different shifts to determine which technicians may be able to handle specific shifts.

Have a pool of part-time people to cover for vacations, holidays, personal days, and sick leave. This reduces the number of times regular staff people must rotate shifts and increases the consistency of the schedule.

Overlap the staff for at least 30 minutes during shift changes so proper case review and updates can occur. This also provides time for the staff to interact with their coworkers and help eliminate the feeling of isolation that sometimes occurs among night workers.

Consistency is extremely important. The ideal situation would be to eliminate shift rotation schedules, but because it is difficult to find people interested in working only nights, rotations have become part of the system. A variety of rotations have been developed. Some are more beneficial to the normal body rhythms, others are detrimental. The most beneficial rotations are slow rotations, in which each person stays on a specific shift 5 to 14 days. Two weeks on a specific shift is best. Slow rotation by phase advance is the rotation night to afternoon to morning. It is considered to be physiologically and emotionally harmful.

Slow rotation by phase delay is the rotation from morning to afternoon to night. It is considered the ideal shift rotation. When the employee rotates

Slow Rotation by Phase Delay
(Rotation every 2 wk or more)

Week	Shift	Sunday	Monday	Tuesday	Wednesday	Thursday	Friday	Saturday
Week 1	7 AM-5 PM	A			7 AM-12 12-5 PM	D		7 AM-5 PM
			7-3 PM G					
	3 PM-1 AM	B			3 PM-8 PM 8 PM-1 AM	E		3 PM-1 AM
			3-11 PM H					
	11 PM-9 AM	C			11 PM-4 AM 4 AM-9 AM	F		11 PM-9 AM
			11-7 AM I					
Week 2	7 AM-5 PM	A			7 AM-12 12-5 PM	D		7 AM-5 PM
			7-3 PM G					
	3 PM-1 AM	B			3 PM-8 PM 8 PM-1 AM	E		3 PM-1 AM
			3-11 PM H					
	11 PM-9 AM	C			11 PM-4 AM 4 AM-9 AM	F		11 PM-9 AM
			11-7 AM I					
Week 3	7 AM-5 PM	A			7 AM-12 12-5 PM	D		7 AM-5 PM
			7-3 PM I					
	3 PM-1 AM	B			3 PM-8 PM 8 PM-1 AM	E		3 PM-1 AM
			3-11 PM G					
	11 PM-9 AM	C			11 PM-4 AM 4 AM-9 AM	F		11 PM-9 AM
			11-7 AM H					
Week 4	7 AM-5 PM	C			7 AM-12 12-5 PM	F		7 AM-5 PM
			7-3 PM I					
	3 PM-1 AM	A			3 PM-8 PM 8 PM-1 AM	D		3 PM-1 AM
			3-11 PM G					
	11 PM-9 AM	B			11 PM-4 AM 4 AM-9 AM	E		11 PM-9 AM
			11-7 AM H					
Week 5	7 AM-5 PM	C			7 AM-12 12-5 PM	F		7 AM-5 PM
			7-3 PM H					
	3 PM-1 AM	A			3 PM-8 PM 8 PM-1 AM	D		3 PM-1 AM
			3-11 PM I					
	11 PM-9 AM	B			11 PM-4 AM 4 AM-9 AM	E		11 PM-9 AM
			11-7 AM G					
Week 6	7 AM-5 PM	C			7 AM-12 12-5 PM	F		7 AM-5 PM
			7-3 PM H					
	3 PM-1 AM	A			3 PM-8 PM 8 PM-1 AM	D		3 PM-1 AM
			3-11 PM I					
	11 PM-9 AM	B			11 PM-4 AM 4 AM-9 AM	E		11 PM-9 AM
			11-7 AM G					

through this shift structure, he or she gains 8 hours of sleep (see chart).

Slow Rotation by Phase Delay

Ten-hour shifts, 4-day work week, every 3-week rotation, Persons A, B, C, D, E, F

Eight-hour shifts, 5-day work week, every 2-week rotation, Persons G, H, I

Weeks 1 and 2.

Person A: Sunday-Tuesday 7AM-5 PM, Wednesday 7 AM-12 noon

Person B: Sunday-Tuesday 3 PM-1 AM, Wednesday 3 PM-8 PM

Person C: Sunday-Tuesday 11 PM-9 AM, Wednesday 11 PM-4 AM

Person D: Wednesday 12 noon-5 PM, Thursday-Saturday 7 AM-5 PM

Person E: Wednesday 8 PM-1 AM, Thursday-Saturday 3 PM-1 AM

Person F: Wednesday 4 AM-9 AM, Thursday-Saturday 11 PM-9 AM

Person G: Monday-Friday 7 AM-3 PM

Person H: Monday-Friday 3 PM-11 PM

Person I: Monday-Friday 11 PM-7 AM

Week 3.

Person A: Sunday-Tuesday 7 AM-5 PM, Wednesday 7 AM-12 noon

Person B: Sunday-Tuesday 3 PM-1 AM, Wednesday 3 PM-8 PM

Person C: Sunday-Tuesday 11 PM-9 AM, Wednesday 11 PM-4 AM

Person D: Wednesday 12 noon-5 PM, Thursday-Saturday 7 AM-5 PM
Person E: Wednesday 8 PM-1 AM, Thursday-Saturday 3 PM-1 AM
Person F: Wednesday 4 AM-9 AM, Thursday-Saturday 11 PM-9 AM
Person G: Monday-Friday 3 PM-11 PM
Person H: Monday-Friday 11 PM-7 AM
Person I: Monday-Friday 7 AM-3 PM

Week 4.
Person A: Sunday-Tuesday 3 PM-1 AM, Wednesday 3 PM-8 PM
Person B: Sunday-Tuesday 11 PM-9 AM, Wednesday 11 PM-4 AM
Person C: Sunday-Tuesday 7 AM-5 PM, Wednesday 7 AM,-12 noon
Person D: Wednesday 8 PM-1 AM, Thursday-Saturday 3 PM-1 AM
Person E: Wednesday 4 AM-9 AM, Thursday-Saturday 11 PM-9 AM
Person F: Wednesday 12 noon-5 PM, Thursday-Saturday 7 AM-5 PM
Person G and Person H: Monday-Friday 11 PM-7 AM
Person I: Monday-Friday 7 AM-3 PM

Week 5 and 6.
Person A: Sunday-Tuesday 3 PM-1 AM, Wednesday 3 PM-8 PM
Person B: Sunday-Tuesday 11 PM-9 AM, Wednesday 11 PM-4 AM
Person C: Sunday-Tuesday 7 AM-5 PM, Wednesday 7 AM-12 noon
Person D: Wednesday 8 PM-1 AM, Thursday-Saturday 3 PM-1 AM
Person E: Wednesday 4 AM-9 AM, Thursday-Saturday 11 PM-9 AM
Person F: Wednesday 12 noon-5 PM, Thursday-Saturday 7 AM-5 PM
Person G: Monday-Friday 11 PM-7 AM
Person H: Monday-Friday 7 AM-3 PM
Person I: Monday-Friday 3 PM-11 pm

There are also rapid rotations, which are shifts that rotate the employee through several shifts during 1 week. Rapid rotations are considered the worst type of schedule. The everyday rotation disrupts the body rhythms, making it very difficult for the employee to be productive.

The next category is the dedicated shift, in which the employee is assigned to a single shift during his or her stay with the practice. This is preferred to any rotation but in many cases not an option.

Optimized shift rotation schedules are schedules designed specifically to meet the normal daily rhythms or circadian cycles of human physiology.

Shift schedules should be evaluated routinely. Employees working night shifts should be monitored for productivity and for the physical and emotional effects of the schedule. This will help prevent employee turnover and accidents caused by fatigue.

It is important to remember that not every schedule will work for every team. There are many options to choose from. It is important to involve those who will be directly affected by any shift structure.

CONCLUSION

The veterinary technician who chooses to work in an emergency and critical care unit may be asked to work a variety of shifts during his or her employment. The shift worker and the employer must understand the physical and psychological strain this type of work can cause. Once this is understood and accepted, the people involved with shift work can take the necessary steps to prevent shift lag. The person responsible for scheduling and the shift workers must act as a team. The veterinary technician must be committed to making an extra effort to obtain a restful sleep. The person responsible for scheduling the shift workers must be committed to providing optimal rotations to prevent disruption to the workers' normal body rhythms.

Maintaining a 24-hour emergency critical care team is very challenging. The schedule must be reassessed and changes made as needed.

BIBLIOGRAPHY

Anderson-Parrado P: Energizing ourselves naturally with some good old-fashioned shut eye, *Better Nutrition* 59(3):28, 1997.

Campbell S: Effects of timed bright-light exposure on shift work adaptation in middle aged subjects, *Sleep* 18(6):408-416, 1995.

Chopra D: *Restful sleep,* New York, 1994, Harmony Books.

Czeisler CA, Johnson MP, Duffy JF, et al: Exposure to bright light and darkness to treat physiologic maladaptation to night work, *N Engl J Med* 322(18):1254, 1990.

Czeisler CA: Rotating shift work schedules that disrupt sleep are improved by applying circadian principles, *Science* 217:460, 1982.

Dearholt SL, Feathers CA: Self-scheduling can work, *Nursing Management* 28(8):47, 1997.

Ehret CF: Future perspectives for the application of chronobiological knowledge in occupational work scheduling, *Invited Testimony for the Investigations and Oversight Subcommittee of the Committee on Science and Technology,* Washington, DC, U.S. House of Representatives, March 24, 1983.

Ehret CF: New approaches to chronohygiene for the shift worker in the nuclear power industry. In Reinberg A et al: *Advances in the biosciences: night and shift work biological and social aspects,* New York, 1981, Pergamon.

Goodkind M: Night shifts can be easier, Stanford University Medical Center News Bureau *Health Tips,* January 1996.

Lewy AJ: Treating chronobiologic sleep and mood disorders with bright light, *Psychiatr Ann* 17(9):664, 1997.

O'Conner J: HRD professionals and shift work: do we have a problem? *Interface: Work/Family,* 1996.

Shift work may impede female fertility, *Medical Tribune,* May 23, 1996.

Slon S: Night moves, *Prevention* 49(6):106, 1997.

Weight gain on the night shift, *Tufts University Diet and Nutrition Letter* 14(8):1, 1996.

Westfall P: Too tired to work? *Safety and Health,* September 1996.

Index

Page numbers followed by "t" indicate tables; italic numbers indicate figures.

I

U

V

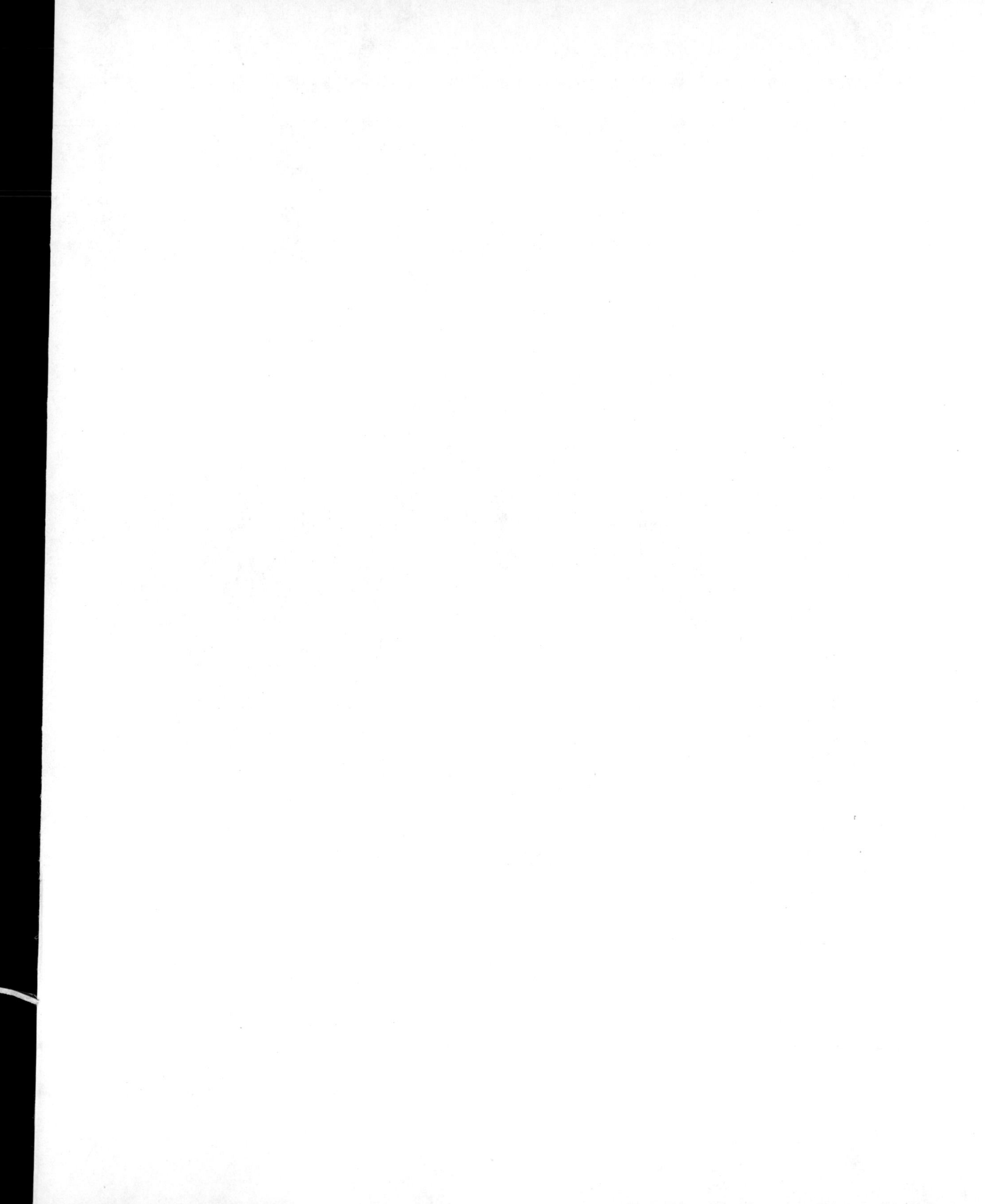